Second Edition

Total Fitness

Exercise, Nutrition, and Wellness

Scott K. Powers

Stephen L. Dodd

UNIVERSITY OF FLORIDA

ALLYN AND BACON

Boston   London   Toronto   Sydney   Tokyo   Singapore

Series Editor: Joseph Burns
Vice President, Editor in Chief: Paul A. Smith
Editorial Assistant: Sara Sherlock
Senior Editorial-Production Administrator: Joe Sweeney
Editorial-Production Service: Schneck-DePippo Graphics
Composition Buyer: Linda Cox
Manufacturing Buyer: Megan Cochran
Cover Administrator: Linda Knowles

Copyright © 1999, 1996 by Allyn & Bacon
A Viacom Company
160 Gould Street
Needham Heights, MA 02494

Library of Congress Cataloging-in-Publication Data
Powers, Scott K. (Scott Kline), 1950–
      Total Fitness: exercise, nutrition, and wellness / Scott K. Powers,
  Stephen L. Dodd. — 2nd. ed.
          p. cm.
      Includes bibliographical references and index.
      ISBN 0-13-095894-8
      1. Exercise. 2. Nutrition. 3. Physical fitness. 4. Health.
    I. Dodd, Stephen L. II. Title.
  RA781.P66 1999
  613.7—dc20   98-50706
                                                            CIP

Printed in the United States of America

10 9 8 7 6 5 4 3 2 1 RRD-RO 00 99 98

PHOTO CREDITS
All photos by Anthony Neste except the following: p.8: Ed Brock/The Stock Market; p.17: Pete Saloutos/Tony Stone Images;
p.67 (left): Robert Harbison; p.115: Courtesy of Biodex Medical; p.151: Rosemary Weller/Tony Stone Images; p.153: Tony
Craddock/Tony Stone Images; p.169: Lawrence Migdale/Tony Stone Images; p.179: Henley & Savage/The Stock Market;
p.193: Bob Daemmrich/Tony Stone Images; p.195: Tom Raymond/Tony Stone Images; p.204: Tom Campbell/Tony Stone
Images; p.206: Janet Durran/Black Star; p.207: The Kansas City Star; p.227: Lori Adams-Peek/Tony Stone Images; p.229:
Gillette/The Stock Market; p.235: Peter Menzel/Stock Boston; p.236: Robert Harbison; p.240: Dick Luria/FPG Int'l.; p.253:
NMSB/Custom Medical Stock Photo; p.255: Alexander Tsiaras/Photo Researchers; p.267 (both): CMSP/Custom Medical
Stock Photo; p.268: Mark Joseph/Tony Stone Images; p.276: Will Faller; p.285: Anthony Blake/Tony Stone Images; p.292:
James Marshall/The Stock Market; p.302: Robert Harbison; p.312: David Higgs/Tony Stone Images; p.321: John
Running/Tony Stone Images; p.328: Geri Enberg/The Stock Market; p.333: Stewart Cohen/Tony Stone Images; p.336 (top):
Ariel Skelley/The Stock Market; p.337: Jon Feingersh/The Stock Market.

To my family,
Betsy, Haney, Will, Mom, and Dad.
Your love and encouragement have always
meant more than you will ever know.

Stephen L. Dodd

To my mother,
who encouraged me to pursue academic endeavors.

Scott K. Powers

CONTENTS

Chapter 3

General Principles of Exercise for Health and Fitness   61

Chapter 4

Exercise Prescription Guidelines: Cardiorespiratory Fitness   73

Chapter 5

Improving Muscular Strength and Endurance 103

Chapter 6

Improving Flexibility   133

Chapter 7

Nutrition, Health, and Fitness   151

Chapter 9

Exercise and the Environment   219

Chapter 10

Exercise for Special Populations   235

Chapter 11

Prevention and Rehabilitation of Exercise-Related Injuries 247

Chapter 12

Prevention of Cardiovascular Disease 265

Chapter 13

Prevention of Cancer   285

Chapter 14

Stress Management and Modifying Unhealthy Behavior   301

Chapter 15

Sexually Transmitted Diseases and Drug Abuse   321

Chapter 16

Life Time Fitness   333

Good health is our most precious possession. Although it is usually only in times of illness or injury that we really appreciate good health, more and more people are realizing that health is not simply the lack of disease. Indeed, there are degrees of health, or, to use the more popular phrase, degrees of "wellness" and it is now clear that lifestyle can have a major impact on our degree of wellness.

Like the first edition, this second edition is intended for an introductory college course in physical fitness and wellness and focuses upon how to alter one's lifestyle to achieve a high degree of physical fitness and wellness. The two major aspects of our daily lives that most affect our level of wellness are exercise and diet. Hence, a major theme of this book is that exercise and diet interact and that both regular exercise and good nutrition are essential to achieve total fitness and wellness.

This text is an effort to provide clear and objective research-based information to college students during their first course in physical fitness and wellness. By providing a research based text we hope to dispel the many myths associated with exercise, nutrition, weight loss, and wellness. Further, we have attempted to provide a "how-to" approach for the evaluation of various wellness components such as fitness levels and nutritional status. We also describe ways to bring about a change in lifestyle (design a fitness program, alter food choices, etc.) which will lead to a higher degree of wellness. Indeed, the title of the book, "Total Fitness: Exercise, Nutrition, and Wellness" is indicative of the philosophy that to be completely fit, one must combine optimal physical activity and proper nutrition to achieve total fitness and wellness.

Why Another Text?

Numerous physical fitness and wellness texts are available today. Our motivation in writing the second edition of this text was to provide a "unique" physical fitness text that not only covers the primary concepts of physical fitness and wellness but also addresses important issues such as exercise-related injuries, exercise and the environment, and exercise for special populations that are often omitted from many texts. Further, in the second edition, we have refined a text that has a strong foundation in both exercise physiology and nutrition. We believe that the combination of the following components make this text unique:

Foundation in Exercise Physiology

First, we believe that it is imperative that a student have an understanding of the basic physiological adaptations which occur in response to both acute exercise and regular exercise training. Without this understanding, it will be impossible to plan, modify and properly execute a "lifetime" exercise program. As active researchers in exercise physiology, it was a challenge to present accurate and detailed information to adequately explain the physiological adaptations during exercise, yet convey this information to college students with limited science background. Based upon positive reviews by dozens of college students and college instructors, we believe that we have accomplished this formidable task.

Strong Emphasis on Nutrition

To discuss physical fitness and wellness without considering the interaction of exercise and good nutrition would be a serious mistake. While many texts present some nutrition information, we have put a major emphasis on a comprehensive coverage of basic nutrition and weight control by dedicating separate chapters to each. In addition, because we feel so strongly that the interaction of nutrition with exercise is important and, an understanding of one almost necessitates an understanding of the other, we have "weaved" a nutritional theme throughout the text. In each chapter, we have included information boxes entitled *"Nutritional Links to Fitness"* which give examples of how nutrition is related to the subject matter of that chapter. This is a unique feature that is not contained in current physical fitness and wellness texts.

Coverage of the Latest Scientific Research on Physical Fitness, Nutrition, and Wellness

We feel strongly that college physical fitness and wellness texts should contain the latest scientific information and include references for scientific studies to support key information about physical fitness, nutrition, or wellness. Without scientific references to support key statements, a text may become another source of opinion and speculation which leads to much misinformation in an already confused arena. Our approach has been to provide current scientific references to document the validity of our facts in every chapter. In addition, some of the material in each chapter is referenced with current reviews on the topic being covered to provide a broad-based source of material for those readers with an in-depth interest in a particular area. We have also provided a "suggested readings" list at the end of each chapter for the reader who wants an even more broad-based source of information.

In regard to new information, we have attempted to present the most current research in the fitness/wellness arena. For example, it is now clear that exercise plays a role in reducing the risk of some cancers, and contributes to a longer life. While there has been speculation about this for years, supporting evidence has only recently become available. In the area of nutrition, scientific data are now suggesting that there may be a new role for vitamins in preventing certain diseases and even in combating the aging process. In addition, while it is well accepted that fat in the diet increases our risk of heart disease, it has recently been shown that dietary fat plays a greater role in weight gain than other nutrients. These are but a few examples of how we have attempted to make this text current. However, with any attempt to present the latest information, there is always the risk of presenting ideas that are not fully substantiated by good research. We have made a concerted effort to avoid this pitfall by using research from highly respected scientific journals and consulting with colleagues who are experts in the field.

Layout and Features

While there are many ways in which textual material can be arranged, it was agreed that the best way to determine the book content would be to ask instructors. We met with focus groups from coast-to-coast in an attempt to determine the most important topics, most desirable layout, features, and supplements. Accordingly, we have included the following coverage, layout and features to enhance learning.

Coverage The text contains more material than can be covered in a typical 15-week semester. This is by design. The text is designed to be comprehensive in order to afford instructors a large degree of freedom to select the material they consider most important for the makeup of their class. The book begins (chapter 1) by defining the major concepts of the text (i.e., physical fitness, health-related fitness, wellness, etc.). One of the unique features of this book is that there is an early coverage of the "how-to" of evaluation early (chapter 2). This provides the opportunity to introduce classes to the practical portion of the material at the beginning of the term and to add other "lecture" topics later in the term. Chapters 3–6 serve as the core of the physical fitness portion of the text as they provide the foundation and techniques for developing exercise programs. Chapters 7 and 8 are dedicated to a comprehensive coverage of nutrition and diet/weight loss. As previously mentioned, the nutritional link to fitness is a common thread throughout the text.

Chapters 9–11 cover special considerations that are important to exercise programs (e.g. environmental issues, special populations, and injuries). The comprehensive coverage of these topics is a unique aspect to the text. Chapters 12–15 give extensive coverage to the "wellness" concepts. The ways in which heart disease, cancer, stress, sexually transmitted diseases, and drug abuse affect our level of wellness is discussed, as well as ways to modify your lifestyle to reduce the health risk from these problems. Finally, chapter 16 illustrates ways in which you can incorporate the concepts presented throughout the text into your lifestyle and make fitness a lifetime commitment.

Writing Style This text uses a writing style which is appropriate for students from all majors. Indeed, no course prerequisites are necessary for reading and understanding the text. Although the fitness concepts discussed in this text are based on scientific research, they are presented in a simple and straightforward style. Illustrations and examples are commonly used to clarify or further explain a concept.

Nutritional Focus The focus of the text stresses the importance of proper nutrition in maintaining physical fitness and wellness. To support this focus, the book contains a detailed chapter on nutrition as well as a chapter covering the relationship between diet, exercise, and weight control. Further, every chapter in the text contains "Nutritional Links to Fitness" boxes that provide additional nutritional knowledge.

Unique Topics This text contains several "unique" chapters not contained in all introductory fitness/wellness texts. For example, this book includes chapters on: a) exercise and the environment, b) exercise for special populations, and c) prevention and rehabilitation of exercise-related injuries. Further, in several chapters we have included an elementary discussion of the "physiology of exercise" designed to improve the students knowledge of how the body operates and responds to regular exercise.

References The latest scientific information has been incorporated into each chapter. Source citations are located in the text by number and a complete reference list is provided at the end of each chapter.

Informational "Boxes" All chapters contains informational boxes called "A Closer Look"

which are designed to add additional details or practical applications of topics covered in the text.

Examples Included in each chapter are practical examples to illustrate specific learning objectives.

Lab Exercises Most chapters contain "easy to follow" lab exercises that covering areas such as personal fitness testing, nutritional evaluations, cardiovascular risk assessment, etc..

Food Appendix Includes an appendix containing the caloric and nutrient content of common foods.

Pedagogical Aids Included are a host of pedagogical aids such as:

- Learning objectives at the beginning of each chapter
- Chapter Summaries
- Study Questions at the end of each chapter
- Suggested Readings at the end of each chapter
- Reference list at the end of each chapter
- Glossary
- Information boxes which highlight key ideas pertaining to the subject matter (entitled "*A Closer Look*")
- Informational boxes which link the importance of nutrition to physical fitness (entitled "*Nutritional Links to Fitness*").

Changes in the Second Edition

There are many changes and new additions to the second edition of this text. Notable changes include:

- New and revised "A Closer Look" boxes in many chapters (i.e. Surgeon General's report on physical activity and health)
- New and revised "Nutritional Links to Fitness" in many chapters
- Many laboratories have been modified to improve clarity and facilitate student use
- Addition of the curl-up test for evaluation of abdominal muscle endurance (see Chapter 2)

- New and updated references in every chapter
- Every chapter has a suggested reading list on the World-wide web

Supplements

The following is a list of supplements included with this text:

Test Bank
Instructors Manual
Transparency Masters
Fitness Evaluation Software
Nutritional Evaluation Software

Acknowledgments

An enormous number of people have made great contributions to the completion of both editions of this text. Ted Bolen of Simon and Schuster was the driving force behind the initiation of this project as well as a major contributor to the first edition of this book. Elisa Adams deserves much credit for her tremendous insight into the subject matter and her unique editing skills. Carla Rivera-Pierola deserves credit for her reviews of both illustrations and supplements. As Senior series editor, Suzy Spivey made a significant contribution to the first edition of this book. Her organization, insight and encouragement were greatly appreciated. Recently, Joseph Burns has joined the book team as publisher. Joe's experience and enthusiasm for the second edition has resulted in many improvements of this edition of the text

There is also a long list of professionals whose reviews of the content and style have shaped every part of this book. We owe them a tremendous debt of gratitude:

Ken Sparks, Cleveland State University; Dave Rider, Bloomsburg University; Mike Manley, Anderson University; Barbara Konopka, Oakland Community College; Roy Wohl, Washburn University; Bridget Cobb, Northwestern State University; Randy Deere, Western Kentucky University; J. Dirk Nelson, Missouri State University; David Paul, Ohio State University; Donna Voth, Simpson College; and Lena Marie Cool, Kellogg Community College.

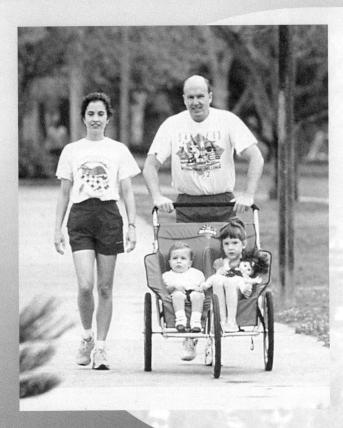

Understanding Health-Related Fitness and Wellness

Learning Objectives

After studying this chapter, you should be able to

1 Describe the health benefits of exercise.

2 Define the terms *coronary artery disease* and *myocardial infarction*.

3 Compare the goals of health-related fitness programs and sport performance conditioning programs.

4 Describe the components of health-related physical fitness.

5 Discuss the wellness concept.

6 Outline the components of wellness.

Congratulations! By reading this chapter, you will take the first step toward improving your physical fitness and maintaining good health. By deciding to improve your personal fitness, you will join millions of people worldwide who are becoming interested in maintaining good health through daily exercise, improved health behaviors, and proper diet.

This book contains the latest scientific information on how to develop and maintain a physical fitness program. A major theme is that good nutrition and exercise work together to improve health and overall well-being. Additional chapters discuss issues such as preventing and treating exercise-related injuries, environmental effects on exercise, stress reduction, and modifying unhealthy behavior. Careful reading of the material throughout will provide answers to hundreds of diet and exercise-related questions.

In this first chapter, we discuss the health benefits of exercise, outline the major components of physical fitness, present the concept of wellness, and introduce exercise goal setting. Understanding the role that exercise plays in the maintenance of good health is a strong motivation for developing and sustaining a lifetime physical fitness program.

Health Benefits of Exercise

Why exercise? Almost all of us ask this question at some time in our lives. The answer is simple: exercise is good for you. Indeed, regular exercise makes us feel better, look better, and provides added vitality and energy to achieve everyday tasks. And perhaps more importantly, it can improve your health (1–7). The importance of regular exercise in promoting good health has been emphasized in a recent report by the Surgeon General (see A Closer Look 1.1).

Exercise Reduces the Risk of Heart Disease

Cardiovascular diseases (i.e., ailments of the heart and blood vessels) are a major cause of death in the United States (see A Closer Look 1.2). In fact, one of every two Americans die of cardiovascular disease (8). It is well established, however, that regular exercise can significantly reduce your risk of developing cardiovascular disease (1–4, 6–10, 26). Many preventive medicine specialists have argued that this fact alone is reason enough to exercise regularly (3, 10, 11). Chapter 12 provides a detailed discussion of exercise and cardiovascular disease.

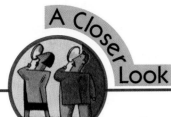

Coronary Heart Disease and Heart Attacks

Coronary heart disease (CHD) is a form of cardiovascular disease that results from a blockage of one or more of the arteries in the heart. The most common cause of coronary artery blockage is the formation of a fatty deposit (called *plaque*) composed of cholesterol, calcium, and fibrous tissue (9). Narrowing of coronary arteries due to plaque build-up can vary from a partial to a severe blockage.

Numerous influences contribute to the development of CHD. Damage to the interior of a coronary artery creates a vulnerable area for the collection of cholesterol, and the formation of plaque begins. The factor(s) that create the original damage to the artery continue to be debated; stress and high blood pressure are potential causes (9). Once the plaque collection begins, elevated blood cholesterol increases the build-up and therefore accelerates the progress of disease.

Blockage of coronary arteries by plaque can reduce the blood flow to the working heart muscle during heavy exercise, thereby depriving the heart of needed oxygen and nutrients. Inadequate heart blood flow can result in chest pain (called *angina*), and advanced CHD can result in complete blockage of a coronary artery. When the heart is deprived of blood flow for several minutes, a heart attack or **myocardial infarction (MI)** occurs, resulting in the death of heart muscle cells. Mild MIs result in the death of only a few heart cells, while severe MIs can destroy hundreds or even thousands of heart cells. Damage to a large portion of the heart reduces its effectiveness as a pump, and in severe cases can result in death.

Exercise Reduces the Risk of Diabetes

Diabetes is a disease characterized by high blood sugar (glucose) levels. Untreated diabetes can result in numerous health problems, including blindness and kidney dysfunction. Regular exercise can reduce the risk of a specific type of diabetes, type II (also called adult-onset diabetes). Specifically, exercise reduces the risk of type II diabetes by improving the regulation of blood glucose (5, 12, 27). More will be said about this in Chapter 12.

Exercise Increases Bone Mass

The primary function of the skeleton is to provide a mechanical lever system of interconnected bones to permit movement and protect internal organs. Given this key role, it is important to maintain strong and healthy bones. The loss of bone mass and strength (called **osteoporosis**) in-

creases the risk of bone fractures. Although osteoporosis can occur in men and women of all ages, it is more common in the elderly, particularly among women.

Is there a link between exercise and maintenance of good bone health? Yes! A key factor in regulating bone mass and strength is mechanical force applied by muscular activity. Indeed, numerous studies have demonstrated that regular exercise increases bone mass and strength in

diabetes A metabolic disorder characterized by high blood glucose levels. Chronic elevation of blood glucose is associated with increased incidence of heart disease, kidney disease, nerve dysfunction, and eye damage.

osteoporosis The loss of bone mass and strength, which increases the risk of bone fractures.

myocardial infarction (MI) Damage to the heart due to a reduction in blood flow, resulting in the death of heart muscle cells.

young adults (13, 14, 28). Further, research on osteoporosis suggests that regular exercise can prevent bone loss in the elderly and is also useful in the treatment of the osteoporotic patient (13).

Exercise Maintains Physical Working Capacity During Aging

Human aging is characterized by a gradual loss of physical working capacity. As we grow older, there is a progressive decline in our ability to perform strenuous activities (i.e., running, cycling, or swimming). Although this process may begin as early as the 20s, the most dramatic changes occur after approximately 60 years of age (1, 15, 16, 29). It is well established that regular exercise training can reduce the rate of decline in physical working capacity during aging (15, 17, 18). This fact is illustrated in Figure 1.1. Notice the differences in physical working capacity between highly trained, moderately trained, and inactive individuals during the aging process. The key point is that although there is a natural decline of physical working capacity with age, regular exercise can reduce the rate of this decline, resulting in an increased ability to enjoy a lifetime of physical recreation. Indeed, perhaps the most important benefit of regular exercise may be the improved quality of life associated with being physically fit.

FIGURE 1.1 The relationship between age, physical activity, and decline in physical working capacity.

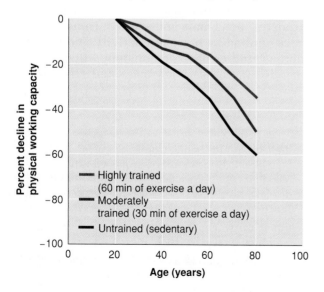

Exercise Increases Longevity

Although controversial, growing evidence suggests that regular exercise (combined with a healthy lifestyle) increases longevity (1, 3, 4, 19, 30). For example, a classic study of Harvard alumni over the past 30 years reported that men with a sedentary lifestyle (i.e., physically inactive) have a 31% greater risk of death from all causes than men who exercise regularly (4). This translates into a longer life span for those who exercise. What factors are responsible for the increased longevity due to regular exercise? The primary factor is that individuals who exercise have a lower risk of both heart attack and cancer (3, 4) (see Chapter 12).

Exercise Does Not Guarantee Good Health

We have seen that there are many good reasons for engaging in regular exercise. While it is well established that exercise can lower risk of CHD, reduce the loss in physical working capacity due to aging, and generally improve the quality of life, exercise alone does not guarantee good health. Indeed, good health (defined as the absence of disease) is the complex interaction of many variables. Factors such as age, gender, genetics, diet, lifestyle, smoking habits, and environment all contribute to the risk of disease (1, 3–7). The interaction between exercise, nutrition, and factors that increase the risk of disease is discussed throughout this text.

Exercise Training for Health-Related Fitness

In general, exercise conditioning programs can be divided into two broad categories defined by their goals: exercise training to improve sport performance and health-related physical fitness. This textbook focuses on health-related fitness.

The overall goal of a total health-related physical fitness program is to optimize the quality of life (1, 2, 10). The specific goals of this type of fitness program are to reduce the risk of disease and to improve total physical fitness so that daily tasks can be completed with less effort and fatigue.

Although some conditioning programs aimed at improving sport performance may reduce the risk of disease, this is not their primary purpose. The single goal of sport conditioning is to improve physical performance in a specific sport. However, the "weekend" athlete who engages in a total health-related physical fitness program could also improve his or her physical performance in many sports. Specifically, a health-related fitness program improves sport performance by increasing muscular strength and endurance, improving flexibility, and reducing the risk of injury, as we will see in the chapters that follow.

Components of Health-Related Physical Fitness

Exercise scientists (i.e., experts in exercise and physical fitness) do not always agree on the basic components of physical fitness. However, most do agree that the five major components of total health-related physical fitness are

1. cardiorespiratory endurance
2. muscular strength
3. muscular endurance

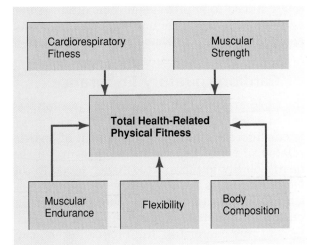

FIGURE 1.2 Components of health-related physical fitness.

4. flexibility
5. body composition

The way that these five components of physical fitness all contribute to "total" health-related physical fitness is illustrated in Figure 1.2. In addition to these, many people also include motor skill performance as a sixth component. Motor skills are those movement qualities, such as agility and coordination, that are required to achieve success in athletics. Although motor skill is important to sport performance, it is not di-

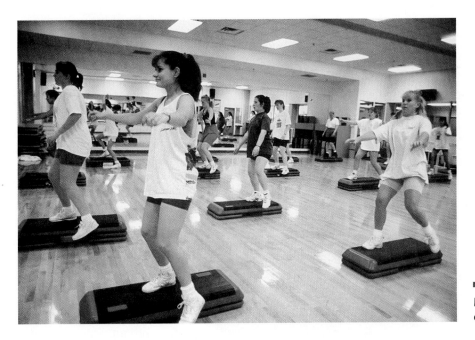

Regular exercise can prevent loss of bone mass.

rectly linked to improvement of health in young adults and is therefore not considered a major component of health-related physical fitness.

Cardiorespiratory Endurance

Cardiorespiratory endurance (sometimes called *aerobic fitness* or *cardiorespiratory fitness*) is considered to be a key component of health-related physical fitness. It is a measure of the heart's ability to pump oxygen-rich blood to the working muscles during exercise. It is also a measure of the muscle's ability to take up and use the delivered oxygen to produce the energy needed to continue exercising. In practical terms, cardiorespiratory endurance is the ability to perform endurance-type exercises (distance running, cycling, swimming, etc.). The individual that has achieved a high measure of cardiorespiratory endurance is generally capable of performing 30 to 60 minutes of vigorous exercise without undue fatigue. Chapter 4 discusses the details of exercise training designed to improve cardiorespiratory fitness.

Muscular Strength

Muscular strength is the maximal ability of a muscle to generate force (20–22). It is evaluated by how much force a muscle (or muscle group) can generate during a single maximal contraction. Practically, this means how much weight that an individual can lift during one maximal effort.

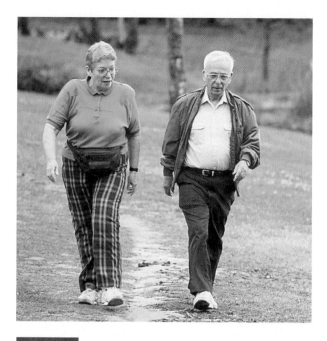

Regular physical activity has been shown to improve longevity.

Muscular strength is important in almost all sports. Sports such as football, basketball, and events in track and field require a high level of muscular strength. Even nonathletes require some degree of muscular strength to function in everyday life. For example, routine tasks around the home, such as lifting bags of groceries and moving furniture, require muscular strength.

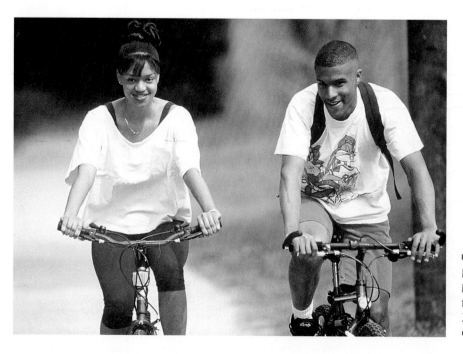

Individuals who have achieved a high level of cardiorespiratory fitness are capable of performing 30–60 minutes of vigorous exercise without undue fatigue.

Weight training (also called *strength training*) results in an increase in the size and strength of muscles. The principles of developing muscular strength are presented in Chapter 5.

Muscular Endurance

Muscular endurance is defined as the ability of a muscle to generate force over and over again. Although muscular strength and muscular endurance are related, they are not the same. These two terms can be best distinguished by examples. An excellent example of muscular strength is a person lifting a heavy barbell during one maximal muscular effort. In contrast, muscular endurance is illustrated by a weight lifter performing multiple lifts or repetitions of a light weight.

Most successfully played sports require muscular endurance. For instance, it is required by tennis players who must repeatedly swing their racquets during a match. Many everyday activities (e.g., waxing your car) also require some level of it. Techniques of developing muscular endurance are discussed in Chapter 5.

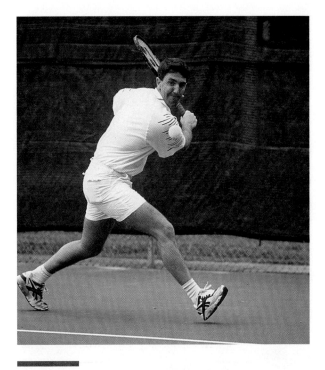

Tennis players require a high level of muscular endurance to play long matches.

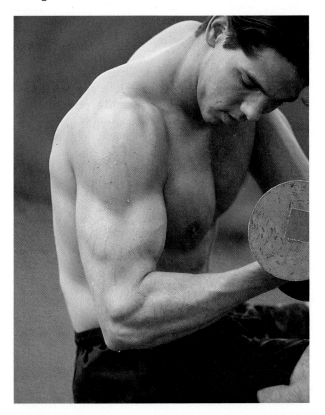

Weight training results in an increase in muscular strength.

Flexibility

Flexibility is the ability to move joints freely through their full range of motion. Flexible individuals can bend and twist at their joints with ease. Without routine stretching, muscles and tendons shorten and become tight; this can retard the range of motion around joints and impair flexibility.

Individual needs for flexibility vary. Certain athletes (such as gymnasts and divers) require great flexibility in order to accomplish complex movements. The average individual requires less flexibility than the athlete; however, everyone needs some flexibility in order to perform activities of daily living. Research suggests that flexibility is useful in preventing some types of muscle–tendon injuries and may be useful in reducing low back pain (23, 24). Some techniques for improving flexibility are discussed in Chapter 6.

muscular strength The maximal ability of a muscle to generate force.

muscular endurance The ability of a muscle to generate force over and over again.

flexibility The ability to move joints freely through their full range of motion.

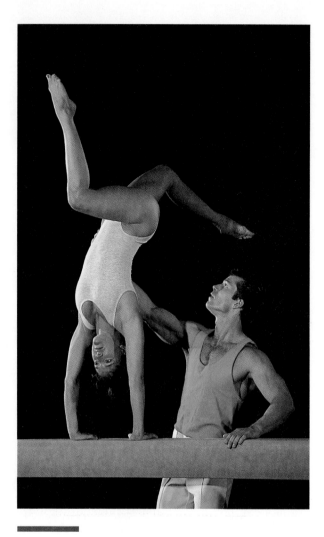

Gymnasts require great flexibility to be successful.

Body Composition

The term **body composition** refers to the relative amounts of fat and lean body tissue (muscle, organs, bone) found in your body. The rationale for including body composition as a component of health-related physical fitness is that having a high percentage of body fat (a condition known as obesity) is associated with an increased risk of CHD. Obesity increases the risk of development of type II diabetes and contributes to joint stress during movement. In general, being "over-fat" elevates the risk of medical problems.

Lack of physical activity has been shown to play a major role in gaining body fat. Conversely, regular exercise is an important factor in promoting the loss of body fat. Assessment of body composition is discussed in Chapter 2, and the relationship between exercise and weight loss is discussed in Chapter 8.

Wellness Concept

Good health is often defined as the absence of disease. In the 1970s and 1980s many exercise scientists and health educators became dissatisfied with this limited definition of good health. These futuristic thinkers believed that health was not only an absence of disease but included physical fitness and emotional and spiritual health as well. This new concept of good health is called **wellness** (2). In a broad sense, the term *wellness* means "healthy living." This state of healthy living is achieved by the practice of a healthy lifestyle which includes regular physical activity, proper nutrition (see Nutritional Links to Health and Fitness 1.1), eliminating unhealthy behaviors (avoiding high-risk activities such as reckless driving, smoking, and drug use), and maintaining good emotional and spiritual health (2). Given the importance of wellness, let's discuss wellness and a healthy lifestyle in more detail.

Wellness: A Healthy Lifestyle

A healthy life style refers to health behaviors aimed at reducing one's risk of disease and accidents, achieving optimal physical health, as well as maximizing emotional, social, intellectual, and spiritual health (2). It can be achieved by eliminating unhealthy behavior to reach a state of wellness. *Wellness* is defined as a state of optimal health which includes physical, emotional, intellectual, spiritual, and social health (Figure 1.3).

Physical Health

Physical health means not only freedom from disease but includes physical fitness as well. Physical fitness can positively affect your health by reducing your risk of disease and improving your quality of life.

Emotional Health

Emotions play an important role in how we feel about ourselves and others. Emotional health (also called *mental health*) includes our social

1.1 *Nutritional* Links to Health and Fitness

Good Nutrition Is Critical to Achieving Physical Fitness and Wellness

A major theme of this book is that good nutrition is essential for developing and maintaining physical fitness and a state of wellness. Good nutrition means that an individual's diet provides all of the components of food (called *nutrients*) needed to promote growth and repair body tissues. Additionally, a proper diet supplies the energy required to meet the body's daily needs.

Consuming too little of any nutrient can impair physical fitness and potentially result in disease (20). Therefore, achieving good nutrition should be a goal of everyone. In many of the chapters that follow, we provide nutritional information in the form of informational boxes such as this one. In addition, Chapter 7 is devoted entirely to nutrition.

Although consuming inadequate nutrients increases your risk of disease, consuming too much food energy (overeating) can be problematic as well. Overeating on a regular basis can result in large amounts of fat gain, resulting in obesity. As mentioned earlier, obesity increases your risk of heart disease and type II diabetes. Chapter 8 discusses the relationship between nutrition, exercise, and weight loss.

---

skills and interpersonal relationships as well. Also included are our levels of self-esteem and our ability to cope with the routine stress of daily living.

FIGURE 1.3 The components of total wellness.

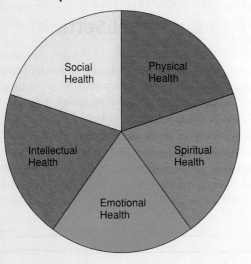

Components of Total Wellness

The cornerstone of emotional health is emotional stability, which describes how well you deal with the day-to-day stresses of personal interactions and the physical environment. Although it is normal to experience some range of emotional highs and lows, the objective of achieving emotional wellness is to maintain emotional stability somewhere between an extreme high and extreme low.

Intellectual Health

Intellectual health can be maintained by keeping your mind active through life-long learning. Although there are many ways to maintain an active mind, attending lectures, engaging in thoughtful discussions with friends or teachers,

body composition The relative amounts of fat and lean body tissue (muscle, organs, bone) found in the body.

wellness A state of healthy living. This state is achieved by the practice of a healthy lifestyle, which includes regular physical activity, proper nutrition, eliminating unhealthy behaviors, and maintaining good emotional and spiritual health.

and reading are obvious ways to promote intellectual health. Maintaining good intellectual health can improve your quality of life by increasing your ability to define and solve problems. Further, continuous learning and thinking can provide you with a sense of fulfillment which accompanies an active mind.

Spiritual Health

Spiritual health is often called the glue that holds an individual together. The term *spiritual* means different things to different people, but regardless of whether you define spiritual health as religious beliefs or the establishment of personal values, it is an important aspect of wellness and is closely linked to emotional health (22).

Optimal spiritual health is often described as the development of spiritual makeup to its fullest potential. This includes the ability to understand the basic purpose in life and to experience love, joy, pain, peace, sorrow, and to care for and respect all living things (22). Anyone who has experienced a beautiful sunset or smelled the first scents of spring can appreciate the pleasure of maintaining optimal spiritual health (22).

Social Health

Social health is defined as the development and maintenance of meaningful interpersonal relationships. This results in the creation of a support network of friends and family. Good social health results in feelings of confidence in social interactions and provides you with a feeling of emotional security.

Interaction of Wellness Components

None of the components of wellness work in isolation; there must be a strong interaction among the five. For example, poor physical health can lead to poor emotional health. Similarly, a lack of spiritual health can contribute to poor emotional health as well as poor physical and intellectual health. These mind–body interactions are illustrated in Figure 1.4. Total wellness can be achieved only by a balance of physical, intellectual, social, emotional, and spiritual health.

Living a Healthy Lifestyle

How does one practice a healthy lifestyle? A good place to begin is with a personal assessment of your health risk status. Laboratory 1.1 is a lifestyle assessment inventory designed to increase your awareness of factors that affect your health. As you work on Laboratory 1.1, keep in mind that you have control over each of these factors, but that awareness alone does not bring about change. A decision to alter your lifestyle to achieve total wellness is necessary and is a decision that only you can make. Make a commitment today to improve the quality of your life by practicing a healthy lifestyle.

Physical fitness, good nutrition and weight control, proper stress management, and healthy behavior are all key components of a lifestyle that leads to wellness. Each of these issues will be discussed in detail in chapters 3 through 16.

Motivation and Exercise Goal Setting

Achieving physical fitness requires time and effort. Unfortunately, many people who begin an exercise program stop before much progress has been achieved. Fitness cannot be achieved in a matter of a few days. In general, 3 to 6 weeks of regular exercise is required for noticeable improvements in muscle tone or muscular endurance. After beginning your personal fitness program, be patient; improvement will come and you will like the changes.

The key to maintaining a long-term exercise program is personal motivation. Motivation, in this case, can be viewed as the *energy required to*

FIGURE 1.4 Interaction of the wellness components.

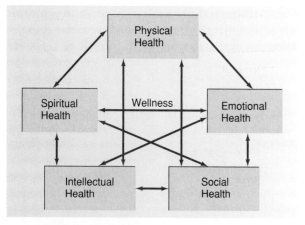

Table 1.1

Key Points in Exercise Goal Setting

Establish achievable goals.

Put goals in writing and in a place where you can see them everyday.

Establish both short-term and long-term goals.

Establish goals that are measurable.

Set target dates for achievement of goals.

After you achieve a goal, establish another achievable goal.

Reward yourself after achievement of each goal.

maintain your drive to engage in daily exercise (22). The motivation to change from a sedentary lifestyle to an active lifestyle requires behavior modification and the establishment of goals. Without question, goal setting is the cornerstone of any successful exercise program. Establishment of realistic goals provides a target for your fitness efforts.

Table 1.1 contains some helpful information concerning exercise goal setting. Note that it is important to establish both short-term and long-term goals. Short-term goals permit you to achieve a goal in a few weeks or months, whereas long-term goals are designed to provide motivation for years to come. Achievement of a short-term goal delivers great personal satisfaction and provides the needed incentive to pursue another fitness goal.

An additional point to notice in Table 1.1 is that goals should be written down. Putting exer-

cise goals on paper is an excellent means of establishing a "contract" with yourself to maintain regular exercise habits. Another important aspect of goal setting is that goals should be measurable. For example, your short-term goal for weight loss might be to lose 5 pounds during a period of six weeks. Because body weight is easily measured, you can assess your progress toward the attainment of your goal by periodic weighing. After achieving a fitness goal, it is important to set new goals to provide the incentive and motivation to continue your fitness program. More guidance in exercise goal setting is provided in chapters 3 and 16.

Physical Fitness and Wellness: A Final Word

In this chapter we discussed the benefits of regular exercise and the importance of a healthy lifestyle to achieve wellness. In the remainder of this book you will be presented with information to help you set goals to increase your physical fitness, enrich your diet, and to improve your health. Simply reading this book, however, will not accomplish these goals. Achieving physical fitness and wellness requires a personal commitment to regular exercise and wise lifestyle choices. Indeed, there is no "magic pill" that you can take to make you healthy or improve your physical fitness. Start today and become an exercise convert; your body will love you for it!

Summary

1. Exercise offers many health benefits. Regular exercise has been shown to reduce risk of CHD and diabetes, increase bone mass, and maintain physical working capacity during normal aging.

2. The five major components of "total" health-related physical fitness are
   1. cardiorespiratory endurance
   2. muscular strength
   3. muscular endurance
   4. flexibility
   5. body composition

3. The term wellness means "healthy living." This state is achieved by the practice of a positive healthy lifestyle, which includes regular physical activity, proper nutrition, eliminating unhealthy behaviors (avoiding high-risk activities such as reckless driving, smoking, and drug use), and maintaining good emotional and spiritual health.

4. Total wellness can be achieved only by a balance of physical, emotional, intellectual, spiritual, and social health. The components of wellness do not work in isolation; there is a strong interaction among the five. For ex-

ample, poor physical health can lead to poor emotional health. Similarly, a lack of spiritual health can contribute to poor emotional health as well as poor physical health.

5. Exercise goal setting is a key component in the maintenance of a lifetime fitness program.

Study Questions

1. Define the term *body composition*.
2. What is cardiorespiratory endurance?
3. Discuss the wellness concept.
4. Define osteoporosis.
5. List and discuss four major health benefits of regular exercise.
6. Discuss fitness training for sport performance versus training for health-related fitness.

7. List and discuss the five components of health-related fitness.
8. Outline the seven key points in exercise goal setting.
9. What causes a myocardial infarction?
10. List and discuss the five components of wellness.

Suggested Reading

American Heart Association. *Heart and stroke facts.* Dallas, TX, 1997.

Blair, S., and M. Moore. Surgeon General's report on physical fitness: The inside story. *ACSM's Health and Fitness Journal* 1:14–18, 1997.

Leeds, M. *Nutrition for healthy living.* WCB-McGraw Hill, Boston, MA, 1998.

Loy, S., P. Andrews, J. Golgert, and B. Yaspelkis. Your 7-step guide to the 150 calorie expenditure. *ACSM's Health and Fitness Journal* 1: 18–32, 1997.

Williams, M. *Lifetime fitness and wellness.* Wm C. Brown, Dubuque, IA, 1996.

Suggested Reading on the World Wide Web

Shape Up America-(http://www.shapup.org/sva/) Latest information about phisical fitness and weight control by ex-Surgeon General, Dr. Everett Koop.

Sympatico:-(http://www.ns.sympatico.ca/healthyway) Articles about fitness and health, book reviews, and links to nutrition, fitness, and wellness topics.

References

1. Bouchard, C., R. Shephard, T. Stephens, J. Sutton, and B. McPherson, eds. *Exercise, fitness, and health: A consensus of current knowledge.* Human Kinetics, Champaign, IL, 1990.
2. Margen, S., et al., eds. *The wellness encyclopedia.* Houghton Mifflin, Boston, 1992.
3. Paffenbarger, R., J. Kampert, I-Min Lee, R. Hyde, R. Leung, and A. Wing. Changes in physical activity and other lifeway patterns influencing longevity. *Medicine and Science in Sports and Exercise* 26:857–865, 1994.
4. Paffenbarger, R., R. Hyde, A. Wing, and C. Hsieh. Physical activity, all cause mortality, longevity of college alumni. *New England Journal of Medicine* 314:605–613, 1986.
5. Helmrich, S., D. Ragland, and R. Paffenbarger. Prevention of non-insulin-dependent diabetes mellitus with physical activity. *Medicine and Science in Sports and Exercise* 26:824–830, 1994.
6. Wood, P. Physical activity, diet, and health: Independent and interactive effects. *Medicine and Science in Sports and Exercise* 26:838–843, 1994.
7. Morris, J. Exercise in the prevention of coronary heart disease: today's best buy in public health. *Medicine and Science in Sports and Exercise* 26:807–814, 1994.
8. American Heart Association. *Heart and stroke facts.* Dallas, TX, 1997.

9. Barrow, M. *Heart talk: Understanding cardiovascular diseases.* Cor-Ed Publishing, Gainesville, FL, 1992.
10. Pollock, M., and J. Wilmore. *Exercise in health and disease.* W. B. Saunders, Philadelphia, 1990.
11. Powell, K., and S. Blair. The public health burdens of sedentary living habits: Theoretical but realistic estimates. *Medicine and Science in Sports and Exercise* 26:851–856, 1994.
12. Rodnick, K., J. Holloszy, C. Mondon, and D. James. Effects of exercise training on insulin-regulatable glucose-transporter protein levels in rat skeletal muscle. *Diabetes* 39:1425–1429, 1990.
13. Rankin, J. Diet, exercise, and osteoporosis. *Certified News (American College of Sports Medicine)* 3:1–4, 1993.
14. Wheeler, D., J. Graves, G. Miller, R. Vander Griend, T. Wronski, S.K. Powers, and H. Park. Effects of running on the torsional strength, morphometry, and bone mass on the rat skeleton. *Medicine and Science in Sports and Exercise* 27:520–529, 1995.
15. Hagberg, J. Effect of training in the decline of VO$_2$ max with aging. *Federation Proceedings* 46:1830–1833, 1987.
16. Fleg, J., and E. Lakatta. Role of muscle loss in the age-associated reduction in VO$_2$ max. *Journal of Applied Physiology* 65:1147–1151, 1988.
17. Hammeren, J., S. Powers, J. Lawler, D. Criswell, D. Martin, D. Lowenthal, and M. Pollock. Exercise training–induced alterations in skeletal muscle oxidative and antioxidant enzyme activity in senescent rats. *International Journal of Sports Medicine* 13:412–416, 1992.
18. Powers, S., J. Lawler, D. Criswell, Fu-Kong Lieu, and D. Martin. Aging and respiratory muscle metabolic plasticity: Effects of endurance training. *Journal of Applied Physiology* 72:1068–1073, 1992.
19. Holloszy, J. Exercise increases average longevity of female rats despite increased food intake and no growth retardation. *Journal of Gerontology* 48:B97–B100, 1993.
20. Powers, S., and E. Howley. *Exercise physiology: Theory and application to fitness and performance.* 3rd ed. Brown and Benchmark, Dubuque, IA, 1994.
21. DeVries, H., and T. Housh. *Physiology of exercise.* 5th ed. Brown and Benchmark, Dubuque, IA, 1994.
22. Williams, M. *Lifetime fitness and wellness.* Wm. C. Brown, Dubuque, IA, 1996.
23. Cady, L., D. Bischoff, E. O'Connell, P. Thomas, and J. Allan. Strength and fitness and subsequent back injuries in fire-fighters. *Journal of Occupational Medicine* 4:269–272, 1979.
24. Cady, L., P. Thomas, and R. Karasky. Programs for increasing health and physical fitness of fire-fighters. *Journal of Occupational Medicine* 2:111–114, 1985.
25. U. S. Department of Health and Human Services. Physical activity and health: A report of the Surgeon General. U. S. Department of Health and Human Services, Centers for Disease Control and Prevention, National Center for Chronic Disease Prevention and Health Promotion, Atlanta, GA, 1996.
26. Williams, P. T. Relationship between distance run per week to coronary heart disease risk factors in 8283 male runners. The National Runners Health Study. *Archives of Internal Medicine* 157: 191–198, 1997.
27. Pan, X. R., et al. Effects of diet and exercise in preventing NIDDM in people with impaired glucose tolerance. *Diabetes Care* 20: 537–544, 1997.
28. Taaffe, D., T. Robinson, C. Snow, and R. Marcus. High impact exercise promotes bone gain in well-trained female athletes. *Journal of Bone and Mineral Research* 12: 255–260, 1997.
29. Nakamura, E. T. Moritani, and A. Kanetaka. Effects of habitual physical exercise on physiological age in men and women aged 20–85 years as estimated using principal component analysis. *European Journal of Applied Physiology* 73: 410–418, 1996.
30. Lee, I., R. Paffenbarger, and C. Hennekens. Physical activity, physical fitness, and longevity. *Aging-Milano* 9: 2–11, 1997.

Lifestyle Assessment Inventory

NAME _____ DATE _____

The purpose of this lifestyle assessment inventory is to increase your awareness of areas in your life that increase your risk of disease, injury, and possibly premature death. A key point to remember is that you have control over each of the lifestyle areas discussed.

Awareness is the first step in making change. After identifying the areas that require modification, use the behavior modification techniques presented in Chapter 14 to bring about positive lifestyle changes.

Directions

Put a check by each statement that applies to you.

A. Physical Fitness

_____ I exercise for a minimum of 20 to 30 minutes at least 3 days per week.

_____ I play sports routinely (2 to 3 times per week).

_____ I walk for 15 to 30 minutes (3 to 7 days per week).

B. Body Fat

_____ There is no place on my body where I can pinch more than 1 inch of fat.

_____ I am satisfied with the way my body appears.

C. Stress Level

_____ I find it easy to relax.

_____ I rarely feel tense or anxious.

_____ I am able to cope with daily stresses better than most people.

D. Car Safety

_____ I have not had an auto accident in the past 4 years.

_____ I always use a seat belt when I drive.

_____ I rarely drive above the speed limit.

E. Sleep

_____ I always get 7 to 9 hours of sleep.

_____ I do not have trouble going to sleep.

_____ I generally do not wake up during the night.

F. Relationships

_____ I have a happy and satisfying relationship with my spouse or boy/girl friend.

_____ I have a lot of close friends.

_____ I have a great deal of family love and support.

G. Diet

_____ I generally eat three balanced meals per day.

_____ I rarely overeat.

_____ I rarely eat large quantities of fatty foods and sweets.

H. Alcohol Use

_____ I consume fewer than two drinks per day.

_____ I never get intoxicated.

_____ I never drink and drive.

I. Tobacco Use

_____ I never smoke (cigarettes, pipe, cigars, etc.).

_____ I am not exposed to second-hand smoke on a regular basis.

_____ I do not use smokeless tobacco.

J. Drug Use

_____ I never use illicit drugs.

_____ I never abuse legal drugs such as diet or sleeping pills.

K. Safe Sex

_____ I always practice safe sex (e.g., always using condoms or being involved in a monogamous relationship).

Scoring

1. **Individual areas:** If you have fewer than three checks in categories A through K, you can improve this area of your lifestyle.
2. **Overall lifestyle:** Add up your total number of checks. Scoring can be interpreted as follows:

   23–29   Very healthy lifestyle

   17–22   Average healthy lifestyle

   ≤16   Unhealthy lifestyle (needs improvement)

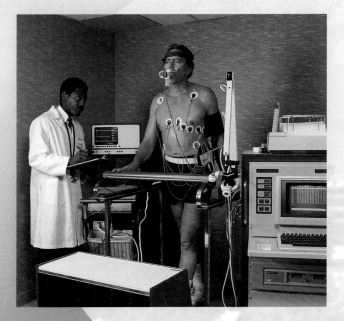

Fitness Evaluation: Self-Testing

Learning Objectives

After studying this chapter, you should be able to

1 Explain the principle behind field testing of cardiorespiratory fitness using the 1.5-mile run test, the 1-mile walking test, the cycle ergometer exercise test, and the step test.

2 Outline the design of the one-repetition maximum test for measurement of muscular strength.

3 Compare the push-up and sit-up tests as a means of evaluating muscular endurance.

4 Define the term *flexibility* and discuss two field tests used to assess it.

5 Discuss why assessment of body composition is important in health-related fitness testing.

6 Explain how body composition is assessed using hydrostatic weighting, the skinfold test, body mass index, and waist-to-hip circumference ratio.

An objective evaluation of your current fitness status is important prior to beginning an exercise training program (1–6). This evaluation provides valuable information concerning your fitness strengths and weaknesses and enables you to set reasonable fitness goals. Further, testing your initial fitness level also provides a benchmark against which you can compare future evaluations. Periodic re-testing (e.g., every 3 to 6 months) provides motivating feedback as your fitness program progresses.

This chapter presents a battery of physical fitness tests that can assess your fitness level. These tests are designed to evaluate each of the major components of health-related physical fitness: cardiorespiratory fitness, muscular strength, muscular endurance, flexibility, and body composition.

Although the risks associated with regular exercise are generally less than the risks associated with living a sedentary lifestyle, it is important to evaluate your health status before engaging in any physical fitness test. A brief discussion of the need for medical clearance prior to beginning an exercise program follows.

Evaluating Health Status

Is a medical exam required before beginning a fitness program? The answer is probably "no" for healthy college-age individuals (1, 2). Although regular medical exams are encouraged for everyone, most people under 29 years of age generally do not require special medical clearance before beginning a low-to-moderate intensity exercise program. However, if you have any concerns about your health, an examination by a physician is prudent prior to starting an exercise program. Laboratory 2.1 is a useful screening questionnaire for people of all ages who are beginning an exercise program. An answer of "yes" to any of the questions in Laboratory 2.1 suggests that a medical problem may exist and that a complete medical exam is required.

Should individuals over 30 years old have a medical exam at the beginning of an exercise program? The most conservative answer is "yes." This is particularly true for obese and/or sedentary individuals. The following general guidelines apply:

18–29 years (men and women): You should have had a medical checkup within the last 2 years and completed Laboratory 2.1.

Nutritional

2.1   Links to Health and Fitness

Can the Content of a Pre-exercise Meal Improve the Results of a Fitness Test?

Many manufacturers of "athletic beverages" and "quick energy" candy bars claim that consumption of their products prior to exercise can improve performance. There is no scientific evidence, however, to support the idea that any type of meal eaten before exercise can improve physical performance (see ref. 13 for a review on this topic). In fact, consumption of high volumes of fluid or large solid meals immediately before exercising can negatively impact performance by creating abdominal discomfort (13). To avoid stomach cramps or other forms of abdominal discomfort during exercise, the pre-exercise meal should be relatively small and eaten at least 2 to 3 hours before exercise. This pre-exercise meal should contain primarily complex carbohydrates (complex sugars such as fruits and breads) and be low in fat. The rationale for this recommendation is based on the fact that carbohydrates are digested rapidly, whereas fat is broken down and absorbed at a slow rate (8). See Chapter 7 for a complete discussion of nutrition and physical fitness.

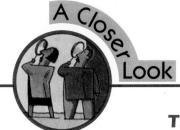

2.1 A Closer Look

The Exercise ECG

The electrocardiogram (ECG, or sometimes EKG) is a common medical test that measures the electrical activity of the heart and can be used to diagnose several types of heart disease (6, 7). Although a resting ECG is useful for determining the heart's function, ECG monitoring during exercise is particularly useful in diagnosing hidden heart problems, because heart abnormalities often appear during periods of emotional or exercise stress (6). An exercise ECG, commonly called an **exercise stress test,** is generally performed on a treadmill while a physician monitors heart rate, blood pressure, and ECG. The test begins with a brief warm-up period followed by a progressive increase in exercise intensity until the patient cannot continue or the physician stops the test for medical reasons. In general, the duration of the test varies as a function of the subject's fitness level. For example, poorly conditioned people may exercise for only 10 to 12 minutes, whereas well-conditioned subjects may work for up to 25 to 30 minutes. Therefore, the exercise stress test not only provides data about your cardiovascular health, but also provides information about cardiorespiratory fitness.

30–39 years (men) and 30–44 years (women): You should have had a medical checkup within the last year and completed Laboratory 2.1.

40 years and above (men): You should have had a medical checkup and a physician-supervised stress test within the last year (see A Closer Look 2.1).

45 years and above (women): You should have had a medical checkup and a physician-supervised stress test within the last year (see A Closer Look 2.1).

Measuring Cardiorespiratory Fitness

As we saw in Chapter 1, cardiorespiratory fitness is the ability to perform endurance-type exercises (e.g., running, cycling, swimming, etc.) and is considered to be a key component of health-related physical fitness. The most accurate means of measuring cardiorespiratory fitness is the laboratory assessment of maximal oxygen consumption (8, 9) (called VO_2 max). In simple terms, VO_2 max is a measure of the endurance capacity of both the cardiorespiratory system and exercising skeletal muscles. Because direct measurement of VO_2 max requires expensive laboratory equipment and is very time consuming, it is impractical for general use. Fortunately, researchers have developed numerous methods for estimating VO_2 max using simple field tests (10–12). In the following paragraphs, we describe several types of field exercise tests designed to evaluate cardiorespiratory fitness.

The 1.5-Mile Run Test

One of the simplest and most accurate means of evaluating cardiorespiratory fitness is the **1.5-mile run test**. This test was popularized by Dr. Kenneth Cooper and works on the physiological principle that people with a high level of cardiorespiratory fitness can run 1.5 miles in less time than less fit individuals (10, 11).

exercise stress test A diagnostic test designed to determine if the patient's cardiovascular system has a normal response to exercise. The test is generally performed on a treadmill while a physician monitors heart rate, blood pressure, and EKG.

1.5-mile run test A fitness test designed to evaluate cardiorespiratory fitness. The objective of the test is to complete a 1.5-mile distance (preferably on a track) in the shortest possible time.

Table 2.1

Fitness Categories for Cooper's 1.5-Mile Run Test to Determine Cardiorespiratory Fitness

Fitness Category	Age (years)					
	13–19	20–29	30–39	40–49	50–59	60+
Men						
Very poor	>15:30	>16:00	>16:30	>17:30	>19:00	>20:00
Poor	12:11–15:30	14:01–16:00	14:46–16:30	15:36–17:30	17:01–19:00	19:01–20:00
Average	10:49–12:10	12:01–14:00	12:31–14:45	13:01–15:35	14:31–17:00	16:16–19:00
Good	9:41–10:48	10:46–12:00	11:01–12:30	11:31–13:00	12:31–14:30	14:00–16:15
Excellent	8:37–9:40	9:45–10:45	10:00–11:00	10:30–11:30	11:00–12:30	11:15–13:59
Superior	<8:37	<9:45	<10:00	<10:30	<11:00	<11:15
Women						
Very poor	>18:30	>19:00	>19:30	>20:00	>20:30	>21:00
Poor	16:55–18:30	18:31–19:00	19:01–19:30	19:31–20:00	20:01–20:30	20:31–21:31
Average	14:31–16:54	15:55–18:30	16:31–19:00	17:31–19:30	19:01–20:00	19:31–20:30
Good	12:30–14:30	13:31–15:54	14:31–16:30	15:56–17:30	16:31–19:00	17:31–19:30
Excellent	11:50–12:29	12:30–13:30	13:00–14:30	13:45–15:55	14:30–16:30	16:30–17:30
Superior	<11:50	<12:30	<13:00	<13:45	<14:30	<16:30

Times are given in minutes and seconds. (> = greater than; < = less than)

From Cooper, K. *The aerobics program for total well-being.* Bantam Books, New York, 1982. Copyright © 1982 by Kenneth H. Cooper. Used by permission of Bantam Books, a division of Bantam Doubleday Dell Publishing Group, Inc.

The 1.5-mile run test is excellent for physically active college-age individuals. Due to its intensity, however, the 1.5-mile run test is not well suited for sedentary people over 30 years of age, severely deconditioned people, individuals with joint problems, and obese individuals.

The objective of the test is to complete a 1.5-mile distance (preferably on a track) in the shortest possible time. The test is best conducted in moderate weather conditions (avoiding very hot or very cold days). For a reasonably physically fit individual, the 1.5-mile distance can be covered by running or jogging. For less fit individuals, the test becomes a run/walk test. A good strategy is to try to keep a steady pace during the entire distance. In this regard, it may be beneficial to perform a practice test in order to determine the optimal pace that you can maintain. Accurate timing of the test is essential, and use of a stop watch is best. Laboratory 2.2 provides instructions for performing the test and recording the score.

Interpreting your test results is simple. Table 2.1 contains norms for cardiorespiratory fitness using the 1.5-mile run test. Find your sex, age group, and finish time on the table and then locate your fitness category on the left side of the table. Consider the following example: Johnny Jones is 21 years old and completes the 1.5-mile run in 13 minutes and 25 seconds (13:25). Using Table 2.1 on page 20 locate Johnny's age group and time column. Note that a finish time of 13:25 for the 1.5-mile run would place Johnny in the "average" fitness category.

The 1-Mile Walk Test

Another field test to determine cardiorespiratory fitness is the **1-mile walk test**, which is particularly useful for sedentary individuals (14–16). It is a weight-bearing test, however, so individuals with joint problems should not participate.

The 1-mile walk test works on the same prin-

Table 2.2

Fitness Classification for 1-Mile Walk Test

Fitness Category	Age (years)			
	13–19	**20–29**	**30–39**	**40+**
Men				
Very Poor	>17:30	>18:00	>19:00	> 21:30
Poor	16:01–17:30	16:31–18:00	17:31–19:00	18:31–21:30
Average	14:01–16:00	14:31–16:30	15:31–17:30	16:01–18:30
Good	12:30–14:00	14:31–16:30	16:31–17:30	14:00–16:00
Excellent	<12:30	<13:00	<13:30	<14:00
Women				
Very Poor	>18:01	>18:31	>19:31	>20:01
Poor	16:31–18:00	17:01–18:30	18:01–19:30	19:31–20:00
Average	14:31–16:30	15:01–17:00	16:01–18:00	18:00–19:00
Good	13:31–14:30	13:31–15:00	14:01–16:00	14:31–17:59
Excellent	<13:00	<13:30	<14:00	<14:30

Because the 1-mile walk test is designed primarily for older or less conditioned individuals, the fitness categories listed here do not include a "superior" category.

ciple as the 1.5-mile run test. That is, individuals with high levels of cardiorespiratory fitness will complete a 1-mile walk in a shorter time than those who are less conditioned. This test is also best conducted in moderate weather conditions, preferably on a track. Subjects should try to maintain a steady pace over the distance. Again, because test scores are based on time, accurate timing is essential.

Laboratory 2.3 provides instructions for performing the test and for recording your score. Table 2.2 contains norms for scoring cardiorespiratory fitness using the 1-mile walk test. Find your age group and finish time on the table and then locate your fitness category on the left side of it.

The Cycle Ergometer Fitness Test

For those with access to a cycle ergometer (a stationary exercise bicycle that provides pedaling resistance via friction applied to the wheel), a **cycle ergometer fitness test** is an excellent means of evaluating cardiorespiratory fitness. It offers advantages over running or walking tests for individuals with joint problems due to the non-weight-bearing nature of cycling. Further, because this type of test can be performed indoors, it has advantages over outdoor fitness tests during very cold or hot weather.

Although numerous types of cycle ergometers exist, the most common type is the friction-braked which incorporates a belt wrapped around the wheel. The belt can be loosened or tightened to provide a change in resistance (pedaling difficulty). The work performed on a cycle ergometer is commonly expressed in units called *kilopond meters per minute* (KPM) or watts. It is not important that you understand the details of these units but you should recognize that KPMs

1-mile walking test A fitness test designed to evaluate cardiorespiratory fitness. The objective of the test is to complete a 1 mile walking distance (preferably on a track) in the shortest possible time.

cycle ergometer fitness test A submaximal exercise test designed to evaluate cardiorespiratory fitness.

Table 2.3

Work Rates for Submaximal Cycle Ergometer Fitness Test

Gender	Age (years)	Pedal Speed (RPM)	Load (watts)
Male	Up to 29	60	150 (900 KPM)
	30 and up	60	50 (300 KPM)
Female	Up to 29 (or poorly conditioned)	60	100 (600 KPM)
	30 and up (or poorly conditioned)	60	50 (300 KPM)

Table 2.4

Cycle Ergometer Fitness Index for Men and Women
Locate your 15-second heart rate in the left-hand column; then find your estimated VO_2 max in the appropriate column on the right. For example, the second column from the left contains the absolute VO_2 max (expressed in ml/min) for male subjects using the 900-KPM work rate. The third column from the left contains the absolute VO_2 max (expressed in ml/min) for women using the 600-KPM work rate, and so on. After determination of your absolute VO_2 max, calculate your relative VO_2 max (ml/kg/min) by dividing your VO_2 max expressed ml/min by your body weight in kilograms (1 kilogram = 2.2 pounds). For example, if your body weight is 70 kilograms and your absolute VO_2 max is 2631 ml/min, your relative VO_2 max is approximately 38 ml/kg/min (i.e., 2631 divided by 70 = 38). After computing your relative VO_2 max, use Table 2.5 to identify your fitness category.

Estimated Absolute VO_2 Max (ml/min)

15-Second Heart Rate	Men: 900 KPM Workrate	Women: 600 KPM Workrate	Men or Women: 300 KPM Workrate
28	3560	2541	1525
29	3442	2459	1475
30	3333	2376	1425
31	3216	2293	1375
32	3099	2210	1325
33	2982	2127	1275
34	2865	2044	1225
35	2748	1961	1175
36	2631	1878	1125
37	2514	1795	1075
38	2397	1712	1025
39	2280	1629	—
40	2163	1546	—
41	2046	1463	—
42	1929	1380	—
43	1812	1297	—
44	1695	1214	—
45	1578	1131	—

Table 2.5

Cardiorespiratory Fitness Norms for Men and Women Based on Estimated VO_2 Max Values Determined by the Bicycle Ergometer Fitness Test

After determining your relative VO_2 max (ml/kg/min), find your appropriate fitness category.

Age Group (years)	Fitness Categories Based on VO_2 max (ml/kg/min)					
	Very Poor	Poor	Average	Good	Excellent	Superior
Men						
13–19	<35	36–39	40–46	47–53	54–59	>60
20–29	<33	34–38	39–45	46–52	53–58	>59
30–39	<32	33–37	38–43	44–49	50–53	>54
40–49	<30	31–36	37–41	42–48	49–52	>53
50–59	<28	29–32	33–38	39–45	46–49	>50
60+	<24	25–29	30–34	35–39	40–44	>45
Women						
13–19	<28	29–34	35–40	41–44	45–52	>52
20–29	<30	31–33	34–38	39–42	43–51	>51
30–39	<28	29–31	32–36	37–42	43-45	>45
40–49	<25	26–28	29–34	35–39	40–42	>42
50–59	<23	24–25	26–30	31–34	35–38	>38
60+	<22	23–24	25–29	30–34	35–36	>36

Modified from Golding, L., C. Myers, and W. Sinning. *Y's way to physical fitness: The complete guide to fitness testing and instruction.* 3rd ed. Human Kinetics, Champaign, IL, 1989.

and watts are measurement units that represent how much work is performed. For example, a work load of 300 KPM (50 watts) on the cycle ergometer would be considered a submaximal (a light load) work rate for almost everyone, whereas a load of 3000 KPM (500 watts) would represent a high work rate for even highly conditioned individuals.

The cycle ergometer fitness test is conducted as follows:

1. Warm up for 3 minutes while pedaling the cycle at 60 revolutions per minute with no load against the pedals.

2. After completion of the warm-up, begin the fitness test. Set the load on the cycle ergometer according to Table 2.3 and perform 5 minutes of exercise.

3. During the last minute of exercise, measure your heart rate for 15 seconds. This can be achieved by palpation of the pulse in your wrist (radial artery) or by gentle palpation of the pulse in your neck (carotid artery). Note that accurate measurement of heart rate is critical for this test to be a valid assessment of cardiorespiratory fitness.

This type of submaximal cycle test works on the principle that individuals with high cardiorespiratory fitness levels have a lower exercise heart rate at a standard work load than less fit individuals (8, 12).

After completing the test, use your 15-second heart rate count to find your estimated VO_2 max in Table 2.4. For example, a 21-year-old woman with a 15-second heart rate of 36 would have an estimated VO_2 max of 39 ml/kg/min (see A Closer Look 2.2 on page 25 for a discussion of VO_2 max units). Now use Table 2.5 to find the corresponding fitness category. A VO_2 max of 39 ml/kg/min for a 21-year-old woman would place her in the "excellent" cardiorespiratory fitness category. Laboratory 2.4 permits recording of your score on this test.

The Step Test

An alternative test to determine your cardiorespiratory fitness level is the **step test**. The step test works on the principle that individuals with a high level of cardiorespiratory fitness will have a lower heart rate during recovery from 3 minutes of standardized exercise (bench stepping) than less conditioned individuals (4, 8). Although the step test is not considered the best field method to estimate cardiorespiratory fitness, it does have advantages in that it can be performed indoors and can be used by people at all fitness levels. Further, the step test does not require expensive equipment and can be performed in a short amount of time.

Step height for both men and women should be approximately 18 inches. In general, locker

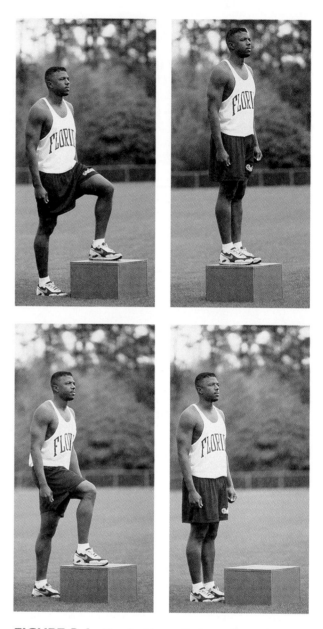

FIGURE 2.1 Step test to evaluate cardiorespiratory fitness.

Friction-braked cycle ergometer (exercise cycle).

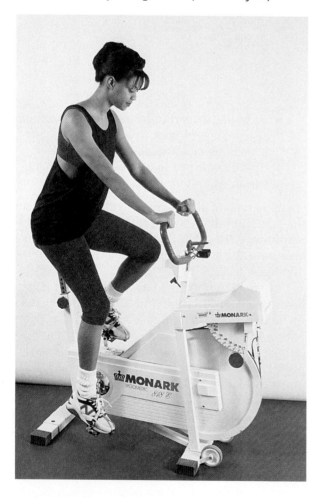

room benches or sturdy chairs can be used as stepping devices. The test is conducted as follows:

1. Select a partner to assist you in the step test. Your partner is responsible for timing the test and assisting you in maintaining the proper stepping cadence. The exercise cadence is 30 complete steps (up and down) per minute during a 3-minute exercise period, which can be maintained by a metronome or voice cues from your friend ("up, up, down, down").

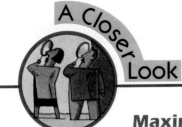

2.2 A Closer Look

Maximum Oxygen Uptake (VO$_2$ max)

As discussed earlier, VO$_2$ max is the maximal capacity to transport and utilize oxygen during exercise and is considered to be the most valid measurement of cardiorespiratory fitness (8, 9). In cardiorespiratory fitness testing, it is common to express VO$_2$ max as a function of body weight (called relative VO$_2$ max). This means that the "absolute" VO$_2$ max (expressed in milliliters per minute; commonly written as ml/min) is divided by the subject's body weight in kilograms (1 kilogram = 2.2 pounds). Therefore, relative VO$_2$ max is expressed in milliliters (ml) of oxygen consumed per minute per kilogram of body weight (ml/kg/min). Expressing VO$_2$ max relative to body weight is particularly appropriate when describing an individual's fitness status during weight-bearing activities such as running, walking, climbing steps, or ice skating (8).

The higher the relative VO$_2$ max, the greater the cardiorespiratory fitness. For example, a 20-year-old female college student with a relative VO$_2$ max of 53 ml/kg/min would be classified in the "superior" cardiorespiratory fitness category. In contrast, a 20-year-old woman with a VO$_2$ max of 29 ml/kg/min would be classified in the "very poor" fitness category (17) (see Table 2.5).

Subjects counting heart rate for 15 seconds using the radial or carotid artery. Palpation of the radial (wrist) or carotid artery (neck) is a simple means of determining heart rate. The procedure is performed as follows. Locate your radial or carotid artery using your index finger. After finding your radial or carotid pulse, count the number of heart beats (pulses) that occur during a 15-second period. Heart rate for 1 minute is computed by multiplying the number of heart beats counted in 15 seconds by 4. For example, a 15-second heart rate count of 30 beats would indicate that the heart rate was 120 beats/min (i.e. 30 x 4 = 120). When palpating the carotid artery, take care to apply limited pressure on the neck. Application of too much force on the carotid artery will result in a reflexic lowering of your heart rate and therefore bias heart rate measurement.

Thus you need to make one complete step cycle every 2 seconds (i.e., set the metronome at 60 tones/min and step up and down with each sound). Note that it is important that you straighten your knees during the "up" phase of the test (see Figure 2.1).

2. After completing the test, sit quietly in a chair or on the step bench. Find your pulse and count your heart rate for 30-second periods during the following recovery times:

1 to 1.5 minutes post exercise

2 to 2.5 minutes post exercise

3 to 3.5 minutes post exercise

Your partner should assist you in timing the recovery period and recording your recovery heart rates. Note that the accuracy of this test de-

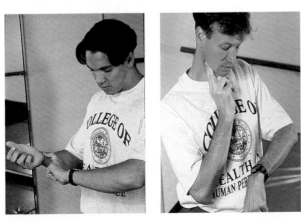

step test A submaximal exercise test designed to evaluate cardiorespiratory fitness. The step test works on the principle that individuals with a high level of cardiorespiratory fitness will have a lower heart rate during recovery from 3 minutes of standardized exercise (bench stepping) than less-conditioned individuals.

pends on the faithful execution of 30 steps per minute during the test and the valid measurement of heart rate during the appropriate recovery times.

Laboratory 2.5 provides a place to record your recovery heart rates and fitness category. To determine your fitness category, add the three 30-second heart rates obtained during recovery; this is called the **recovery index**. Table 2.6 contains norms for step test results in a college-age population (18–25 years). For example, a male student with a recovery index of 165 beats would be classified as having average cardiorespiratory fitness.

Cardiorespiratory Fitness: How Do You Rate?

After completing the cardiorespiratory fitness test of your choice, the next step is to interpret your results and set goals for improvement. If your cardiorespiratory fitness test score placed you in the "very poor" or "poor" classification, your current fitness level is below average compared with that of other healthy men or women of similar age in North America. On the other hand, a fitness test score in the "good" category means that your current cardiorespiratory fitness level is above average for your gender and age group. The fitness category "excellent" means that your level of cardiorespiratory conditioning is well above average. The "superior" rating is reserved for those individuals whose cardiorespiratory fitness level ranks in the top 15% of people in their age group. A key point here is that regardless of how low your current cardiorespiratory fitness level may be, you can improve by adherence to a regular exercise training program.

As mentioned earlier, testing your initial cardiorespiratory fitness level provides a benchmark against which you can compare future evaluations. Performing additional fitness tests as your fitness level improves is important because this type of positive feedback provides motivation to maintain regular exercise habits (3–5, 18).

recovery index Measurement of heart rate during three 30-second recovery periods following a submaximal step test. (See Chapter 2 for complete details.)

one-repetition maximum (1 RM) test Measurement of the maximum amount of weight that can be lifted one time.

Table 2.6

Norms for Cardiorespiratory Fitness Using the Sum of Three Recovery Heart Rates Obtained Following the Step Test

Fitness Category	3-Minute Step Test Recovery Index	
	Women	Men
Superior	95–120	95–117
Excellent	121–135	118–132
Good	136–153	133–147
Average	154–174	148–165
Poor	175–204	166–192
Very poor	205–233	193–217

Fitness categories are for college-age men and women (ages 18–25 years) at the University of Florida who performed the test on an 18-inch bench.

Evaluation of Muscular Strength

As discussed in Chapter 1, muscular strength is defined as the maximum amount of force you can produce during one contraction. Muscular strength not only is important for success in athletics, but also is useful for the average person in performing routine tasks at work or home. Strength can be measured by the **one-repetition maximum (1 RM) test**, which measures the maximum amount of weight that can be lifted one time.

The 1 RM Test

Although the 1 RM test for muscular strength is widely accepted (6), it has been criticized as unsuitable for use with older individuals or highly deconditioned people. The major concern is the risk of injury. The 1 RM test should therefore be attempted only after several weeks of strength training, which will result in improvements in both skill and strength and reduce the risk of injury during the test. An older or sedentary individual would probably require 6 weeks of exercise training prior to the 1 RM test whereas a physically active college-age student could probably perform the 1 RM test after 1 to 2 weeks of training.

The 1 RM test is designed to test muscular strength in selected muscle groups and is performed in the following manner. Begin with a 5- to 10-minute warm-up using the muscles to be tested. For each muscle group, select an initial weight that you can lift without undue stress. Then gradually add weight until you reach the maximum weight that you can lift one time. If you can lift the weight more than once, add additional weight until you reach a level of resistance such that you can perform only one repetition. Remember that a true 1 RM is the maximum amount of weight that you can lift one time.

Figures 2.2 through 2.5 illustrate four common lifts used to measure strength. Three of these (bench press, biceps curl, and shoulder press) use upper body muscle groups; the fourth lift (leg press) measures leg strength. Table 2.7 contains strength score norms for college-age men and women in each of these lifts. Your muscle strength score is your percentage of body weight lifted in each exercise. To compute your strength score in each lift, divide your 1 RM weight in pounds by your body weight in pounds and then multiply by 100. For example, suppose a 150-pound man has a bench press 1 RM of 180 pounds. This individual's muscle strength score for the bench press is computed as

$$\frac{1 \text{ RM weight}}{\text{body weight}} \times 100 = \text{muscle strength score}$$

therefore,

$$\text{muscle strength score} = \frac{180 \text{ pounds}}{150 \text{ pounds}} \times 100 = 120$$

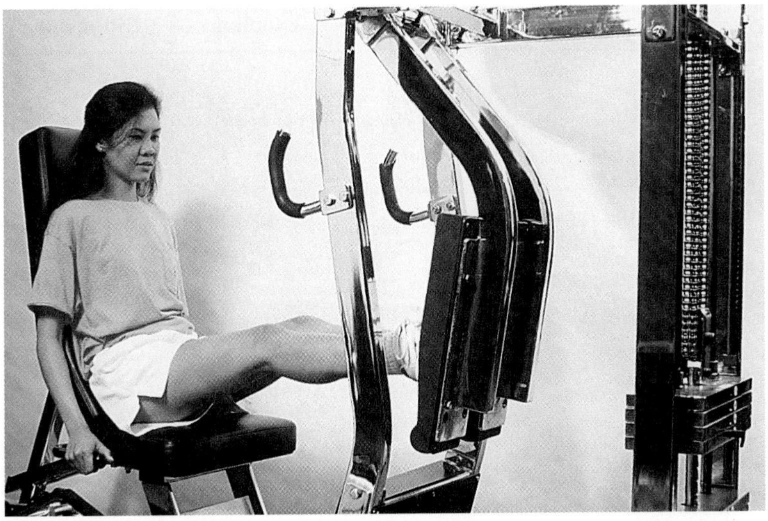

Using Table 2.7, a muscle strength score of 120 on the bench press places a college-age man in the "good" category. You can record your muscle strength scores in Laboratory 2.6.

Muscular Strength: How Do You Rate?

After completion of your muscular strength test, the next step is to interpret your results (Table 2.7) and set goals for improvement. Similar to the fitness categories used for cardiorespiratory fitness, the fitness categories for muscular strength range from very poor (lowest) to superior (highest). If your current strength level is classified as average or below, don't be discouraged; you can improve! A key point in maintaining your motivation to exercise regularly is the establishment of goals. After completion of your initial strength test, record both short-term and long-term goals for improvement. After 6 to 12 weeks of training, perform a retest to evaluate your progress. Reaching a short-term goal provides added incentive to continue your exercise program.

FIGURE 2.3 The bench press to evaluate muscular strength.

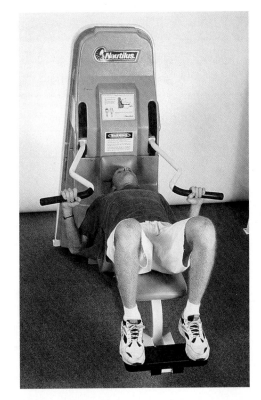

FIGURE 2.2 A leg press to evaluate muscular strength.

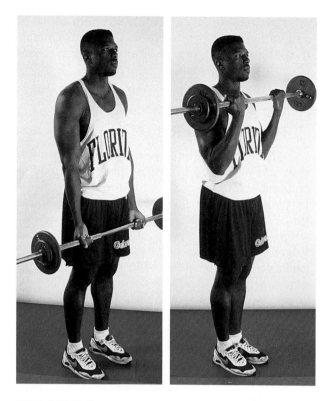

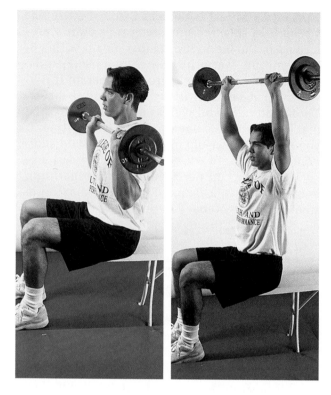

FIGURE 2.4 A biceps curl to evaluate muscular strength.

FIGURE 2.5 The shoulder or "military" press to evaluate muscular strength.

Table 2.7

Norms for Muscle Strength Scores Using a 1 RM Test
In this table, use your muscle strength score to locate your fitness level.

	Fitness Category					
Exercise	Very Poor	Poor	Average	Good	Excellent	Superior
Men						
Bench press	<50	50–99	100–110	111–130	131–149	>149
Biceps curl	<30	30–40	41–54	55–60	61–79	>79
Shoulder press	<40	41–50	51–67	68–80	81–110	>110
Leg press	<160	161–199	200–209	210–229	230–239	>239
Women						
Bench press	<40	41–69	70–74	75–80	81–99	>99
Biceps curl	<15	15–34	35–39	40–55	56–59	>59
Shoulder press	<20	20–46	47–54	55–59	60–79	>79
Leg press	<100	100–130	131–144	145–174	175–189	>189

Norms are from ref. 7.

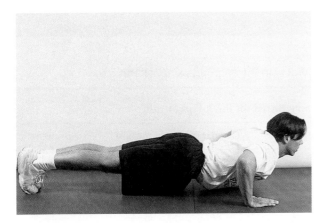

FIGURE 2.6 The standard push-up.

Measurement of Muscular Endurance

Muscular endurance is the ability of a muscle or muscle group to generate force over and over again. Although an individual might have sufficient strength to lift a heavy box from the ground to the back of a truck, he or she might not have sufficient muscular endurance to perform this task multiple times. Because many everyday tasks require submaximal but repeated muscular contractions, muscular endurance is an important facet of health-related physical fitness.

Although numerous methods exist to evaluate muscular strength, two simple tests to assess muscular endurance involve the performance of push-ups and sit-ups or *curl-ups*. Push-ups are a measure of muscular endurance using the shoulder, arm, and chest muscles, whereas sit-ups and curl-ups primarily evaluate abdominal muscle endurance.

The Push-Up Test

The standard **push-up test** to evaluate muscular endurance is performed in the following way. Start by positioning yourself on the ground in push-up position (see Figure 2.6). Your hands should be approximately shoulder width and your legs extended in a straight line with your weight placed on your toes. Lower your body until your chest is within 1 to 2 inches of the ground and raise yourself back to the up position. It is important to keep your back straight and lower your entire body to the ground as a unit.

The push-up test is performed as follows:

1. Select a partner to count your push-ups and assist in the timing of the test (test duration is 60 seconds). Warm up with a few push-ups. Give yourself a 2- to 3-minute recovery period after the warm-up and prepare to start the test.

2. On the command "go," start performing push-ups. Your partner counts your push-ups aloud and informs you of the amount of time remaining in the test period (e.g., at 15-second intervals). Remember only those push-ups that are performed correctly will be counted toward your total; therefore, use the proper form and make every push-up count.

3. After completion of the push-up test, use Table 2.8 to determine your fitness classification, and record your scores in Laboratory 2.7.

The Sit-Up Test

The bent-knee **sit-up test** is probably the best-known field test available to evaluate abdominal muscle endurance (4, 5a). Figure 2.7a on page 31 illustrates the correct position for performance of bent-knee sit-ups. Begin by lying on your back with your arms crossed on your chest. Your knees should be bent at approximately 90-degree angles, with your feet flat on the floor. The com-

push-up test A fitness test designed to evaluate muscular endurance of shoulder and arm muscles.

sit-up test A field test to evaluate abdominal muscle endurance.

Table 2.8

Norms for Muscular Endurance Using the Push-Up Test
Find your age group on the left and then locate your fitness category in the appropriate right-hand column.

Age Group (years)	Fitness Category Based on Push-Ups (1 min)					
	Very Poor	**Poor**	**Average**	**Good**	**Excellent**	**Superior**
Men						
15–19	<20	20–24	25–34	35–44	45–53	>53
20–29	<19	19–23	24–33	34–43	44–52	>52
30–39	<15	15–20	21–24	25–34	35–44	>44
40–49	<12	12–14	15–19	20–29	30–39	>39
50–59	<8	8–11	12–15	16–24	25–34	>34
60+	<5	5–7	8–9	10–19	20–29	>29
Women						
15–19	<5	6–9	10–12	13–14	15–19	>19
20–29	<4	4–8	9–10	11–12	13–18	>18
30–39	<3	4–7	8–11	12–13	14–16	>16
40–49	<2	3–5	6–9	10–12	13–15	>15
50–59	1	2–3	4–5	6–9	10–11	>11
60+	0	1–2	2–3	4–5	6–8	>8

Men's norms are modified from Pollock, M., J. Wilmore, and S. Fox. *Health and fitness through physical activity.* John Wiley and Sons, New York, 1978. Women's norms are unpublished data from the University of Florida.

plete sit-up is performed by bringing your chest up to touch your knees and returning to the original lying position.

Note that although the abdominal muscles are very active during the performance of a bent-leg sit-up, leg muscles such as hip flexors also play a role. Therefore, this test evaluates not only abdominal muscle endurance but hip muscle endurance as well (26).

Sit-up tests are generally considered to be relatively safe fitness tests, but two precautions should be mentioned. First, avoid undue stress on your neck during the "up" phase of the exercise. That is, let your abdominal muscles do the work; do not whip your neck during the sit-up movement. Second, avoid hitting the back of your head on the floor during the "down" phase of the sit-up. Performance of the test on a padded mat is helpful.

The protocol for the sit-up test is as follows:

1. Select a partner to count your sit-ups, to hold your feet on the floor by grasping your ankles, and to assist in the timing of the test.

2. Warm up with a few sit-ups. Give yourself a 2- to 3-minute recovery period after the warm-up and prepare to start the test.

3. On the command "go," start performing sit-ups and continue for 60 seconds. Your partner should count your sit-ups aloud and inform you of the time remaining in the test period (perhaps by called-out 15-second intervals). Remember that only sits-ups performed correctly will be counted toward your total.

4. After completing the sit-up test, use Table 2.9a to determine your fitness classification. Record your scores in Laboratory 2.7.

The Curl-Up Test

As mentioned earlier, although sit-up tests utilize abdominal muscles, leg muscles are also recruited to move the trunk upward. Use of these leg muscles can be eliminated by performing a partial sit-up or a curl-up. The curl-up differs from the sit-up in that the trunk is not raised more than 30–40 degrees above the mat (attained when the shoulders are lifted approximately 6–10 inches above the mat; see Figure 2.7b) (25, 26). There are two advantages of the curl-up over the sit-up. First, the curl-up recruits only abdominal muscles, whereas the sit-up test involves both abdominal muscles and hip flexors. Second, research suggests that the curl-up provides less stress on the lower back than the conventional sit-up (28). For these reasons, the **curl-up test** is growing in popularity and is often used instead

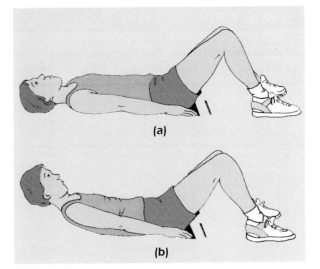

FIGURE 2.7b The proper position and movement pattern for the performance of a curl-up.

FIGURE 2.7a The proper position for the performance of sit-ups.

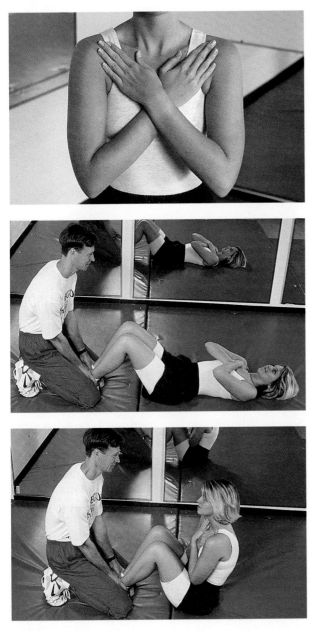

of the sit-up to evaluate abdominal muscle endurance.

The protocol for the curl-up test is as follows:

1. Select a partner to count your curl-ups; lie on your back with knees bent 90 degrees.

2. Extend your arms so that your fingertips touch a strip of tape perpendicular to the body (Figure 2.7b). A second strip of tape is located toward the feet and parallel to the first (8 centimeters or 3.15 inches apart). The curl-up is accomplished by raising your trunk (i.e., curling upward) until your fingertips touch the second strip of tape and then returning to the starting position.

3. The curl-up test is not timed and is performed at a slow and controlled cadence of 20 curl-ups per minute. This cadence is guided by the aid of a metronome set at 40 beats per minute (curl-up on one beat and down on the second).

4. On the command "go" start performing curl-ups in cadence with the metronome. Perform as many curl-ups as you can to a maximum of 75 without missing a beat. See Table 2.9b on page 33 to determine your fitness category and record your score in Laboratory 2.7.

curl-up test A field test to evaluate abdominal muscle endurance.

Table 2.9a

Norms for Muscular Endurance Using the 1-Minute Sit-Up Test
Find your age group on the left and then locate your fitness category in the appropriate column on the right.

Age Group (years)	Fitness Category Based on Sit-Ups (1 min)					
	Very Poor	Poor	Average	Good	Excellent	Superior
Men						
17–29	<17	17–35	36–41	42–47	48–50	>50
30–39	<13	13–26	27–32	33–38	39–48	>48
40–49	<12	12–22	23–27	28–33	34–43	>43
50–59	<8	8–16	17–21	22–28	29–38	>38
60+	<6	6–12	13–17	18–24	25–35	>35
Women						
20–29	<14	14–28	29–32	33–35	36–47	>47
30–39	<11	11–22	23–28	29–34	35–45	>45
40–49	<9	9–18	19–23	24–30	31–40	>40
50–59	<6	6–12	13–17	18–24	25–35	>35
60+	<5	5–10	11–14	15–20	21–30	>30

Modified from Pollock, M., J. Wilmore, S. Fox. *Health and fitness through physical activity.* John Wiley and Sons, New York, 1978.

Muscular Endurance: How Do You Rate?

The fitness categories for muscular endurance range from very poor (lowest) to superior (highest). If your muscular endurance test score placed you in the "very poor" or "poor" classification, your present muscular endurance level is below average compared with other men and women of your age group. On the other hand, a fitness test score in the "good" category means that your current muscular endurance is above average. The fitness category "excellent" means that your muscular endurance level is well above average. Finally, the fitness category labeled "superior" is reserved for those individuals whose muscular endurance ranks in the top 15% of men and women in your age group.

If you scored poorly on either the push-up or sit-up test, do not be discouraged. Establish your goals and begin doing sit-ups and push-ups on a regular basis (see Chapter 5 for the exercise prescription for muscular strength). Your ability to perform both sit-ups and push-ups will increase within the first 3 to 4 weeks of training and will continue to improve for weeks to come.

Assessment of Flexibility

Flexibility, the ability to move joints freely through their full range of motion, can decrease over time due to tightening of muscles and/or tendons. Loss of flexibility can occur due to both muscle disuse and muscular training. The key to maintaining flexibility is a program of regular stretching exercises (see Chapter 6).

Individual needs for flexibility are variable. Some athletes, such as gymnasts, require great flexibility in order to perform complex movements in competition (3, 5, 9, 18). In general, the nonathlete requires less flexibility than the athlete. Some flexibility, however, is required for everyone in order to perform common activities of daily living or recreational pursuits.

It is important to appreciate that flexibility is joint-specific. That is, a person might be flexible in one joint but lack flexibility in another. Although there is no single test that is representative of total body flexibility, measurements of trunk and shoulder flexibility are commonly evaluated.

Table 2.9b

Norms for Muscular Endurance Using the Curl-Up Test

Find your gender and age group on the left and locate the fitness category closest to your score on the right.

Age Group (years)	Fitness Category Based on Curl-Ups Performed				
	Poor	Average	Good	Excellent	Superior
Men					
<35	15	30	45	60	75
35–44	10	25	40	50	60
>45	5	15	25	40	50
Women					
<35	10	25	40	50	60
35–44	6	15	25	40	50
>45	4	10	15	30	40

Modified from Faulkner, R. A., et al. A partial curl-up protocol for adults based on two procedures. *Canadian Journal of Sports Sciences* 14:135–141, 1989.

Trunk Flexibility

The **sit and reach test** measures the ability to flex the trunk, which means stretching the lower back muscles and the muscles in the back of the thigh (hamstrings). Figure 2.8 illustrates the sit and reach test using a sit and reach box. The test is performed in the following manner.

Start by removing your shoes and sitting upright with your feet flat against the box. Keeping your feet flat on the box and your legs straight, extend your hands as far forward as possible and

FIGURE 2.8 The sit and reach test to evaluate flexibility.

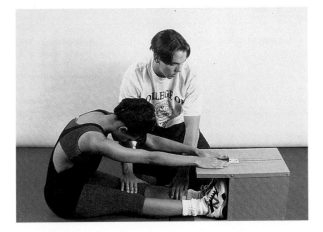

hold this position for 3 seconds. Repeat this procedure three times. Your score on the sit and reach test is the distance, measured in inches, between the sit and reach box and the tips of your fingers during the best of your three stretching efforts.

Note that a brief warm-up period consisting of a few minutes of stretching is recommended prior to performance of the test. To reduce the possibility of injury, participants should avoid rapid or jerky movements during the test. It is often useful to have a partner help by holding your legs straight during the test and to assist in the recording of your score. After completing the test, consult Table 2.10 to locate your flexibility fitness category, and record your scores in Laboratory 2.8.

Shoulder Flexibility

As the name implies, the shoulder flexibility test evaluates shoulder range of motion (flexibility). The test is performed in the following man-

sit and reach test A fitness test that measures the ability to flex the trunk (i.e., stretching the lower back muscles and the muscles in the back of the thigh).

Table 2.10

Physical Fitness Norms for Trunk Flexion Using the Sit and Reach Test
Note that these norms are for both men and women (ages 18–50 years). Units for the sit and reach score are inches and indicate the distance of your finger tips from the edge of the sit and reach box. Negative numbers indicate that you cannot reach your toes, whereas positive numbers indicate the number of inches that you can reach past your toes.

Sit and Reach Score	Fitness Classification
–6 to –15	Very poor
–1 to –5	Poor
0 to +1	Average
+2 to +3	Good
+3 to +5	Excellent
+6 or above	Superior

Modified from Golding, L., C. Myers, and W. Sinning. *Y's way to physical fitness: The complete guide to fitness testing and instruction.* 3rd ed. Human Kinetics, Champaign, IL, 1989.

ner. While standing, raise your right arm and reach down your back as far as possible (see Figure 2.9). At the same time, extend your left arm behind your back and reach upward toward your right hand. The objective is to try to overlap your fingers as much as possible. Your score on the shoulder flexibility test is the distance, measured in inches, of finger overlap.

Measure the distance of finger overlap to the nearest inch. For example, an overlap of 3/4 inch would be recorded as 1 inch. If your fingers fail to overlap, record this score as minus one (–1). Finally, if your fingertips barely touch, record this score as zero (0).

After completing the test with the right hand up, repeat the test in the opposite direction (left arm up). Note that it is common to be more flexible on one side than on the other.

A brief warm-up period consisting of a few minutes of stretching is recommended prior to performance of the shoulder flexibility test. Again, to prevent injury, avoid rapid or jerky movements during the test. After completion of the test, consult Table 2.11 to locate your shoulder flexibility category, and record your scores in Laboratory 2.8.

FIGURE 2.9 The trunk extension test to evaluate flexibility.

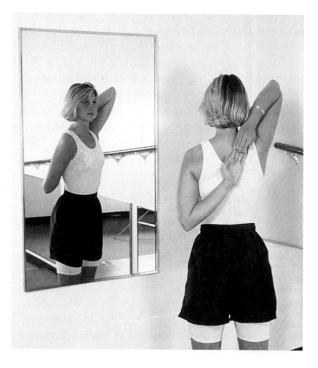

Table 2.11

Physical Fitness Norms for Shoulder Flexibility
Note that these norms are for both men and women of all ages. Units for the shoulder flexibility test score are inches and indicate the distance between the fingers of your right and left hands.

Right Hand Up Score	Left Hand Up Score	Fitness Classification
<0	<0	Very poor
0	0	Poor
+1	+1	Average
+2	+2	Good
+3	+3	Excellent
+4	+4	Superior

From Fox, E.L., Kirby, T.E., and Fox, A.R. *Bases of Fitness.* Copyright © 1987. All rights reserved. Adapted by permission of Allyn and Bacon. Norms from ref. 4.

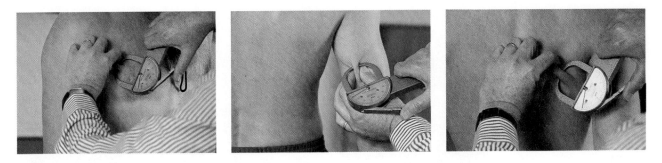

FIGURE 2.10 Skinfold measurement sites for men.

Flexibility: How Do You Rate?

It is not uncommon for both active and inactive individuals to be classified as average or below for both trunk flexion and shoulder flexibility. In fact, only individuals who regularly perform stretching exercises are likely to possess flexibility levels that exceed the average. Regardless of your current flexibility classification, your flexibility goal should be to reach a classification of above average (i.e., good, excellent, or superior).

Assessment of Body Composition

Recall that a high percentage of body fat is associated with an increased risk of heart disease and other diseases. It is therefore not surprising that several methods of assessing body composition have been developed. A technique considered to be the gold standard for laboratory assessment of body fat in humans is **hydrostatic weighing** and involves weighing the individual both on land and in a tank of water (6, 8, 27). The two body weights are then entered into a simple formula to calculate the percent of body fat. Unfortunately, underwater weighing is very time consuming and requires expensive equipment. Thus, this procedure is rarely employed to assess body composition in collegiate physical fitness courses. A rapid and inexpensive method to assess body composition is measurement of subcutaneous fat or fat beneath the skin (called *the skinfold test*).

The Skinfold Test

Subcutaneous fat is measured using an instrument called a skinfold caliper. The **skinfold test** relies on the fact that over 50% of body fat lies just beneath the skin (6, 8, 19). Therefore, measurement of representative samples of subcutaneous fat provides a means of estimating overall body fatness. Skinfold measurements to determine body fat are reliable but generally have a ±3% to 4% margin of error (6, 8).

One of the most accurate skinfold tests to estimate body fatness requires three skinfold measurements for both men and women (20). The anatomical sites to be measured in men (chest, triceps, and subscapular skinfolds) are illustrated in Figure 2.10 and the measurement sites for women (triceps, suprailium, and abdominal skinfolds) are illustrated in Figure 2.11. Note that for standardization, all measurements should be made on the right side of the body.

1. To make each measurement, hold the skinfold between the thumb and index finger and slowly release the tension on the skinfold calipers so as to pinch the skinfold within 1/2 inch of your fingers. Continue to hold the skinfold with your fingers and fully release the tension on the calipers; then, simply read

hydrostatic weighing A method of determining body composition that involves weighing the individual both on land and in a tank of water.

skinfold test A field test to estimate body composition. The test works on the principle that over 50% of the body fat lies just beneath the skin. Therefore, measurement of representative samples of subcutaneous fat provides a means of estimating overall body fatness.

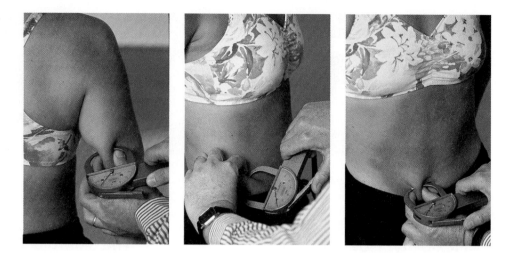

FIGURE 2.11 Skinfold measurement sites for women.

the number (the skinfold thickness in millimeters) from the gauge. Release the skinfold and allow the tissue to relax. Repeat this procedure three times and average the sum of the three measurements.

2. After completing the three skinfold measurements, total the measurements and use Tables 2.12 and 2.13 to determine the percent body fat for women and men, respectively. After obtaining your percent body fat, refer to Table 2.14 (21) to determine the body composition fitness category, and record your score in Laboratory 2.9.

Estimation of Body Composition: Field Techniques

Several quick and inexpensive field techniques exist to evaluate body composition and the risk of heart disease associated with over-fatness (18, 22–24). Here we describe some of the more popular procedures currently in use.

Waist-to-Hip Circumference Ratio Recent evidence suggests that the waist-to-hip circumfer-ence ratio is an excellent index for determining the risk of disease associated with high body fat (24). The rationale for this technique is that a high percentage of fat in the abdominal region is associated with an increased risk of disease (such as heart disease or hypertension). Therefore, an individual with a large fat deposit in the abdominal region would have a high waist-to-hip ratio and would have a higher risk of disease than someone with a lower waist-to-hip ratio. The procedure for assessment of **waist-to-hip circumference ratio** is as follows:

1. Both waist and hip circumference measurements should be made while standing, using a nonelastic tape. It is important that bulky clothing not be worn during the measurement, because it could bias the circumference measurement. During measurement, the tape should be placed tightly around the body but should not press into the skin. Record your measurements to the nearest millimeter or sixteenth of an inch.

2. Perform the waist measurement first. Begin by placing the tape at the level of the umbilicus (see Figure 2.12A). Make your measurement at the end of a normal expiration.

3. To make the hip measurement, place the tape around the maximum circumference of the buttocks (Figure 2.12B).

4. After completing the measurements, divide the waist circumference by the hip circumference to determine the waist-to-hip ratio. Use Table 2.15 to determine the hip-to-waist ratio rating. Your goal in terms of waist-to-hip ratio classification should be to reach the optimal classification that places you in the lowest risk category for heart disease.

waist-to-hip circumference ratio An index for determining the risk of disease associated with high body fat. The rationale for this technique is that a high percentage of fat in the abdominal region is associated with an increased risk of disease (e.g., heart disease or hypertension). Therefore, an individual with a large fat deposit in the abdominal region would have a high waist-to-hip ratio and would have a higher risk of disease than someone with a lower waist-to-hip ratio.

Table 2.12

Percent Fat Estimate for Women
Sum of Triceps, Abdomen, and Suprailium Skinfolds

Sum of Skinfolds (mm)	Age (years)								
	18–22	23–27	28–32	33–37	38–42	43–47	48–52	53–57	>57
8–12	8.8	9.0	9.2	9.4	9.5	9.7	9.9	10.1	10.3
13–17	10.8	10.9	11.1	11.3	11.5	11.7	11.8	12.0	12.2
18–22	12.6	12.8	13.0	13.2	13.4	13.5	13.7	13.9	14.1
23–27	14.5	14.6	14.8	15.0	15.2	15.4	15.6	15.7	15.9
28–32	16.2	16.4	16.6	16.8	17.0	17.1	17.3	17.5	17.7
33–37	17.9	18.1	18.3	18.5	18.7	18.9	19.0	19.2	19.4
38–42	19.6	19.8	20.0	20.2	20.3	20.5	20.7	20.9	21.1
43–47	21.2	21.4	21.6	21.8	21.9	22.1	22.3	22.5	22.7
48–52	22.8	22.9	23.1	23.3	23.5	23.7	23.8	24.0	24.2
53–57	24.2	24.4	24.6	24.8	25.0	25.2	25.3	25.5	25.7
58–62	25.7	25.9	26.0	26.2	26.4	26.6	26.8	27.0	27.1
63–67	27.1	27.2	27.4	27.6	27.8	28.0	28.2	28.3	28.5
68–72	28.4	28.6	28.7	28.9	29.1	29.3	29.5	29.7	29.8
73–77	29.6	29.8	30.0	30.2	30.4	30.6	30.7	30.9	31.1
78–82	30.9	31.0	31.2	31.4	31.6	31.8	31.9	32.1	32.3
83–87	32.0	32.2	32.4	32.6	32.7	32.9	33.1	33.3	33.5
88–92	33.1	33.3	33.5	33.7	33.8	34.0	34.2	34.4	34.6
93–97	34.1	34.3	34.5	34.7	34.9	35.1	35.2	35.4	35.6
98–102	35.1	35.3	35.5	35.7	35.9	36.0	36.2	36.4	36.6
103–107	36.1	36.2	36.4	36.6	36.8	37.0	37.2	37.3	37.5
108–112	36.9	37.1	37.3	37.5	37.7	37.9	38.0	38.2	38.4
113–117	37.8	37.9	38.1	38.3	39.2	39.4	39.6	39.8	39.2
118–122	38.5	38.7	38.9	39.1	39.4	39.6	39.8	40.0	40.0
123–127	39.2	39.4	39.6	39.8	40.0	40.1	40.3	40.5	40.7
128–132	39.9	40.1	40.2	40.4	40.6	40.8	41.0	41.2	41.3
133–137	40.5	40.7	40.8	41.0	41.2	41.4	41.6	41.7	41.9
138–142	41.0	41.2	41.4	41.6	41.7	41.9	42.1	42.3	42.5
143–147	41.5	41.7	41.9	42.0	42.2	42.4	42.6	42.8	43.0
148–152	41.9	42.1	42.3	42.4	42.6	42.8	43.0	43.2	43.4
153–157	42.3	42.5	42.6	42.8	43.0	43.2	43.4	43.6	43.7
158–162	42.6	42.8	43.0	43.1	43.3	43.5	43.7	43.9	44.1
163–167	42.9	43.0	43.2	43.4	43.6	43.8	44.0	44.1	44.3
168–172	43.1	43.2	43.4	43.6	43.8	44.0	44.2	44.3	44.5
173–177	43.2	43.4	43.6	43.8	43.9	44.1	44.3	44.5	44.7
178–182	43.3	43.5	43.7	43.8	44.0	44.2	44.4	44.6	44.8

From Jackson, A., and M. Pollock. Practical assessment of body composition. *Physician and Sports Medicine* 13:76–90, 1985.

Table 2.13

Percent Fat Estimate for Men
Sum of Triceps, Chest, and Subscapula Skinfolds

Sum of Skinfolds (mm)	Age (years)								
	<22	23–27	28–32	33–37	38–42	43–47	48–52	53–57	>57
8–10	1.5	2.0	2.5	3.1	3.6	4.1	4.6	5.1	5.6
11–13	3.0	3.5	4.0	4.5	5.1	5.6	6.1	6.6	7.1
14–16	4.5	5.0	5.5	6.0	6.5	7.0	7.6	8.1	8.6
17–19	5.9	6.4	6.9	7.4	8.0	8.5	9.0	9.5	10.0
20–22	7.3	7.8	8.3	8.8	9.4	9.9	10.4	10.9	11.4
23–25	8.6	9.2	9.7	10.2	10.7	11.2	11.8	12.3	12.8
26–28	10.0	10.5	11.0	11.5	12.1	12.6	13.1	13.6	14.2
29–31	11.2	11.8	12.3	12.8	13.4	13.9	14.4	14.9	15.5
32–34	12.5	13.0	13.5	14.1	14.6	15.1	15.7	16.2	16.7
41–43	16.0	16.6	17.1	17.6	18.2	18.7	19.3	19.8	20.3
44–46	17.1	17.7	18.2	18.7	19.3	19.8	20.4	20.9	21.5
47–49	18.2	18.7	19.3	19.8	20.4	20.9	21.4	22.0	22.5
50–52	19.2	19.7	20.3	20.8	21.4	21.9	22.5	23.0	23.6
53–55	20.2	20.7	21.3	21.8	22.4	22.9	23.5	24.0	24.6
56–58	21.1	21.7	22.2	22.8	23.3	23.9	24.4	25.0	25.5
59–61	22.0	22.6	23.1	23.7	24.2	24.8	25.3	25.9	26.5
62–64	22.9	23.4	24.0	24.5	25.1	25.7	26.2	26.8	27.3
65–67	23.7	24.3	24.8	25.4	25.9	26.5	27.1	27.6	28.2
68–70	24.5	25.0	25.6	26.2	26.7	27.3	27.8	28.4	29.0
71–73	25.2	25.8	26.3	26.9	27.5	28.0	28.6	29.1	29.7
74–76	25.9	26.5	27.0	27.6	28.2	28.7	29.3	29.9	30.4
77–79	26.6	27.1	27.7	28.2	28.8	29.4	29.9	30.5	31.1
80–82	27.2	27.7	28.3	28.9	29.4	30.0	30.6	31.1	31.7
83–85	27.7	28.3	28.8	29.4	30.0	30.5	31.1	31.7	32.3
86–88	28.2	28.8	29.4	29.9	30.5	31.1	31.6	32.2	32.8
89–91	28.7	29.3	29.8	30.4	31.0	31.5	32.1	32.7	33.3
92–94	29.1	29.7	30.3	30.8	31.4	32.0	32.6	33.1	33.4
95–97	29.5	30.1	30.6	31.2	31.8	32.4	32.9	33.5	34.1
98–100	29.8	30.4	31.0	31.6	32.1	32.7	33.3	33.9	34.4
101–103	30.1	30.7	31.3	31.8	32.4	33.0	33.6	34.1	34.7
104–106	30.4	30.9	31.5	32.1	32.7	33.2	33.8	34.4	35.0
107–109	30.6	31.1	31.7	32.3	32.9	33.4	34.0	34.6	35.2
110–112	30.7	31.3	31.9	32.4	33.0	33.6	34.2	34.7	35.3
113–115	30.8	31.4	32.0	32.5	33.1	33.7	34.3	34.9	35.4
116–118	30.9	31.5	32.0	32.6	33.2	33.8	34.3	34.9	35.5

From Jackson, A., and M. Pollock. Practical assessment of body composition. *Physician and Sports Medicine* 13:76–90, 1985.

Table 2.14

Body Composition Fitness Categories for Men and Women

Percent Body Fat	Body Composition Fitness Category
Men	
<10%	Low body fat
10–20%	Optimal range of body fat
21–25%	Moderately high body fat
26–31%	High body fat
>31%	Very high body fat
Women	
<15%	Low body fat
15–25%	Optimal range of body fat
26–30%	Moderately high body fat
31–35%	High body fat
>35%	Very high body fat

Data from Lohman (21).

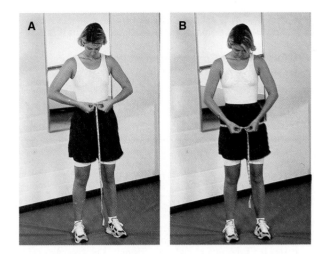

FIGURE 2.12 Illustration of the waist-to-hip circumference measurement.

Body Mass Index Although many limitations exist, research has shown that the **body mass index** (BMI) is a useful technique for placing people into categories of normal or too much body fat (22, 24). The BMI is simply the ratio of the body weight (kilograms; kg) divided by the height (in meters) squared (m^2):

BMI = weight (kg)/height (m^2)

(Note: 1 kg = 2.2 pounds and 1 m = 39.25 inches.)

For example, if an individual weighs 64.5 kg and is 1.72 m tall, the BMI would be computed as follows:

$$64.5 \text{ kg}/(1.72 \text{ m})^2 = 64.5/2.96 = 21.8$$

After calculation of your BMI, use Table 2.16 to determine your degree of body fatness. The concept behind the BMI is that individuals with low percent body fat will have a low BMI. For example, men and women with a BMI of less than 25 and 27, respectively, are classified as being non-obese. In contrast, men and women with a BMI of greater than 40 are considered to be extremely obese.

Height/Weight Tables The Metropolitan Life Insurance Company has published a height/weight table designed to determine whether a person is overweight due to too much body fat. Although the idea that a simple table could be used to determine the ideal body weight is attractive, several problems exist with this procedure. The major problem with this approach is that the tables do not indicate how much of the body weight is fat. For example, an individual can exceed the ideal body weight on such a chart by being either heavily muscled or overfat. Therefore, this approach to determination of an "ideal body weight" is not recommended.

Body Composition: How Do You Rate?

The fitness categories presented for body composition differ from those presented earlier for the other components of health-related physical fitness. While "superior" was the highest fitness level presented that could be achieved for cardiorespiratory, strength, and muscular endurance fitness, in terms of body composition fitness, the classification of "optimal" is the highest standard. Regardless of the body composition test employed to assess body fat, any category

body mass index A useful technique for categorizing people with respect to their degree of body fat. The body mass index (BMI) is simply the ratio of the body weight (kilograms; kg) divided by the height squared (meters^2).

Table 2.15

Waist-to-Hip Circumference Ratio Rating Scale

Classification (risk of disease)	Men	Women
High risk	>1.0	>0.85
Moderately high risk	0.90–1.0	0.80–0.85
Optimal low risk of disease	<0.90	<0.80

Modified from Van Itallie, T. Topography of body fat: Relationship to risk of cardiovascular and other diseases. In: T. Lohman, et al., eds. Human Kinetics, *Anthropometric standardization reference manual.* Champaign, IL, 1988.

Table 2.16

Body Mass Index Classification of the Degree of Body Fatness

Degree of Obesity	BMI (weight/height^2)	
	Men	Women
Optimal body fat	<25	<27
Moderately high body fat	25–30	27–30
High body fat	31–40	31–40
Very high body fat	>40	>40

Adapted from DiGirolamo, M. Body composition—roundtable. *Physician and Sports Medicine* (March):144–162, 1986.

other than optimal is considered unsatisfactory for health-related fitness. Therefore, your goal should be to reach and maintain an optimal body composition.

The rationale for the concept of optimal body composition is as follows. Research suggests that a range of 10% to 20% body fat is an optimal health and fitness goal for men; the optimal range for women is 15% to 25%. These ranges in body fat provide little risk of disease associated with body fatness and permit individual differences in physical activity patterns and diet. Body fat levels above the optimal range are associated with

an increased risk of disease and are therefore undesirable.

What is less obvious is that a body fat percentage that is lower than the recommended optimal range is also undesirable. Indeed, percentages of body fat below the optimal range may also increase the risk of health problems. This is because extremely low percentages of body fat are often associated with poor nutrition and a loss of muscle mass. This is clearly undesirable. The relationship between diet, exercise, and body composition is discussed in detail in Chapter 8.

Summary

1. Prior to beginning a fitness program (or performing a fitness evaluation), you should evaluate your health status.

2. An objective evaluation of your current fitness status is important before beginning an exercise training program. Further, periodic retesting can provide feedback about your training progress.

3. Cardiorespiratory endurance is the ability of the heart to pump oxygen-rich blood to exercising muscles; this translates into the ability to perform endurance-type exercise. Field tests to evaluate cardiorespiratory fitness include the 1.5-mile run test, the 1-mile walk test, the submaximal cycle exercise test, and the step test.

4. Muscular strength is the maximum amount of force you can produce during one contraction. The most popular method of evaluating muscular strength is the one-repetition maximum (1 RM) test.

5. Muscular endurance is the ability of a muscle group to generate force over and over again. Two commonly used methods of evaluating muscular endurance are the push-up and sit-up tests.

6. Flexibility is defined as the ability to move joints freely through their full range of motion. Although flexibility is joint-specific, two popular means of evaluating flexibility are the sit and reach test and the shoulder flexibility test.

7. Body composition is an important component of health-related physical fitness because a high percentage of body fat is associated with an increased risk of disease.

In the field, the amount of body fat can be estimated using skinfold measurements, assessment of the body mass index, or examination of the waist-to-hip circumference ratio.

Study Questions

1. Describe the following field tests used to evaluate cardiorespiratory fitness: the 1.5-mile run test, the 1-mile walk test, the cycle ergometer exercise test, and the step test.

2. Discuss the one-repetition maximum (1 RM) test for measurement of muscular strength. What safety concerns are associated with this test?

3. Explain how the push-up and sit-up tests are used to evaluate muscular endurance.

4. Discuss the concept that flexibility is joint-specific.

5. Identify two field tests used to examine flexibility.

6. Define the term *recovery index.*

7. Discuss the following techniques to assess body composition: hydrostatic weighing and the skinfold test.

8. How can measurement of the waist-to-hip circumference ratio and body mass index be used to assess body composition?

Suggested Reading

Williams, M. *Lifetime fitness and wellness.* Wm. C. Brown, Dubuque, IA, 1996.
Sparling, P. Field testing for abdominal muscular fitness; speed versus cadence sit-ups. *ACSM's Health and Fitness Journal* 1(4): 30–33, 1997.
Lohman, T., et al. Body fat measurement goes high-tech: Not all are created equal. *ACSM's Health and Fitness Journal* 1(1): 30–35, 1997.

Suggested Reading on the World Wide Web
Fitness Tests: Explained (http://arnie.pec.BrockU.CA/~hsac/tests/tests.html) Fitness tests for aerobic power, anaerobic power, flexibility, and body composition.

References

1. American College of Sports Medicine. *Guidelines for exercise testing.* Lea and Febiger, Philadelphia, 1995.

2. American College of Sports Medicine. *Resource manual for exercise testing and prescription.* Lea and Febiger, Philadelphia, 1998.

3. Corbin, C., and R. Lindsey. *Concepts of physical fitness.* Wm. C. Brown, Dubuque, IA, 1994.

4. Getchell, B. *Physical fitness: A way of life.* Allyn and Bacon, Needham Heights, MA, 1997.

5. Barrow, M. *Heart talk: understanding cardiovascular diseases.* Cor-Ed Publishing, Gainesville, FL, 1992.

5a. McGlynn, G. *Dynamics of fitness: A practical approach.* Wm. C. Brown, Dubuque, IA, 1996.

6. Pollock, M., and J. Wilmore. *Exercise in health and disease.* W. B. Saunders, Philadelphia, 1990.

7. Pollock, M., J. Wilmore, and S. Fox. *Health and fitness through physical activity.* John Wiley and Sons, New York, 1978.

8. Powers, S., and E. Howley. *Exercise physiology: Theory and application to fitness and performance.* 3rd ed. Brown and Benchmark, Dubuque, IA, 1997.

9. DeVries, H., and T. Houch. *Physiology of exercise.* Brown and Benchmark, Dubuque, IA, 1994.

10. Cooper, K. *The aerobics program for total well-being.* M. Evans, New York, 1982.

11. Cooper, K. *The aerobics way.* Bantam Books, New York, 1977.

12. Fox, E. A simple technique for predicting maximal aerobic power. *Journal of Applied Physiology* 35:914–916, 1973.

13. Lamb, D., and M. Williams. *Ergogenics: Enhancement of performance in exercise and sport.* Vol. 4. Brown and Benchmark, Dubuque, IA, 1991.

14. Rippe, J., A. Ward., J. Porcari, and P. Freedson. Walking for fitness and health. *Journal of the American Medical Association* 259:2720–2724, 1988.

15. Rippe, J. Walking for fitness: A roundtable. *Physician and Sports Medicine* 14:144–159, 1986.

16. Ward, A., and J. Rippe. *Walking for health and fitness.* J. B. Lippincott, Philadelphia, 1988.

17. Golding, L., C. Myers, and W. Sinning. *Y's way to physical fitness: The complete guide to fitness testing and instruction.* 3rd ed. Human Kinetics, Champaign, IL, 1989.

18. Howley, E., and B. D. Franks. *Health fitness: Instructors handbook.* Human Kinetics, Champaign, IL, 1997.

19. Williams, M. *Lifetime fitness and wellness.* Wm. C. Brown, Dubuque, IA, 1996.

20. Jackson A., and M. Pollock. Practical assessment of body composition. *Physician and Sports Medicine* 13:76–90, 1985.

21. Lohman, T. The use of skinfold to estimate body fatness in children and youth. *Journal of Alliance for Health, Physical Education, Recreation, and Dance* 58:98–102, 1987.

22. DiGirolamo, M. Body composition—roundtable. *Physician and Sports Medicine* (March):144–162, 1986.

23. Roche, A., ed. *Body composition assessment in youth and adults.* Ross Laboratories, Columbus, OH, 1985.

24. Van Itallie, T. Topography of body fat: Relationship to risk of cardiovascular and other diseases. In: T. Lohman et al., eds. *Anthropometric standardization reference manual.* Champaign, IL, Human Kinetics, 1988.

25. Faulkner, R., et al. A partial curl-up protocol for adults based on two procedures. *Canadian Journal of Sports Sciences* 14:135–141, 1989.

26. Sparling, P. Field testing for abdominal muscular fitness; speed versus cadence sit-ups. *ACSM's Health and Fitness Journal* 1 (4): 30–33, 1997.

27. Lohman, T., et al. Body fat measurement goes high-tech: Not all are created equal. *ACSM's Health and Fitness Journal* 1(1): 30–35, 1997.

28. Axler, C., and S. McGill. Low back loads over a variety of abdominal exercises: Searching for the safest abdominal challenge. *Medicine and Science in Sports and Exercise* 29: 804–810, 1997.

Health Status Questionnaire

NAME _____ DATE _____

The following questions are part of an exercise screening questionnaire originally developed by the Connecticut Mutual Life Insurance Company and modified by the authors. If you answer "yes" to any of the following questions, you should have a thorough medical exam prior to beginning an exercise program.

1. Have you ever had chest pains or a sensation of pressure in your chest that occurred during or immediately following exercise?

2. Do you get chest discomfort when climbing stairs, walking against a cold wind, or during any physical activity?

3. Does your heart ever beat unevenly or irregularly or seem to flutter or skip beats?

4. Do you ever have sudden bursts of very rapid heart action or periods of slow heart action without apparent cause?

5. Do you take any prescription medicine on a regular basis?

6. Has your doctor ever told you that you have heart problems?

7. Do you have any respiratory problems such as asthma, or do you experience shortness of breath during light physical activity?

8. Do you have arthritis or any condition affecting your joints or back that makes exercise painful?

9. Do you have any of the following risk factors for heart disease: (a) high blood pressure; (b) high blood cholesterol; (c) overweight by more than 30%; (d) smoking; or (e) any close relatives (father, mother, brother, etc.) that have had a history of heart disease prior to 55 years of age?

Measurement of Cardiorespiratory Fitness: The 1.5-Mile Run Test

NAME _____ DATE _____

Directions

The objective of the test is to complete the 1.5 mile distance as quickly as possible. The run can be completed on an oval track or any properly measured course. You should attempt this test only if you have met the medical clearance criteria discussed in Chapter 2 of the text.

Prior to beginning the test, perform a 5- to 10-minute warm-up. If you become extremely fatigued during the test, slow your pace—do not overstress yourself! If you feel faint, nauseated, or experience any unusual pains in your upper body, stop and notify your instructor!

On completion of the test, cool down and record your time and fitness category (see Table 2.1).

Test 1

Date:_____

Ambient conditions

*Temperature:_____   *Relative humidity:_____

Finish time:_____   Fitness category:_____

Test 2

Date:_____

Ambient conditions

*Temperature:_____   *Relative humidity:_____

Finish time:_____   Fitness category:_____

Test 3

Date:_____

Ambient conditions

*Temperature:_____   *Relative humidity:_____

Finish time:_____   Fitness category:_____

*The purpose of recording the temperature and relative humidity is to provide a record of the amount of heat stress during the test. High heat and relative humidity could have a negative impact on your test score.

Measurement of Cardiorespiratory Fitness: The 1-Mile Walk Test

NAME _____ DATE _____

Directions

The objective of the test is to complete the 1-mile distance as quickly as possible. The walk can be completed on an oval track or any properly measured course. You should attempt this test only if you have met the medical clearance criteria discussed in Chapter 2 of the text.

Prior to beginning the test, perform a 5- to 10-minute warm-up. If you become extremely fatigued during the test, slow your pace—do not overstress yourself! If you feel faint or nauseated, or experience any unusual pains in your upper body, stop and notify your instructor!

On completion of the test, cool down and record your time and fitness category (see Table 2.2).

Test 1

Date: _____

Ambient conditions

Temperature: _____ Relative humidity: _____

Finish time: _____ Fitness category: _____

Test 2

Date: _____

Ambient conditions

Temperature: _____ Relative humidity: _____

Finish time: _____ Fitness category: _____

Test 3

Date: _____

Ambient conditions

Temperature: _____ Relative humidity: _____

Finish time: _____ Fitness category: _____

Submaximal Cycle Test to Determine Cardiorespiratory Fitness

NAME _____ DATE _____

Directions

Warm up for 3 minutes using unloaded pedaling. Set the appropriate load for your age and gender (see Chapter 2 for load-setting instructions) and begin. Exercise for a 5-minute period. Count your pulse during a 15-second period between minutes 4.5 and 5 of the test.

   Cool down for 3 to 5 minutes using unloaded pedaling. Record your 15-second heart rate below and compute your relative VO_2 max using Table 2.4. After calculating your relative VO_2 max, locate your fitness category in Table 2.5.

Test 1

Date:_____

Heart rate (15-s count) during minute 5 of test:_____

Fitness category:_____

Test 2

Date:_____

Heart rate (15-s count) during minute 5 of test:_____

Fitness category:_____

Test 3

Date:_____

Heart rate (15-s count) during minute 5 of test:_____

Fitness category:_____

Step Test to Determine Cardiorespiratory Fitness

NAME _____ DATE _____

Directions

Perform 30 complete step ups and downs per minute using an 18-inch step over a 3-minute period. On completion of 3 minutes of exercise, sit quietly and count your recovery heart rate during the following time periods: 1 to 1.5 minutes posttest; 2 to 2.5 minutes posttest; and 3 to 3.5 minutes posttest. Record your heart rates below and use Table 2.6 to determine your fitness category.

Test 1

Date:_____

Recovery heart rate postexercise (beats)

1–1.5 min_____

2–2.5 min_____

3–3.5 min_____

Total _____ (recovery index)

Fitness category:_____

Test 2

Date:_____

Recovery heart rate postexercise (beats)

1–1.5 min_____

2–2.5 min_____

3–3.5 min_____

Total _____ (recovery index)

Fitness category:_____

Test 3

Date:_____

Recovery heart rate postexercise (beats)

1–1.5 min_____

2–2.5 min_____

3–3.5 min_____

Total _____ (recovery index)

Fitness category:_____

Measurement of Muscular Strength: The 1 RM Test

NAME _____ DATE _____

Directions

After performance of your 1 RM test, compute your muscular strength scores as follows:

$$\frac{1 \text{ RM weight}}{\text{body weight}} \times 100 = \text{muscle strength score}$$

Record your muscular strength scores below and use Table 2.7 to determine your fitness category.

Age:_____ **Body weight:**_____**pounds**

Test 1

Date:_____

Exercise	1 RM (lbs)	Muscular Strength Score	Fitness Category
Bench press	_____	_____	_____
Biceps curl	_____	_____	_____
Shoulder press	_____	_____	_____
Leg press	_____	_____	_____

Test 2

Date:_____

Exercise	1 RM (lbs)	Muscular Strength Score	Fitness Category
Bench press	_____	_____	_____
Biceps curl	_____	_____	_____
Shoulder press	_____	_____	_____
Leg press	_____	_____	_____

Measurement of Muscular Endurance: The Push-Up, Sit-Up, and Curl-Up Tests

NAME _____ DATE _____

Directions

After completion of the push-up and sit-up tests, record your scores and fitness classifications (see Tables 2.8, 2.9a, and 2.9b).

Age:_____

Test 1

Date:_____

Number of push-ups (1 min):_____   Fitness category:_____

Number of sit-ups (1 min):_____   Fitness category:_____

Number of curl-ups:_____   Fitness category:_____

Test 2

Date:_____

Number of push-ups (1 min):_____   Fitness category:_____

Number of sit-ups (1 min):_____   Fitness category:_____

Number of curl-ups:_____   Fitness category:_____

Assessment of Flexibility: Trunk Flexion (Sit and Reach Test) and the Shoulder Flexibility Test

NAME _____ DATE _____

Directions

After completion of the sit and reach test and shoulder flexibility test, record your scores and fitness classifications (see Tables 2.10 and 2.11).

Test 1

Date:_____

Sit and reach score (inches):_____   Fitness category:_____

Shoulder flexibility (inches):_____   Fitness category:_____

Test 2

Date:_____

Sit and reach score (inches):_____   Fitness category:_____

Shoulder flexibility (inches):_____   Fitness category:_____

Assessment of Body Composition

NAME _____ DATE _____

Directions

In the spaces below, record your body composition raw data and fitness classification obtained using the skinfold test, body mass index, and/or the waist-to-hip circumference test (see Tables 2.12 – 2.16).

Test 1

Date:_____

Skinfold Test

Sum of three skinfolds (mm):_____

Percent body fat:_____

Fitness category:_____

Body Mass Index

Body mass index score:_____

Fitness category:_____

Waist-to-Hip Circumference Ratio

Waist-to-hip circumference ratio:_____

Fitness category:_____

Test 2

Date:_____

Skinfold Test

Sum of three skinfolds (mm):_____

Percent body fat:_____

Fitness category:_____

Body Mass Index

Body mass index score:_____

Fitness category:_____

Waist-to-Hip Circumference Ratio

Waist-to-hip circumference ratio:_____

Fitness category:_____

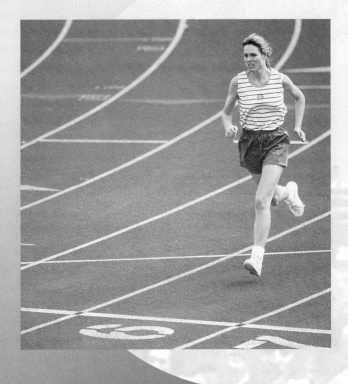

3

General Principles of Exercise for Health and Fitness

After studying this chapter, you should be able to do the following:

1 Discuss the following concepts of physical fitness: overload principle; specificity of exercise; principle of recuperation; and reversibility of training effects.

2 Outline the physiological objectives of a warm-up and cool-down.

3 Identify the general principles of exercise prescription.

4 Discuss the concepts of progression and maintenance of exercise training.

5 Explain why individualizing the workout is an important concept for the development of an exercise prescription.

6 Explain how the "threshold for health benefits" differs from the "threshold of training."

$\mathbb{R}$esearch in exercise science has provided guidelines for the development of a safe and efficient program to improve personal fitness (1–9). The purpose of this chapter is to provide you with an overview of general principles for improving your physical fitness. The basic concepts contained within this chapter can be applied to both men and women as well as individuals of all ages and fitness levels. The individual components of health-related physical fitness are covered in chapters 4, 5, and 6 which detail the development of cardiorespiratory fitness, muscular strength/endurance, and flexibility, respectively.

Principles of Exercise Training to Improve Physical Fitness

Although the specifics of exercise training programs should be tailored to the individual, the general principles of physical fitness are the same for everyone. In the following section we describe the training concepts of overload, specificity, recuperation, and reversibility.

Overload Principle

The **overload principle** is a key component of all conditioning programs (1–9). In order to improve physical fitness, the body or specific muscles must be stressed. For example, for a skeletal muscle to increase in strength, the muscle must work against a heavier load than normal. In this case we achieve an overload by increasing the intensity of exercise (i.e., by using heavier weights). However, note that overload can also be achieved by increasing the duration of exercise. For instance, to increase muscular endurance, a muscle must be worked over a longer duration than normal (by performing a higher number of exercise repetitions). Another practical example of the overload principle applied to health-related physical fitness is the improvement of flexibility. To increase the range of motion at a joint, we must stretch the muscle to a longer length than normal or hold the stretch for a longer time.

Although improvement in physical fitness requires application of overload, this does not mean that exercise sessions must be exhausting.

The often-heard quote, "No pain, no gain," is not completely accurate. In fact, improvement in physical fitness can be achieved without punishing training sessions (5).

Principle of Progression

The **principle of progression** is an extension of the overload principle. It states that overload should be increased gradually during the course of a physical fitness program. This concept is illustrated in Figure 3.1. Note that the overload of a training program should generally be increased slowly during the first 4 to 6 weeks of the exercise program. After this initial period, the overload can be increased at a steady but progressive rate during the next 18 to 20 weeks of training. It is important that the overload not be increased too slowly or too rapidly if optimum fitness improvement is to result. Progression that is too slow will result in limited improvement in physical fitness. Increasing the exercise overload too rapidly may result in chronic fatigue and injury. Muscle or joint injuries that occur because of too much exercise are called *overuse injuries.* Exercise-induced injuries can come from either short bouts of high-intensity exercise or long bouts of low-intensity exercise (see Chapter 11 for care and prevention of injuries).

What is a safe rate of progression during an exercise training program? A definitive answer to

FIGURE 3.1 The progression and maintenance of exercise training during the first several months after beginning an exercise program. (From Pollock, M.L., Wilmore, J.H., and Fox, S.M., III. Prentice-Hall, New York, 1978. Copyright © 1978. Reprinted by permission of Allyn & Bacon.)

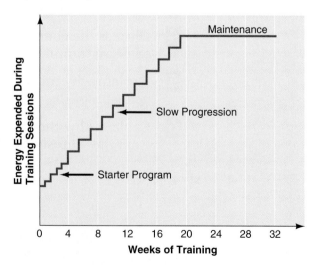

this question is not possible because individuals vary in their tolerance for exercise overload. However, a common sense guideline for improvement of physical fitness and avoiding overuse injuries is the **ten percent rule** (6). In short, this rule says that the training intensity or duration of exercise should not be increased more than ten percent per week. For example, a runner running 20 minutes per day could increase his or her daily exercise duration to 22 minutes per day (10% of 20 = 2) the following week.

When an individual reaches his or her desired level of physical fitness (that is, you have reached your goal as defined by one of the fitness tests described in Chapter 2), it is no longer necessary to increase the training intensity or duration. Indeed, once a desired level of fitness has been achieved, physical fitness can be maintained by regular exercise at a constant level (see Figure 3.1). Exercising to sustain a certain level of physical fitness is referred to as a *maintenance program.*

Specificity of Exercise

Another key concept of training is the **principle of specificity.** That is, the exercise training effect is specific to those muscles involved in the activity (10). You would not expect your arms to become trained following a 10-week jogging program!

Specificity of training also applies to the types of adaptations that occur in the muscle. For example, strength training results in an increase in muscle strength but does not greatly improve the endurance of the muscle. Therefore, strength training is specific to improving muscular strength (11). Similarly, endurance exercise training results in an improvement in muscular endurance without altering muscular strength (12).

Consider the following simple illustration of exercise specificity. Suppose you want to improve your ability to run a distance of 3 miles. In this case, specific training should include running 3 or more miles several times a week. This type of training would improve muscular endurance in your legs but would not result in large improvements in leg strength (10).

Principle of Recuperation

Because the principle of overload requires exercise stress to improve physical fitness, it follows that exercise training places a stress on the body. During the recovery period between exercise training sessions, the body adapts to the exercise stress by increasing endurance or becoming stronger. Therefore, a period of rest is essential to achieve maximal benefit from exercise. This needed rest period between exercise training sessions is called the **principle of recuperation** (see Figure 3.2).

Concept of specificity. Running promotes improvements in muscular endurance.

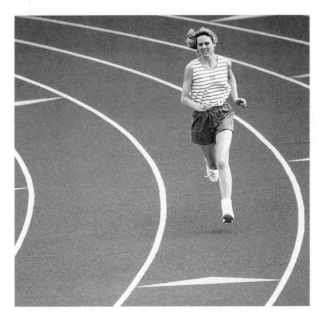

overload principle A basic principle of physical conditioning. The overload principle states that in order to improve physical fitness, the body or specific muscles must be stressed. For example, for a skeletal muscle to increase in strength, the muscle must work against a heavier load than normal.

principle of progression A principle of training which dictates that overload should be increased gradually during the course of a physical fitness program.

ten percent rule A rule of training that states that the training intensity or duration of exercise should not be increased more than 10% per week.

principle of specificity The principle that the exercise training effect is specific to those muscles involved in the activity.

principle of recuperation The principle of recuperation states that the body requires recovery periods between exercise training sessions in order to adapt to the exercise stress. Therefore, a period of rest is essential to achieve maximal benefit from exercise.

Principle of Recuperation

Exercise Training Session

↓

Adequate Rest Period

↓

Exercise Training Session

FIGURE 3.2 Principle of recuperation requires that adequate rest periods separate exercise training sessions.

How much rest is required between heavy exercise training sessions? One or two days is adequate for most individuals (6). Failure to get enough rest between sessions may result in a fatigue syndrome referred to as **overtraining.** Overtraining may lead to chronic fatigue and/or injuries. A key question is, how do you diagnose overtraining? Sore and stiff muscles or a feeling of general fatigue the morning after an exercise training session, sometimes called a "workout hangover," is a common symptom. The cure is to increase the duration of rest between workouts, reduce the intensity of workouts, or both. Although too much exercise is the primary cause of the overtraining syndrome, failure to consume a well-balanced diet can contribute to the feeling of a workout hangover (see Nutritional Links to Health and Fitness 3.1).

Reversibility of Training Effects

Although rest periods between exercise sessions are essential for maximal benefit from exercise, long intervals between workouts (that is, several days or weeks) can result in a reduction in fitness levels (14). Maintenance of physical fitness requires regular exercise sessions. In other words, physical fitness cannot be stored. The loss of fitness due to inactivity is an example of the **principle of reversibility.** The old adage, "What you don't use, you lose," is true when applied to physical fitness.

How quickly is fitness lost when training is stopped? The answer depends on which component of physical fitness you are referring to. For example, after cessation of strength training, the loss of muscular strength is relatively slow (11, 15). In contrast, after you stop performing endurance exercise, the loss of muscular endurance is relatively rapid (14). Figure 3.3 illustrates this point. Note that 8 weeks after stopping strength training, only 10% of muscular strength is lost (15). In contrast, note that 8 weeks after cessation of endurance training, 30% to 40% of muscular endurance is lost (14).

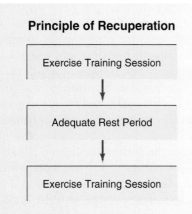

3.1   Nutritional Links to Health and Fitness

Diet and the Workout Hangover

Can a poor diet contribute to fatigue and overtraining? Yes! Failure to consume the recommended amounts of carbohydrates, fats, proteins, vitamins, and minerals can lead to chronic fatigue (13). Of particular importance to people engaged in a regular exercise training program is dietary carbohydrates. Because heavy exercise uses carbohydrates as a primary fuel source (6), diets low in carbohydrates can result in a depletion of muscle carbohydrate stores and can lead to a feeling of chronic fatigue. To maintain muscle carbohydrate stores, these nutrients should comprise 60% of the total energy contained in your diet (6,13). See Chapter 7 for a complete discussion of diet and nutrition for physical fitness.

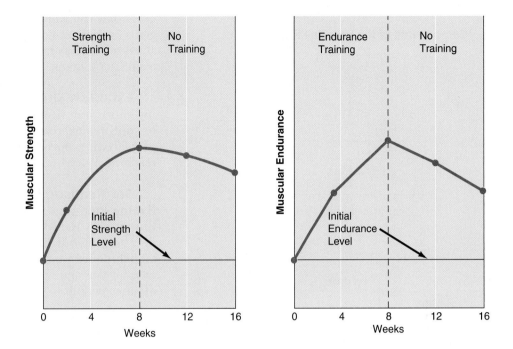

FIGURE 3.3 Retention of muscular strength and muscular endurance after training is stopped.

General Principles of Exercise Prescription

Doctors often prescribe medications to treat certain diseases, and for every individual there is an appropriate dosage of medicine to cure an illness. Similarly, for each individual, there is a correct dosage of exercise to effectively promote physical fitness, called an **exercise prescription** (5, 8). Exercise prescriptions should be tailored to meet the needs of the individual (1–9, 16). It should include fitness goals, mode of exercise, a warm-up, a primary conditioning period, and a cool-down (Figure 3.4). The following sections provide a general introduction to each of these components.

Fitness Goals

As mentioned in Chapter 1, establishing short-term and long-term fitness goals is an important part of an exercise prescription. Goals serve as motivation to start an exercise program. Further, attaining your fitness goals improves self-esteem and provides the incentive needed to make a lifetime commitment to regular exercise.

A logical and common type of fitness goal is a performance goal. You can establish performance goals in each component of health-related physi-

cal fitness. Table 3.1 on page 66 illustrates a hypothetical example of how Susie Jones might establish short-term and long-term performance goals using fitness testing (see Chapter 2) to determine when she has reached her objective. The column labeled "current status" contains Susie's fitness ratings based on tests performed prior to starting her exercise program. After consultation with her instructor, Susie has established short-term goals that she hopes to achieve within the first 8 weeks of training. Note that the short-term goals are not "fixed in stone" and can be modified if the need arises. Susie's long-term goals are fitness levels that she hopes to reach within the first 18 months of training. Similar to short-term goals, long-term goals can be modified to meet changing needs or circumstances.

overtraining Failure to get enough rest between exercise training sessions. Overtraining may lead to chronic fatigue and/or injuries.

principle of reversibility The loss of fitness due to inactivity.

exercise prescription The correct dosage of exercise to effectively promote physical fitness. Exercise prescriptions should be tailored to meet the needs of the individual and include fitness goals, mode of exercise, a warm-up, a primary conditioning period, and a cool-down.

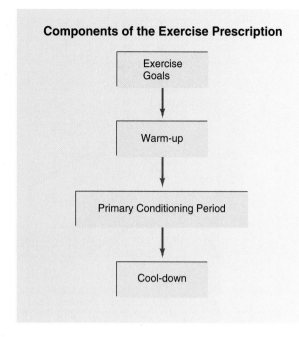

Components of the Exercise Prescription

Exercise Goals

↓

Warm-up

↓

Primary Conditioning Period

↓

Cool-down

FIGURE 3.4 Components of the exercise prescription.

In addition to performance goals, consider establishing exercise adherence goals. That is, set a goal to exercise a specific number of days per week. Exercise adherence goals are important because fitness will improve only if you exercise regularly!

In writing your personal fitness goals, consider the following guidelines:

Set Realistic Goals The most important rule in setting goals is that you must establish realistic ones. After a thorough self-evaluation and consultation with your instructor, set fitness goals that you can reach. Because failure to reach goals is discouraging, establishment of realistic short-term goals is critical to the success of your exercise program.

Establish Short-Term Goals First Reaching short-term fitness goals is a great motivation to continue exercising. Therefore, establishment of realistic short-term goals is critical. After reaching a short-term goal, establish a new one.

Set Realistic Long-Term Goals In establishing long-term goals consider your physical limitations. Heredity plays an important role in determining our fitness limits. Therefore, in establishing long term goals, set goals that are realistic for you and not based on performance scores of other people.

Establish Lifetime Maintenance Goals In addition to short-term and long-term goals, consider establishing a fitness maintenance goal. A maintenance goal is established when your fitness goals have been met and your focus becomes remaining physically active and fit.

List Goals in Written Form A key to meeting goals is to write them down and put them in a place where you can see them every day. Goals can be forgotten if they are not verifiable in writing. Further, remember that all goals should be periodically reevaluated and modified if necessary. Just because goals are in writing does not mean that they cannot be changed.

Recognize Obstacles to Achieving Goals If you do not make your fitness goals a serious priority, you will keep putting them off until they

Table 3.1

Illustration of Short-Term and Long-Term Performance Goals
The fitness categories are the five components of health-related physical fitness. The current status, short-term, and long-term goals are the fitness norms presented in Chapter 2.

Fitness Category	Current Status	Short-Term Goal	Long-Term Goal
Cardiorespiratory fitness	Poor	Average	Excellent
Muscular strength	Poor	Average	Excellent
Muscular endurance	Very poor	Average	Good
Flexibility	Poor	Average	Good
Body composition	High fat	Moderately high	Optimal

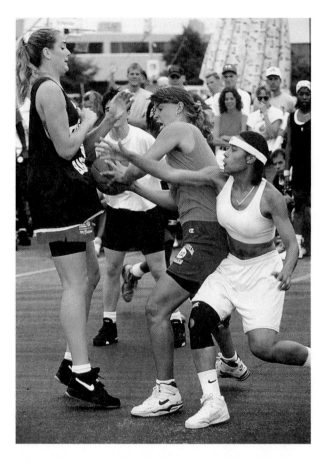

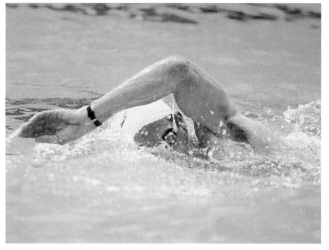

Examples of low-impact and high-impact activities. Swimming is considered to be a low-impact activity, whereas basketball is considered to be a high-impact activity.

no longer exist. Once you begin your fitness program, be prepared to make mistakes (e.g., skip workouts and lose motivation) and backslide some (e.g., fitness level declines). This is normal. However, once you realize that you have stopped making progress toward your goals, you must get back on track and start making progress again as soon as you can.

The importance of fitness goals cannot be overemphasized. Goals provide structure and motivation for a personal fitness program. Keys to maintaining a lifelong fitness program are discussed again in Chapter 16.

Mode of Exercise

Every exercise prescription includes at least one **mode of exercise**—that is, a specific type of exercise to be performed. For example, to improve cardiorespiratory fitness, you could select from a wide variety of exercise modes, such as running, swimming, or cycling. Key factors to consider when selecting an exercise mode are enjoyment, availability of the activity, and risk of injury.

Physical activities can be classified as being either high impact or low impact based on the amount of stress placed on joints during the activity. Activities that place a large amount of pressure on joints are called high-impact activities, whereas low-impact activities are less stressful. Because of the strong correlation between high-impact modes of exercise and injuries, many fitness experts recommend low-impact activities for fitness beginners or for those individuals susceptible to injury (such as participants who are older or overweight). Examples of some high-impact activities include running, basketball, and high-impact aerobic dance. Low-impact activities include walking, cycling, swimming, and low-impact aerobic dance.

mode of exercise The specific type of exercise to be performed. For example, to improve cardiorespiratory fitness, one could select from a wide variety of exercise modes, including running, swimming, or cycling.

Warm-Up

A **warm-up** is a brief (5- to 15-minute) period of exercise that precedes the workout. It generally involves light calisthenics or a low-intensity form of the actual mode of exercise and often includes stretching exercises as well (see Chapter 6). The purpose of a warm-up is to elevate muscle temperature and increase blood flow to those muscles that will be engaged in the workout (3, 6, 17). A warm-up can also reduce the strain on the heart imposed by rapidly engaging in heavy exercise and may reduce the risk of muscle and tendon injuries (17).

Primary Conditioning Period: The Workout Plan

The major components of the exercise prescription that make up the primary conditioning period are the mode of exercise (described earlier), frequency, intensity, and duration (see Figure 3.5). The **frequency of exercise** is the number of times per week that you intend to exercise. In general, the recommended frequency of exercise to improve most components of health-related physical fitness is three to five times per week (5, 18–20).

The **intensity of exercise** is the amount of physiological stress or overload placed on the body during the exercise. The method for determining the intensity of exercise varies with the type of exercise performed. For example, because heart rate increases linearly with energy expenditure (effort) during exercise, measurement of heart rate has become a standard means of determining exercise intensity during training to improve cardiorespiratory fitness. Although heart rate can also be used to gauge exercise intensity during strength training, the number of exercise repetitions that can be performed before muscular fatigue occurs is more useful for monitoring stress during weight lifting. For instance, a load that can be lifted only five to eight times before complete muscular fatigue is an example of high-intensity weight lifting. In contrast, a load that can be lifted 50 to 60 times without resulting in muscular fatigue is an illustration of low-intensity weight training.

Finally, flexibility is improved by stretching muscles beyond their normal lengths. Intensity of stretching is monitored by the degree of tension or discomfort felt during the stretch. Low-intensity stretching results in only minor tension (or limited discomfort) on the muscles and tendons. In contrast, high-intensity stretching places great tension or moderate discomfort on the muscle groups being stretched.

Another key component of the exercise prescription is the **duration of exercise** (i.e. the amount of time invested in performing the primary workout). Note that the duration of exercise does not include the warm-up or cool-down. In general, research has shown that 20 to 30 minutes per exercise session (performed at least three times per week) is the minimum amount of time required to significantly improve physical fitness (see ref. 5 for a review).

Cool-Down

The **cool-down** (sometimes called a *warm-down*) is a 5- to 15-minute period of low-intensity exercise that immediately follows the primary conditioning period. For instance, a period of slow walking might be used as a cool-down following a running workout. A cool-down period accomplishes several goals (see Figure 3.6). First, one primary purpose of a cool-down is to allow blood to be returned from the muscles back toward the heart (3–6). During exercise, large amounts of blood are pumped to the working muscles. On cessation of exercise, blood tends to remain in large blood vessels (called *pooling*) located around the exercised muscles. Failure to redistribute pooled blood after exercise could result in your feeling lightheaded or even fainting. Prevention of blood pooling is best accomplished by

FIGURE 3.5 The primary conditioning period includes the mode of exercise and the frequency, intensity, and duration of the workout.

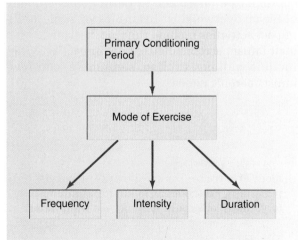

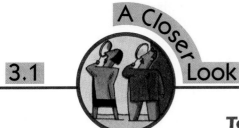

low-intensity exercise using those muscles utilized during the workout.

Finally, some fitness experts argue that post-exercise muscle soreness may be reduced as a result of a cool-down (21). Although a cool-down period may not eliminate muscular soreness entirely, it seems possible that the severity of exercise-induced muscle soreness may be reduced in people who perform a proper cool-down (21).

FIGURE 3.6 Purposes of a cool-down.

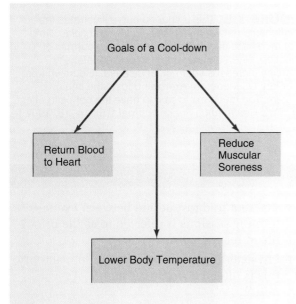

Individualizing the Workout

A key point to remember about exercise prescriptions is that the prescription should be tailored to the needs and objectives of the individual. Although the same general principles of exercise training apply to everyone, no two people are the same. Therefore, the exercise prescription should consider such factors as the individual's general health, age, fitness status, musculoskeletal condition, and body composition. More will be said about individualizing workouts in later chapters.

warm-up A brief (5 to 15 minute) period of exercise that precedes the workout. The purpose of a warm-up is to elevate muscle temperature and increase blood flow to those muscles that will be engaged in the workout.

frequency of exercise The number of times per week that one intends to exercise.

intensity of exercise The amount of physiological stress or overload placed on the body during exercise.

duration of exercise The amount of time invested in performing the primary workout.

cool-down The cool-down (sometimes called a *warm-down*) is a 5 to 15 minute period of low-intensity exercise that immediately follows the primary conditioning period.

How Much Exercise Is Enough?

An often asked question is, "How much exercise is enough?" The answer depends on your specific exercise goals. Figure 3.7 illustrates the concept that there are two separate thresholds of exercise training. The minimum level of physical activity required to achieve some of the health benefits of exercise is called the **threshold for health benefits.** Recent studies have demonstrated that some health benefits can be achieved by very low levels of physical activity (gardening, slow walking, and so on) when these activities are performed regularly and for a considerable duration (expending at least 2000 calories per week) (18, 20, 22). For example, 9 to 12 hours of gardening may be required to expend 2000 calories. Note, however, that although low physical activity may improve health, it does not generally improve the components of health-related physical fitness; that is, physical fitness is not improved. The minimum dose of exercise required to improve health-related physical fitness is called the *threshold of training.* Each component of physical fitness has its own threshold for improvement. Details for each of the health-related aspects of fitness are discussed in chapters 4 through 6.

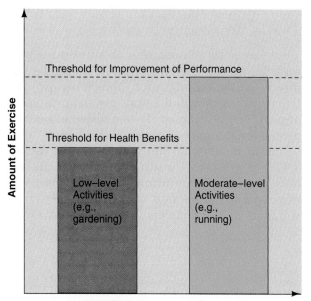

FIGURE 3.7 Two thresholds for exercise benefits exist: one for health and one for performance.

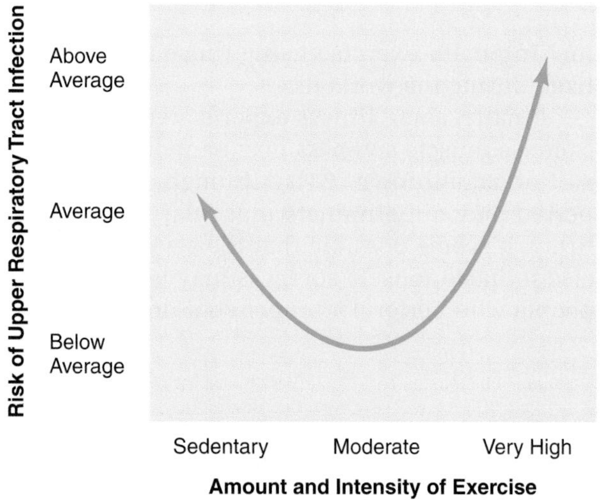

FIGURE 3.8 This *J*-shaped curve illustrates the relationship between physical activity and colds. Note that moderate physical activity reduces your risk of infection, whereas long-duration or high-intensity exercise increases your risk of disease. (Redrawn from Nieman, D., Moderate exercise boosts the immune system: Too much exercise can have the opposite effect. *ACSM's Health and Fitness Journal* 1(5): 14–18, 1997.)

Summary

1. The overload principle is the most important principle of exercise training. In order to improve physical fitness, the body or muscle used during exercise must be overloaded.

2. The principle of progression states that overload should be increased gradually during the course of a physical fitness program.

3. The required rest period between exercise training sessions is referred to as the principle of recuperation.

4. Physical fitness can be lost due to inactivity; this is often called the principle of reversibility.

5. The components of the exercise prescription include fitness goals, mode of exercise, the warm-up, the workout, and the cool-down.

6. All exercise training programs need to be tailored to meet the objectives of the individual. Therefore, the exercise prescription should consider the individual's age, health, fitness status, musculoskeletal condition, and body composition.

7. The minimum dose of exercise required to improve health-related physical fitness is called the threshold of training. The minimum level of physical activity required to achieve some of the health benefits of exercise is called the threshold of health benefits.

Study Questions

1. Define the following terms: *overtraining* and *principle of recuperation.*

2. What is the general purpose of a cool-down and a warm-up?

3. Describe and discuss the components of the exercise prescription.

4. How does the principle of progression apply to the exercise prescription?

5. Discuss the overload principle.

6. Define the *threshold for health benefits and the threshold of training.*

7. What happens to physical fitness if you stop training?

8. Explain why the exercise prescription should be individualized.

Suggested Reading

Clarkson, P. Oh, those aching muscles: Causes and consequences of delayed onset muscle soreness. *ACSM's Health and Fitness Journal* 1(3): 12–17, 1997.

Nieman, D. Moderate exercise boosts the immune system: Too much exercise can have the opposite effect. *ACSM's Health and Fitness Journal* 1(5): 14–18, 1997.

Williams, M. *Lifetime fitness and wellness.* Wm. C. Brown, Dubuque, IA, 1996.

Suggested Reading on the World Wide Web

Shape Up America (http://www.shapup.org/sva/) Latest information about physical fitness and weight control by ex-Surgeon General, Dr. Everett Koop.

Sympatico: (http://www.ns.sympatico.ca/healthyway) Articles about fitness and health, book reviews, and links to nutrition, fitness, and wellness topics.

International Association of Fitness Professionals-IDEA (http://www.fit.org/idea/index.html) Provides education, professional development for fitness instructors, personal trainers, and business owners on exercise training and development of healthy lifestyle programs.

American Council on Exercise (ACE) (http://www.acefitness.org/) A nonprofit organization that provides information on the certification of fitness professionals, plus education.

References

1. Getchell, B. *Physical fitness: A way of life.* Allyn and Bacon, Needham Heights, MA, 1997.

2. Hockey, R. *Physical fitness: The pathway to healthful living.* Times Mirror/Mosby, St. Louis, 1996.

3. Howley, E., and B. D. Franks. *Health fitness: Instructors handbook.* Human Kinetics, Champaign, IL, 1997.

4. Fleck, S. and W. Kraemer. *Designing resistance training programs.* Human Kinetics, Champaign, Il, 1997.

threshold for health benefits The minimum level of physical activity required to achieve some of the health benefits of exercise.

5. Pollock, M., and J. Wilmore. *Exercise in health and disease.* W. B. Saunders, Philadelphia, 1990.

6. Powers, S., and E. Howley. *Exercise physiology: Theory and application to fitness and performance.* 2nd ed. Brown and Benchmark, Dubuque, IA, 1997.

7. Williams, M. *Lifetime fitness and wellness.* Wm. C. Brown, Dubuque, IA, 1996.

8. American College of Sports Medicine. *Guidelines for exercise testing and prescription.* Lea and Febiger, Philadelphia, 1991.

9. Corbin, C., and R. Lindsey. *Concepts of physical fitness and wellness.* Brown and Benchmark, Dubuque, IA, 1997.

10. Roberts, J., and J. Alspaugh. Specificity of training effects resulting from programs of treadmill running and bicycle ergometer riding. *Medicine and Science in Sports* 4:6–10, 1972.

11. Abernethy, P., J. Jurimae, P. Logan, A. Taylor, and R. Thayer. Acute and chronic response of skeletal muscle to resistance exercise. *Sports Medicine* 22–28, 1994.

12. Powers, S., D. Criswell, J. Lawler, L. Ji, D. Martin, R. Herb, and G. Dudley. Influence of exercise and fiber type on antioxidant enzyme activity in rat skeletal muscle. *American Journal of Physiology* 266:R375–R380, 1994.

13. Lamb, D., and M. Williams. *Ergogenics: Enhancement of performance in exercise and sport.* Vol. 4. Brown and Benchmark, Madison, WI, 1991.

14. Coyle, E., W. Martin, D. Sinacore, M. Joyner, J. Hagberg, and J. Holloszy. Time course of loss of adaptations after stopping prolonged intense endurance training. *Journal of Applied Physiology* 57:1857–1864, 1984.

15. Costill, D., and A. Richardson. *Handbook of sports medicine: Swimming.* Blackwell Publishing, London, 1993.

16. McGlynn, G. *Dynamics of fitness: A practical approach.* Wm. C. Brown, Dubuque, IA, 1996.

17. DeVries, H., and T. Housh. *Exercise physiology.* 5th ed. Brown and Benchmark, Dubuque, IA, 1994.

18. Bouchard, C., R. Shephard, T. Stephens, J. Sutton, and B. McPherson, eds. *Exercise, fitness, and health: A consensus of current knowledge.* Human Kinetics, Champaign, IL, 1990.

19. Barrow, M. *Heart talk: Understanding cardiovascular diseases.* Cor-Ed Publishing, Gainesville, FL, 1992.

20. Morris, J. Exercise in the prevention of coronary heart disease: Today's best buy in public health. *Medicine and Science in Sports and Exercise* 26:807–814, 1994.

21. Fox, E., R. Bowers, and M. Foss. *The physiological basis for exercise and sport.* Brown and Benchmark, Madison, WI, 1993.

22. Paffenbarger, R., J. Kampert, I-Min Lee, R. Hyde, R. Leung, and A. Wing. Changes in physical activity and other lifeway patterns influencing longevity. *Medicine and Science in Sports and Exercise* 26:857–865, 1994.

23. Nieman, D. Moderate exercise boosts the immune system: Too much exercise can have the opposite effect. *ACSM's Health and Fitness Journal* 1(5): 14–18, 1997.

24. Nieman, D. Immune response to heavy exertion. *Journal of Applied Physiology* 82: 1385–1394, 1997.

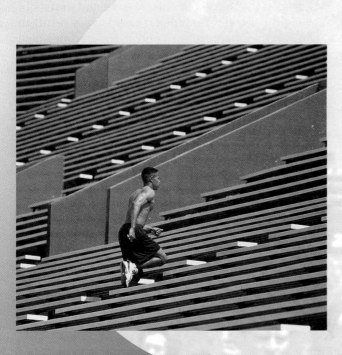

4

Exercise Prescription Guidelines: Cardiorespiratory Fitness

Learning Objectives

After studying this chapter, you should be able to

1 Explain the benefits of developing cardiorespiratory fitness.

2 Identify the three energy systems involved in the production of adenosine triphosphate for muscular contraction.

3 Discuss the role of the circulatory and respiratory systems during exercise.

4 Define VO_2 max.

5 Identify the major changes that occur in skeletal muscles, the circulatory system, and the respiratory system in response to aerobic training.

6 Explain the purpose of a warm-up.

7 List several modes of training used to improve cardiovascular fitness.

8 Discuss the benefits of a cool-down at the completion of a workout.

9 Outline the general components of an exercise prescription designed to improve cardiorespiratory fitness.

10 Design an exercise program for improving cardiorespiratory endurance.

Much of the current interest in cardiorespiratory training began in 1968 with the publication of Dr. Kenneth Cooper's best-selling fitness book, *Aerobics* (1). After the book's appearance, the term **aerobics** became a common term to describe all forms of low-intensity exercise designed to improve cardiorespiratory fitness (such as jogging, walking, cycling, and swimming). Because aerobic exercise has proven effective in promoting weight loss (2) and reducing the risk of cardiovascular disease (3), many exercise scientists consider cardiorespiratory fitness to be one of the most important components of health-related physical fitness.

In the first three chapters of this book we have discussed the health benefits of exercise, fitness assessment, and the general principles of exercise training. In the next three chapters we will describe how to design a comprehensive, scientifically based exercise program to promote health-related physical fitness. This chapter describes techniques to promote cardiorespiratory fitness. Before we discuss the exercise prescription for cardiovascular fitness, however, let's discuss the benefits of cardiorespiratory fitness and some basic concepts concerning how your body works during aerobic exercise.

Benefits of Cardiorespiratory Fitness

The benefits of cardiorespiratory fitness are many. A key advantage is that people with high levels of cardiorespiratory fitness have a lower risk of heart disease and increased longevity. Other health benefits include a reduced risk of type II diabetes, lower blood pressure, and increased bone density in weight-bearing bones (4).

Another positive factor associated with developing cardiorespiratory fitness is that as fitness improves, energy for work and play increases. This translates into your being able to perform more work with less fatigue. Indeed, people with high levels of cardiorespiratory fitness often state that one of the reasons they exercise is because they feel better as a result.

Development of cardiorespiratory fitness through regular exercise has been shown to improve self-esteem (5). This improvement probably comes from several factors. First, starting and maintaining a regular exercise program provides a strong sense of accomplishment. Second, regular exercise improves muscle tone and assists in weight control. Combined, these factors result in an improved appearance and therefore improved self-esteem. Finally, studies have shown that people with high levels of cardiorespiratory fitness sleep better than less fit individuals (6). Fit individuals tend to sleep longer without interruptions (i.e., they enjoy a more restful sleep) compared with less fit people. This exercise-related improved sleep results in a better night's rest and a more complete feeling of being mentally restored.

Physiological Basis for Developing Cardiorespiratory Fitness

Energy to Perform Exercise

Where do muscles get the energy to contract during exercise? The answer is, from the chemical energy released by the breakdown of food (such as carbohydrates, proteins, and fat). However, food energy cannot be used directly for energy by the muscles. Instead, the energy released from the breakdown of foodstuffs is used to manufacture another biochemical compound, called **adenosine triphosphate** (ATP), a high-energy compound that is synthesized and stored in small quantities in muscle and other cells. The breakdown of ATP results in a release of energy that

aerobics A common term to describe all forms of low-intensity exercise designed to improve cardiorespiratory fitness (e.g., jogging, walking, cycling, and swimming). Because aerobic exercise has proved effective in promoting weight loss and reducing the risk of cardiovascular disease, many exercise scientists consider cardiorespiratory fitness to be one of the most important components of health-related physical fitness.

adenosine triphosphate (ATP) A high-energy compound that is synthesized and stored in small quantities in muscle and other cells. The breakdown of ATP results in a release of energy that can be used to fuel muscular contraction. ATP is the only compound in the body that can provide this immediate source of energy.

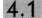

4.1 Links to Health and Fitness

Creatine Monohydrate: A Real Ergogenic Aid?

Recently, many athletes and body builders have begun taking creatine, a supplement that they think will increase muscle mass and endurance. Creatine is a compound synthesized in the body and contained in foods such as meat and fish. It is stored by the body in skeletal muscle and much of it has phosphate added to form phosphocreatine. It is this form, phosphocreatine, that is used to help resynthesize energy (ATP) during short-term, intense exercise. In fact, the depletion of creatine during intense exercise has been shown to be related to the onset of fatigue. Thus, the idea behind supplementation with creatine monohydrate (supplement form for best absorption) is to increase endurance in short-term, intense exercise. Recently, it has been shown that creatine monohydrate does increase total creatine in muscle (21). In addition, several studies (22, for review) have shown that creatine supplementation enhances endurance during repeated bouts of short-term, in-

tense exercise (bouts lasting <20 seconds). Another touted claim of many creatine users is the possibility that creatine increases muscle mass. This possibility has not been thoroughly investigated with scientific studies. Although body weight does increase with creatine supplementation, the likely source of the weight gain is an increase in body water due to the water that is stored with creatine in muscle. In addition, weight gain usually occurs in approximately one week—much too quick for increased muscle protein synthesis. Thus, creatine supplementation may be effective in delaying muscle fatigue during repeated bouts of short-term, intense exercise. However, its effect of increasing muscle mass by increasing muscle protein is unlikely. One important caveat is that the long-term effects of prolonged supplementation with creatine are unknown. Therefore, it would be unwise to use such a substance.

can be used to fuel muscular contraction. It is the only compound in the body that can provide this immediate source of energy. Therefore, for muscles to contract during exercise, a supply of ATP must be available.

Two "systems" in muscle cells can produce ATP. One of these does not require oxygen and is called the **anaerobic** (without oxygen) system. The second system requires oxygen and is called the **aerobic** (with oxygen) system. Let's discuss the anaerobic system first.

Anaerobic ATP Production Most of the anaerobic ATP production in muscle occurs in a metabolic process called *glycolysis*, which breaks down carbohydrates (sugars) in the cell. The end result of glycolysis is the anaerobic production of ATP and often the formation of lactic acid. Because lactic acid is often a by-product of glycolysis, this pathway for ATP production is often called the **lactic acid system**. The lactic acid system can only use carbohydrates as an energy

source. Carbohydrates are supplied to muscles from blood sugar (*glucose*) and from muscle stores of glucose (called *glycogen*).

Conceptually, it is convenient to think of the lactic acid system as the energy pathway that produces ATP at the beginning of exercise and during short-term (30–60 seconds) high-intensity exercise. For instance, most of the ATP required

anaerobic Means "without oxygen"; as pertains to energy-producing biochemical pathways in cells that do not require oxygen to produce energy.

aerobic Means "with oxygen"; as pertains to energy-producing biochemical pathways in cells that use oxygen to produce energy.

lactic acid A by-product of glucose metabolism. Produced primarily during intense exercise (i.e., greater than 50%–60% of maximal aerobic capacity). Results in inhibition of muscle contraction and, therefore, fatigue.

to sprint 400 meters (which may require 60–80 seconds) would be derived from the lactic acid system. During this type of intense exercise, muscles produce large amounts of lactic acid because the lactic acid system is at high speed. The accumulation of lactic acid in muscles results in fatigue and explains the decline in running speed of a 400-meter runner struggling toward the finish line.

Aerobic ATP Production Exercise lasting longer than 60 seconds requires ATP production from the aerobic system. Therefore, activities of daily living and many types of exercise depend on aerobic ATP production.

Whereas the lactic acid system uses only carbohydrate as a food source, aerobic metabolism can use all three foodstuffs (fats, carbohydrates, and protein) to produce ATP. In a healthy individual consuming a balanced diet, however, proteins play a limited role as an energy source during exercise; therefore, carbohydrates and fats are the primary sources. In general, at the beginning of exercise, carbohydrate is the principal foodstuff broken down during aerobic ATP production. During prolonged exercise (i.e., greater than 20 minutes' duration), there is a gradual shift from carbohydrate to fat as an energy source. This process is illustrated in Figure 4.1.

The Energy Continuum Although it is common to speak of aerobic versus anaerobic exercise, in reality, the energy to perform many types of exercise comes from both sources. Figure 4.2A illustrates the anaerobic–aerobic energy continuum as a function of the exercise duration. Anaerobic energy production dominates during short-term exercise, whereas aerobic energy production is greatest during long-term exercise. For example, maximal exercise of 10 seconds' duration uses anaerobic energy sources almost exclusively. On the other end of the energy spectrum, notice that aerobic energy production dominates during 2 hours of continuous exercise. Running a maximal-effort 800-meter race (exercise of 2–3 minutes' duration) is an example of an exercise duration that uses almost an equal amount of aerobic and anaerobic energy sources.

Figure 4.2B applies the anaerobic–aerobic energy continuum to various sports activities. Let's consider a few examples. Weight lifting, gymnastics, and football are illustrations of sports that use anaerobic energy production almost exclusively. Boxing and skating (1500 meters) are examples of sports that require an equal contribution of anaerobic and aerobic energy production. Finally, cross-country skiing and jogging are examples of activities in which aerobic energy production dominates.

Exercise and the Cardiorespiratory System

The term *cardiorespiratory system* refers to the cooperative work of the circulatory and respiratory systems. Together, they are responsible for the delivery of oxygen and nutrients as well as for the removal of waste products (e.g., carbon dioxide) from tissues. Exercise poses a major challenge to the cardiorespiratory system by increasing the muscular demand for oxygen and nutrients. The cardiorespiratory system must meet this demand to allow the individual to continue exercising. In the following sections we present a brief overview of cardiorespiratory function during exercise.

The Circulatory System

The circulatory system is a closed loop composed of the heart and blood vessels. The pump in this system is the heart, which, by contracting, generates pressure to move blood through the

FIGURE 4.1 Changes in carbohydrate and fat utilization during 90 minutes of aerobic exercise.

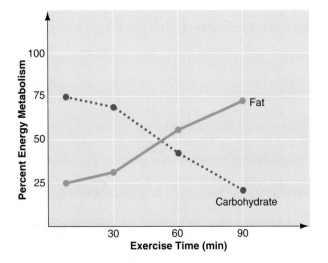

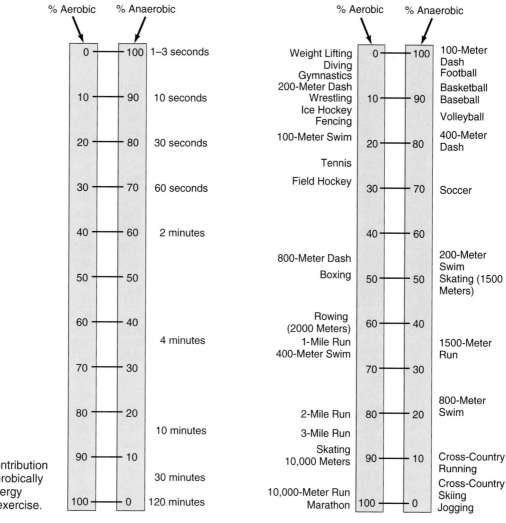

FIGURE 4.2 Contribution of anaerobic and aerobically produced ATP to energy metabolism during exercise.

system. Figure 4.3 illustrates that the heart can be considered two pumps in one. The right side pumps oxygen-depleted (deoxygenated) blood through the lungs (called the **pulmonary circuit**), while the left side pumps oxygen-rich (oxygenated) blood to tissues throughout the body (called the **systemic circuit**). Let's consider these two circuits in more detail.

In the systemic circuit, blood carrying oxygen leaves the heart in **arteries** which branch to form microscopic vessels called *arterioles*; arterioles eventually develop into beds of smaller vessels called *capillaries*. **Capillaries** are thin-walled vessels that permit the exchange of gases (oxygen and carbon dioxide) and nutrients between the blood and tissues. After this exchange, blood passes from the capillaries into microscopic vessels called *venules*. As venules move back toward the heart, they increase in size and form **veins,** which carry oxygen-depleted blood back to the heart.

pulmonary circuit The blood vascular system which circulates blood from the right side of the heart, through the lungs, and back to the left side of the heart.

systemic circuit The blood vascular system which circulates blood from the left side of the heart, throughout the body, and back to the right side of the heart.

arteries The blood vessels that transport blood away from the heart.

capillaries Thin-walled vessels that permit the exchange of gases (oxygen and carbon dioxide) and nutrients to occur between the blood and tissues.

veins Blood vessels that transport blood toward the heart.

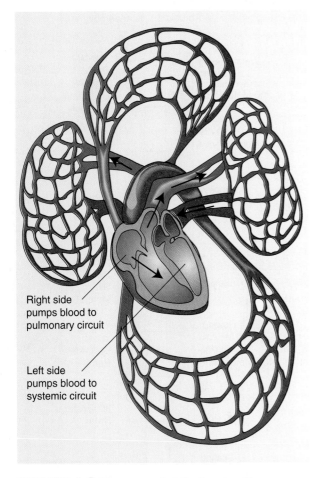

FIGURE 4.3 The concept of the heart as "two pumps in one." (From Wilmore, J.H. and Costill, D.L. *Physiology of Sport and Exercise* (p. 173). Champaign, IL: Human Kinetics Publishers. Copyright © 1994 by Jack H. Wilmore and David L. Costill. Reprinted with permission.)

Right side pumps blood to pulmonary circuit

Left side pumps blood to systemic circuit

Venous blood (i.e., blood carried by veins) from all parts of the body returns to the right side of the heart and is pumped through the lungs. There oxygen is loaded into the blood, and carbon dioxide is removed from the blood into the lungs. The oxygen-rich blood is then returned to the left side of the heart and pumped to all body tissues by the systemic circuit.

The amount of blood the heart pumps per minute is called **cardiac output**. Cardiac output is the product of the **heart rate** (number of heart beats per minute) and the **stroke volume** (how much blood is pumped per heart beat, generally expressed in milliliters). During exercise, cardiac output can be increased by increasing either heart rate or stroke volume or both. Stroke volume does not increase beyond light work rates (i.e., low-

intensity exercise). Therefore, at moderate work rates and above, the rise in cardiac output is achieved by increases in heart rate alone. (Changes in cardiac output in response to exercise will be discussed later in this chapter.)

Maximal cardiac output declines in both men and women after approximately 20 years of age, primarily due to a decrease in maximal heart rate. The decrease in maximal heart rate (HR max) with age can be estimated by the formula:

HR max = 220 – age (years)

According to this formula, a 20-year-old individual would have a maximal HR of 200 beats per minute (220 – 20 = 200), whereas a 60-year-old would have a maximal HR of 160 beats per minute (220 – 60 = 160).

Blood Pressure

Blood is moved through the circulatory system by pressure generated by the heart. The pressure that blood exerts against the walls of arteries

FIGURE 4.4 Measuring blood pressure using a sphygmomanometer.

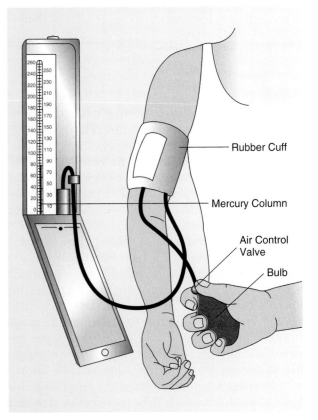

Rubber Cuff

Mercury Column

Air Control Valve

Bulb

is called *blood pressure*. Measurement of arterial blood pressure is generally attained by a device called a *sphygmomanometer* (Figure 4.4). During contraction of the heart (called *systole*) arterial blood pressure reaches its highest value. Blood pressure during systole is called **systolic blood pressure**; the normal resting systolic blood pressure for a young male adult is approximately 120 mm Hg (women may register 10–20 mm Hg lower). During the relaxation phase of the heart (called *diastole*), blood pressure declines and reaches its lowest value. Blood pressure during diastole is called **diastolic blood pressure**; normal diastolic blood pressure for a young male adult is approximately 80 mm Hg (again, women may register 10–20 mm Hg lower). It is important to measure both systolic and diastolic blood pressure because it is the combination of these two pressures that determines your mean (average) arterial pressure.

The walls of arteries are elastic, and they expand during the contraction of the heart. The increase in blood pressure during systole causes a pulsation in the arteries which can be felt by placing your finger (not your thumb) on the skin near a major artery. One pulse represents one heart beat. This technique can be used to count your heart rate during or after exercise (discussed in Chapter 2).

Approximately 20% of all adults living in the United States (7) have abnormally high blood pressure, or **hypertension**. Systolic blood pressure above 140 mm Hg and diastolic blood pressure above 90 mm Hg are considered to be the "threshold" values for hypertension. Hypertension is a serious health problem because it increases the risk of heart attack and stroke (8). As we saw in Chapter 1, regular exercise has been shown to reduce blood pressure in many individuals. Therefore, physicians often prescribe light exercise for hypertensive patients in an effort to lower their blood pressure.

The Respiratory System

The primary purpose of the respiratory system (also called the *pulmonary system*) is to provide a means of replacing oxygen and removing carbon dioxide from the blood. This is achieved by bringing oxygen-rich air into the lungs, which we do by breathing. Oxygen then moves from the lungs into the blood, and carbon dioxide moves from the blood into the lungs and is then exhaled.

Maximal Cardiorespiratory Function: VO₂ max

The body's maximum ability to transport and utilize oxygen during exercise (called **VO₂ max** or *maximal aerobic capacity*) was introduced in Chapter 2. VO₂ max is considered by many exercise physiologists to be the most valid measurement of cardiorespiratory fitness. Indeed, graded exercise tests designed to measure VO₂ max are often conducted by fitness experts to determine an individual's cardiorespiratory fitness. These tests require expensive equipment to measure oxygen consumption and are usually conducted on a treadmill or stationary exercise cycle. This type of test is often called an incremental exercise test.

Figure 4.5 illustrates the change in oxygen consumption (called *oxygen uptake*) at every exercise intensity (work rate) during a typical incremental exercise test. Note that oxygen uptake increases in a straight line with respect to work rate until VO₂ max is reached; thus, VO₂ max represents a "physiological ceiling" for the ability of the cardiorespiratory system to transport oxygen and for the muscles to utilize it.

Physiological Responses to Exercise

Now that we have an idea how the cardiovascular, respiratory, and energy-producing systems function, let's discuss the specifics of how these systems respond to exercise.

cardiac output The amount of blood the heart pumps per minute.

heart rate Number of heart beats per minute.

stroke volume The amount of blood pumped per heart beat (generally expressed in milliliters).

systolic blood pressure The pressure of the blood in the arteries at the level of the heart during the contractile phase of the heart (systole).

diastolic blood pressure The pressure of the blood in the arteries at the level of the heart during the resting phase of the heart (diastole).

hypertension (high blood pressure) Usually considered to be a blood pressure of greater than 140 for systolic or 90 for diastolic.

VO₂ max The highest oxygen consumption achievable during exercise. Practically speaking, VO₂ max is a laboratory measure of the endurance capacity of both the cardiorespiratory system and exercising skeletal muscles.

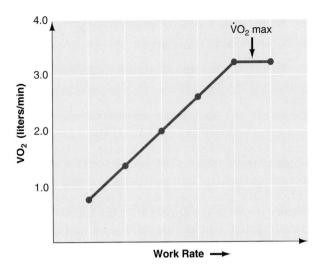

FIGURE 4.5 The relationship between exercise intensity (work rate) and VO_2. VO_2 max is the highest oxygen uptake that can be obtained during heavy exercise.

Circulatory Responses Exercise increases the body's need for oxygen. To meet this need, blood flow (and therefore oxygen delivery) to working muscle must increase in proportion to the demand. Increased oxygen transport to skeletal muscle is accomplished by increasing cardiac output and redistributing blood flow toward working muscle. The change in cardiac output, heart rate, and blood pressure in response to exercise of varying intensities is illustrated in Figure 4.6. Note that both heart rate and cardiac output increase in a straight line as exercise intensity increases.

The fact that heart rate increases as a function of exercise intensity is useful for monitoring the intensity of exercise or the amount of physiological stress. For instance, a person riding a bicycle or running can stop exercising and quickly check heart rate (the pulse) to measure how hard he or she is working. Because it is easy to check heart rate during exercise, this has become the standard means of determining exercise intensity. Also, notice in Figure 4.6 that both heart rate and cardiac output reach a plateau when VO_2 max is achieved. Again, VO_2 max represents a physiological ceiling of the body's ability for delivery and utilization of oxygen in exercising muscles.

Finally, let's consider the changes in blood pressure in response to exercise of varying intensity (see Figure 4.6). The key point in Figure 4.6 is that systolic blood pressure increases as the exercise intensity rises; in contrast, note that diastolic blood pressure remains relatively un-

changed from the resting state. The rise in systolic blood pressure with higher exercise intensity provides the increased driving pressure to push blood toward the exercising muscles.

Respiratory Responses The responsibility of the respiratory system during exercise is to maintain constant arterial oxygen and carbon dioxide levels. Therefore, because exercise increases oxygen consumption and carbon dioxide production, the breathing rate must increase to bring more oxygen into the body and to remove carbon dioxide. Notice in Figure 4.7 that breathing (called *ventilation*) increases in proportion to exercise intensity up to approximately 50% of VO_2 max. At higher work rates, breathing increases rapidly, resulting in an increased delivery of oxygen and removal of carbon dioxide.

Responses of the Energy-Producing Systems Recall that the energy needed to perform many types of exercise comes from both anaerobic and aerobic sources and that anaerobic exercise dominates in high-intensity exercise, whereas aerobic energy production is greatest in low-intensity exercise. The relationship between exercise intensity and anaerobic energy production is discussed in detail in A Closer Look 4.1.

FIGURE 4.6 Changes in blood pressure, cardiac output, and heart rate as a function of exercise intensity.

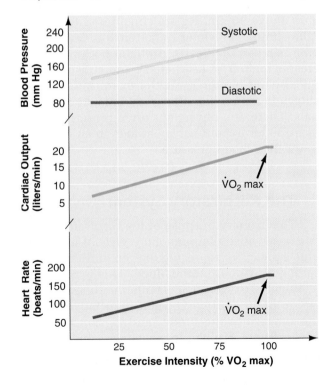

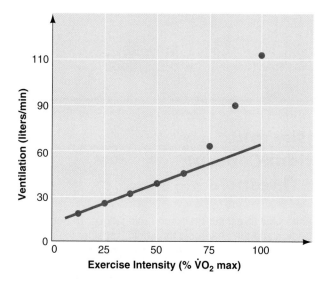

FIGURE 4.7 The ventilatory response to exercise. Each point on the graph represents the amount of ventilation required at a specific exercise intensity. Points lying on the straight line indicate exercise work rates below the anaerobic threshold (see A Closer Look 4.1 on page 82 for an explanation).

Exercise Prescription for Cardiorespiratory Fitness

After assessing your health status and evaluating your current cardiorespiratory fitness level (see Chapter 2), you are ready to develop your exercise prescription to improve your cardiorespiratory fitness. As we have discussed, the exercise training session is composed of three primary elements: warm-up, workout (primary conditioning period), and cool-down.

Warm-Up

Every workout should begin with a warm-up. The major purposes of a warm-up are to increase heart rate and body temperature and to elevate blood flow to the muscles. A warm-up usually consists of 5 to 15 minutes of slow-paced exercise. This allows a gradual warming of the muscles and connective tissue before engaging in vigorous exercise. Although some fitness instructors recommend stretching during the warm-up period (and we have listed stretching as part of the warm-up in chapters 2 and 3), we suggest that stretching exercises are optional during the warm-up and probably should be emphasized fol-

lowing the cool-down period. The rationale is that stretching is probably most effective after the muscles are warmed from the workout.

A warm-up routine for someone who will be jogging for the cardiorespiratory workout might consist of the following steps:

1. 1 to 3 minutes of light calisthenics
2. 1 to 3 minutes of walking at a pace that elevates heart rate by 20 to 30 beats/min above rest
3. 2 to 4 minutes of stretching (optional; see Chapter 6 for details)
4. 2 to 5 minutes of jogging at a slow pace to gradually elevate the heart rate toward the desired target heart rate (discussed later in the section on intensity).

If the workout is to consist of exercise modes other than jogging, the same general warm-up routine could be followed by substituting other exercise modes, as in steps 2 and 4. For instance, if cycling is the primary mode of exercise, low-intensity cycling exercise would take the place of walking and jogging in steps 2 and 4.

Workout: Primary Conditioning Period

The components of an exercise prescription to improve cardiovascular fitness include the mode, frequency, intensity, and duration of exercise (9a). Let's discuss each of these factors briefly.

Mode Several modes of exercise can be used to improve cardiorespiratory fitness. Some of the most common are walking, jogging, cycling, and swimming. In general, any activity that uses a large muscle mass (e.g., the legs) in a slow, rhythmical pattern can be used to improve cardiorespiratory fitness. See Table 4.1 on page 83 for a list of numerous activities that have been shown to improve cardiorespiratory fitness.

There are several key factors to consider when choosing an exercise mode. First, the activity must be fun! Choose an exercise mode that you enjoy. Your chances of sticking with an exercise program are much greater if you choose an activity that you like. A second consideration is that the type of exercise you choose must be convenient and accessible. For example, don't choose swimming if the nearest pool is 50 miles from your home. Similarly, don't choose cycling if you don't have use of a bicycle. A final factor is

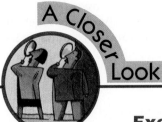

4.1

A Closer Look

Exercise Intensity and Lactic Acid Production: Concept of the Anaerobic Threshold

High-intensity exercise results in an increased production of lactic acid. The relationship between exercise intensity and blood levels of lactic acid is illustrated in Figure 4.8. Note that blood levels of lactic acid during exercise remain low until an exercise intensity of 50% to 60% of VO_2 max is achieved. However, exercise above 50% to 60% of VO_2 max results in a rapid accumulation of blood lactic acid. The exercise intensity that results in an increased rate of muscle lactic acid accumulation is called the **anaerobic threshold** (9).

During exercise above the anaerobic threshold, muscles begin to produce large amounts of lactic acid, resulting in muscular fatigue. This explains why exercise below the anaerobic threshold can be tolerated for a long period, whereas exercise above the

anaerobic threshold results in rapid fatigue. To better understand the anaerobic threshold, consider the following illustration. Many of us have gone running or cycling and have experimented with the maximal speed that we can maintain during this exercise. Experience has taught us that there is a maximal running speed we can tolerate for the full duration of our exercise session. This maximal speed represents an exercise intensity close to but below the anaerobic threshold. Any attempt to pick up the pace to a speed above the anaerobic threshold results in muscle fatigue, and we must slow our pace. Therefore, prolonged exercise sessions (i.e., 20–60 minutes' duration) aimed at improving cardiorespiratory fitness are generally performed at exercise intensities below the anaerobic threshold.

FIGURE 4.8 The relationship between blood lactic acid concentration and exercise intensity. Points lying on the straight line indicate exercise work rates below the anaerobic threshold (see A Closer Look 4.1 for explanation).

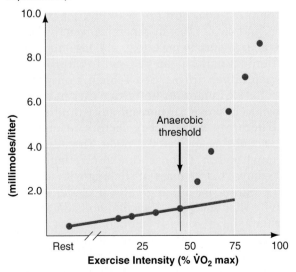

the risk of injury. High-impact activities such as running present a greater risk of injury than low-impact activities such as cycling and swimming. A common sense rule when choosing an exercise mode is that if you tend to be injury-prone, choose a low-impact activity. In contrast, if you rarely experience exercise-related injuries, feel free to choose either a high- or low-impact activity mode.

Historically, most exercise prescriptions for improving cardiorespiratory fitness have used only one activity mode. However, there is a current trend toward using **cross training** (i.e., a variety of activity modes) for training the cardiorespiratory system. Many fitness experts feel that participating in only one mode of exercise is boring and leads to more exercise dropouts. Further, cross training may also reduce the frequency of injury. (Cross training is discussed in detail later in this chapter.)

Table 4.1

Popular Activities That Promote Cardiorespiratory Fitness

Aerobic dance
Bicycling
Calisthenics (heavy)
Cross country skiing
Rope skipping
Rowing
Running
Skating (ice or roller)
Stair climber
Swimming
Walking

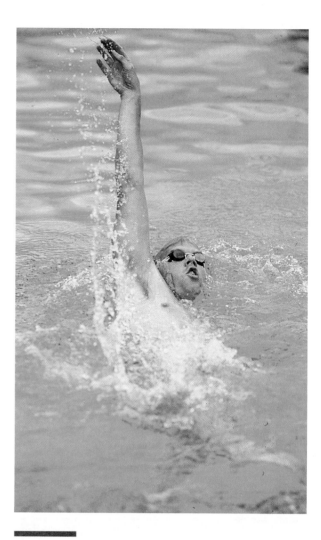

Walking, jogging, cycling, and swimming are popular modes of exercise that can be used to improve cardiorespiratory fitness.

Frequency Although cardiorespiratory fitness gains can be achieved with as few as two exercise sessions per week, the general recommendation for exercise frequency is three to five sessions per week to achieve near-optimal gains in cardiorespiratory fitness and minimal risk of injury (10). If training is injury-free, the frequency can be increased to 5 days per week if desired. It is, however, unlikely that even greater health or fitness benefits will accrue from exercising more than 5 days per week.

Intensity Improvements in cardiorespiratory fitness occur when the training intensity is approximately 50% of VO_2 max (this work rate is often called the **training threshold**). Although improvements in cardiorespiratory fitness can be achieved by exercising at VO_2 max, most people could only exercise for 1 to 2 minutes at that intensity. Thus, the recommended range of exercise intensity for improving health-related physical fitness is between 50% and 85% VO_2 max.

Recall that training intensity can be monitored indirectly by measurement of heart rate (see Chapter 2). The heart rate which corresponds to an exercise intensity sufficient to improve health-related physical fitness is called the **target heart rate (THR).** The most popular method of determining THR is the percentage of maximal heart rate (HR max) method. This method works on the principle that exercise intensity (i.e., % VO_2 max) can be estimated by measurement of exercise

anaerobic threshold The work intensity during graded, incremental exercise at which there is a rapid accumulation of blood lactic acid. This usually occurs at 50% to 60% of VO_2 and contributes to muscle fatigue.

cross training The use of a variety of activity modes for training the cardiorespiratory system.

training threshold The training intensity above which there is an improvement in cardiorespiratory fitness. This intensity is approximately 50% of VO_2 max.

target heart rate (THR) The range of heart rates that corresponds to an exercise intensity of approximately 50% to 85% VO_2 max. This is the range of training heart rates that results in improvements in aerobic capacity.

heart rate. To compute your THR using this method, simply multiply your HR max by both 90% and 70% to arrive at the high and low ends of your THR range. For example, the maximal HR of a 20-year-old college student can be estimated by the formula

$$HR \ max = 220 - 20 = 200 \ beats/min$$

The THR is then computed as

$$200 \ beats/min \times 0.70 = 140 \ beats/min$$

$$200 \ beats/min \times 0.90 = 180 \ beats/min$$

$$THR = 140 \ to \ 180 \ beats/min$$

In this example, the THR to be maintained during a workout to improve cardiorespiratory fitness is between 140 and 180 beats/min; this range of exercise intensities is sometimes called *the training sensitive zone.*

The reasoning behind using 70% and 90% of your maximal heart rate to compute your target rate is based on the relationship between percent HR max and percent VO_2 max (see Table 4.2). Note that 70% of HR max represents the heart rate associated with an exercise intensity of approximately 50% VO_2 max (the lower end of the training sensitive zone), and that 90% of HR max

represents approximately 85% VO_2 max (the upper end of the recommended training sensitive zone).

Finally, it is important to remember that your THR will change as you get older due to the decrease in maximal heart rate. This point is illustrated in Figure 4.9. For instance, while the THR for a 20-year-old college student is between 140 and 180 beats/min, the THR for a 60-year-old is 108 to 139 beats/min.

Duration Recall that the duration of exercise does not include the warm-up or cool-down. In general, exercise durations that have been shown to be most effective in improving cardiorespiratory fitness are between 20 and 60 minutes (10). The reason for this large "window" of duration is that the time required to obtain training benefits depends on both the individual's initial level of fitness and the training intensity. For example, a poorly conditioned individual may only require 20 to 30 minutes of daily exercise at his or her THR to improve cardiorespiratory fitness. In contrast, a highly trained person may require daily exercise sessions of 40 to 60 minutes' duration to improve cardiorespiratory fitness.

Another key point to understand is that improvement of cardiorespiratory fitness by engaging in low-intensity exercise requires a longer daily training duration than high-intensity exercise. For example, an individual training at 50% of VO_2 max may require a daily exercise duration of 40 to 50 minutes to improve cardiorespiratory fitness. In contrast, the same person exercising at 70% of VO_2 max may require only 20 to 30 minutes of daily exercise to achieve the same effect. A summary of the guidelines to improve cardiorespiratory fitness is illustrated in Figure 4.10.

Safety: Improving Cardiorespiratory Fitness without Injury

What is the optimal combination of exercise intensity, duration, and frequency to promote cardiorespiratory fitness while minimizing risk of injury? The answer to this question is illustrated in Figure 4.11. The optimal exercise intensity to improve cardiorespiratory fitness without increasing the risk of injury is between 60% and 80% of VO_2 max (73–87% HR max). Further, note that the optimal frequency and duration are 3 to 4 days/week and 20 to 60 minutes/day, respectively.

Table 4.2

The Relationship between Target Heart Rate, Percent HR Max, and the Percent of VO_2 Max for an Individual 20 Years of Age

THR (beats/minute*)	% VO_2 max	% HR max
186	90	93
180	85	90
173	80	87
166	75	83
160	70	80
153	65	76
146	60	73
140	55	70
134	49	67

*Heart rate based on a HR max of 200 beats/min.
Source: Adapted from Fox, E., R. Bowers, and M. Foss. *The physiological basis for exercise and sport.* Brown and Benchmark, Dubuque, IA, 1989.

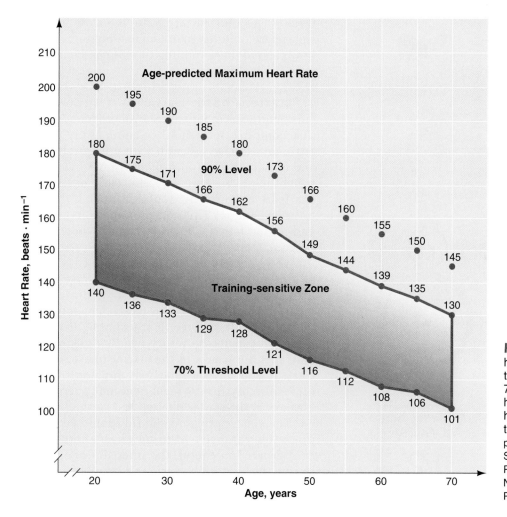

FIGURE 4.9 Target heart rate zones for ages 20 through 70. The zones cover 70% to 90% of maximum heart rate with the maximal heart rate shown across the top for each age. (Used with permission from Fitness and Sports Medicine: A Health-Related Approach, by David C. Nieman. Bull Publishing Co., Palo Alto, CA, 1995.)

Cool-Down

Every training session should conclude with a cool-down (5–15 minutes of light exercises and stretching). A primary purpose of a cool-down is to promote blood return to the heart, thereby preventing blood from pooling in the arms and legs, which could result in dizziness and/or fainting. A cool-down may also decrease the muscle soreness and cardiac irregularities that sometimes appear after a vigorous workout. Although cardiac irregularities are rare in healthy individuals, it is prudent to cool down and reduce the risk.

A general cool-down of at least 5 minutes (of light exercise such as walking and calisthenics) should be followed by 5 to 30 minutes of flexibility exercises. In general, stretching exercises should focus on the muscles used during training. The type and duration of the stretching session depends on your flexibility goals (see Chapter 6).

Starting and Maintaining a Cardiorespiratory Fitness Program

Two key elements in any fitness program are the specific short-term and long-term goals. Without these, motivation to continue training is hard to maintain. Many fitness experts agree that the lack of goals is a major contributor to the high dropout rates seen in many organized fitness programs (11). It pays to establish both short-term and long-term fitness goals *before* you start your training program.

If your training plans include running, walking, aerobic dance, or other weight-bearing activities, it is important to exercise in good shoes. Unfortunately, good running, walking, or aerobics shoes are not cheap (costs range from $50–$150).

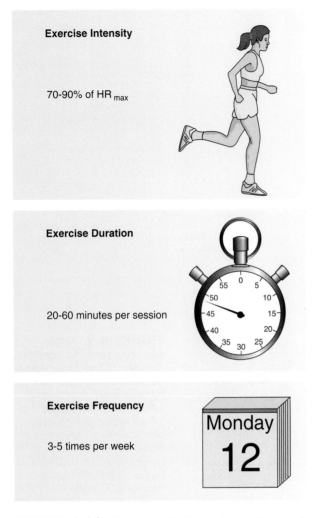

Exercise Intensity

70-90% of HR $_{max}$

Exercise Duration

20-60 minutes per session

Exercise Frequency

3-5 times per week

Monday
12

FIGURE 4.10 The suggested intensity, duration, and frequency of exercise necessary to improve cardiovascular fitness.

However, investing in good shoes is important for both comfort and injury prevention. Look for a well-cushioned shoe with the following features: soft comfortable upper material; adequate toe room (as indicated by comfort); well-padded heel and ankle collar; firm arch support; and a heel lift (a wedge that raises the heel about 1/2 inch higher than the sole). Many athletic shoe stores have well-trained sales personnel to assist you in the selection process.

Developing an Individualized Exercise Prescription

Regardless of your initial fitness level or your choice of exercise mode, the exercise prescription to improve cardiovascular fitness usually has three stages: the starter phase, the slow progression phase, and the maintenance phase. Let's see how each of these training phases can be tailored to individual needs.

Starter Phase The quickest way to extinguish enthusiasm for an exercise program is to try to accomplish too much too soon. Many people begin an exercise program with great excitement and anticipation of improved fitness levels and weight loss. Unfortunately, this early excitement can lead to exercising too hard during the first training session! This can promote sore muscles and undue fatigue. Therefore, start your fitness program slowly.

The objective of the starter phase is to gradually permit the body to adapt to exercise and to avoid soreness, injury, and personal discouragement. It usually lasts 2 to 6 weeks, depending on your initial fitness level. For example, if you are in a poor cardiorespiratory fitness category, you may spend 6 weeks in the starter phase. In contrast, if you have a relatively high initial cardiorespiratory fitness level, you may spend only 2 weeks in the starter phase.

The starter program should include a warm-up, a low-intensity training phase, and then a cool-down. In general, the intensity of exercise during the starter phase should be relatively low (up to 70% of HR max). The following are key points to remember during the starter phase of an exercise program:

1. Start at an exercise intensity that is comfortable for you.
2. Don't increase your training duration or intensity if you are not comfortable.
3. Be aware of new aches or pains. Pain is a symptom of injury and indicates that rest is required to allow the body to repair itself (see Chapter 11 for a discussion of injury prevention and treatment).

Slow Progression Phase The slow progression phase may last 12 to 20 weeks, with exercise progression being more rapid than during the starter phase. The intensity can be gradually elevated, and the frequency and duration of exercise increased, depending on fitness goals and the presence or absence of injuries. In general, this stage should reach an exercise frequency of 3 to 4 times/week and an exercise duration of at least 30 minutes per session. Exercise intensity should range between 70% and 90% HR max, depending on your personal fitness goals.

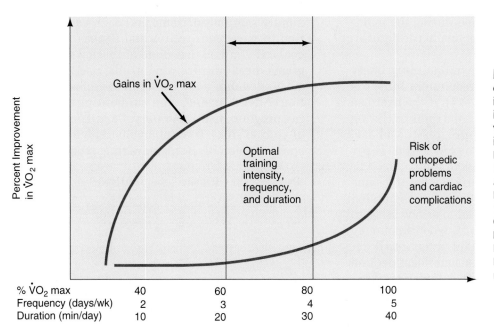

FIGURE 4.11 The effects of increasing frequency, intensity, and duration on the improvements in VO$_2$ max versus the increased risk of injury. (Source: Powers, S., and E. Howley. *Exercise physiology: Theory and application to fitness and performance.* Wm. C. Brown, Dubuque, IA, 1994. Copyright © 1994 Wm. C. Brown Communications, Inc. Reprinted by permission of Times Mirror Higher Education Group, Inc., Dubuque, Iowa. All rights reserved.)

Maintenance Phase The average college-age student will generally reach the maintenance phase of the exercise prescription after 16 to 28 weeks of training. At this stage you should have achieved your fitness goal and are no longer interested in increasing your training load. The objective now becomes to maintain this level of fitness. As the old saying goes, "Fitness is not something you can put in the bank." To maintain cardiorespiratory fitness, you must continue to train on a regular basis. The key question now is,

Nutritional

4.2 Links to Health and Fitness

Fuels for Endurance Exercise

The predominant fuels used during endurance training are fats and carbohydrates. Everyone has a great deal of energy stored as fat. However, carbohydrate reserves are small and can be depleted. Depletion of carbohydrate stores can lead to muscle fatigue. The following example illustrates the average amount of energy stored as fat and carbohydrate for a typical, college-aged man and woman.

	MAN	WOMAN
Body weight (lbs.)	160	110
% Body fat	15	25
Pounds of fat	24	27.5
Kcal from stored fat	84,000	96,250
Kcal from stored carbohydrate	1,700	1,200

Based on an energy expenditure of 3000 kcals/day for an individual engaged in a vigorous exercise training program, this chart illustrates that there is enough stored fat to supply the energy needs of the body for approximately a month! However, the body cannot use fat as the sole source of energy. Carbohydrates must also be used for fuel, as indicated by the axiom, "Fat burns in the flame of carbohydrate." Thus, a problem may arise because carbohydrate stores can be almost depleted within a day in an active individual on a low kcal/carbohydrate diet. This example shows the importance of consuming adequate amounts of carbohydrates if you lead an active lifestyle. Without sufficient carbohydrate in the diet, endurance exercise can lead to depletion of carbohydrate stores and chronic fatigue.

How much training is required during the maintenance phase to prevent a decline in cardiorespiratory fitness?

Several studies have shown that the primary factor in maintaining cardiorespiratory fitness is the intensity of exercise (12–14). If the exercise intensity and duration remain the same as during the final weeks of the slow progression phase, frequency can be reduced to as few as 2 days per week without a significant loss in fitness. In addition, if frequency and intensity remain the same as during the final weeks of the slow progression phase, duration can be reduced to as few as 20 to 25 minutes per day. In contrast, when frequency and duration are held constant, a one-third decrease in intensity results in a significant decline in cardiorespiratory fitness. To summarize, if exercise intensity is maintained, the exercise frequency and duration necessary to maintain a given level of cardiorespiratory fitness are substantially less than that required to improve fitness levels.

Sample Exercise Prescriptions As mentioned, the exercise prescription must be tailored to the individual. The key factor to consider when designing a personal training program is your current fitness level. Programs designed for people with good or excellent cardiorespiratory fitness levels start at a higher level and progress more rapidly, compared with programs designed for people in poor condition. Tables 4.3 through 4.5 illustrate three sample cardiorespiratory training programs designed for college-aged people who are beginning a fitness program. Table 4.3 contains an exercise prescription that might be appropriate for people in very poor or poor cardiorespiratory fitness. Table 4.4 on page 90 illustrates a sample program designed for people in good or average cardiorespiratory fitness, while Table 4.5 on page 91 contains a program aimed at people with a cardiorespiratory rating of excellent or above. Note that these programs are merely sample programs and each can be modified to meet your individual fitness levels and goals. If you feel that none of these training programs meet your training needs, use Laboratory 4.1 to develop your personal exercise prescription. After designing your cardiorespiratory training program, use Laboratory 4.2 to keep a record of your exercise training habits. The following is an illustration of a typical training record:

Date	Activity	Duration	Exercise Heart Rate	Comments

Training Techniques

Endurance training is a generic term that refers to any mode of exercise aimed at improving cardiorespiratory fitness. Over the years, numerous endurance training techniques have evolved. In the next section, we discuss several common ones.

Cross Training

As previously mentioned, cross training is a popular form of training that uses several different training modes. It may mean running on one day, swimming on another day, and cycling on another day. One advantage of this type of training is that cross training reduces the boredom of performing the same kind of exercise day after day. Further, it may reduce the incidence of injuries by avoiding overuse of the same body parts. The disadvantage of cross training is the lack of training specificity. For example, daily jogging does not improve swimming endurance because the arm muscles are not trained during jogging. Similarly, swimming does not improve jogging endurance. In general, to improve endurance in a particular activity, training should utilize exercises similar to that activity.

Long, Slow Distance Training

Long, slow distance training, or continuous training, requires a steady, submaximal exercise intensity (i.e., the intensity is generally around 70% HR max). It is one of the most popular cardiorespiratory training techniques and can be ap-

long, slow distance training The term utilized to indicate continuous exercise which requires a steady, submaximal exercise intensity (i.e., the intensity is generally around 70% HR max).

interval training Repeated bouts or intervals of relatively intense exercise. The duration of the intervals can be varied, but a 1- to 5-minute duration is common. Each interval is followed by a rest period, which should be equal to or slightly greater than the interval duration.

Table 4.3

Sample Cardiorespiratory Exercise Program Designed for People in the Very Poor or Poor Fitness Category

General guidelines:
1. Begin each session with a warm-up.
2. Don't progress to the next level until you feel comfortable with your current level of exercise.
3. Monitor your heart rate during each training session.
4. End each session with a cool-down.
5. Be aware of aches and pains. If you are injury prone, choose an activity mode that is low impact, and limit your exercise duration to 20 to 30 minutes per day.

Week No.	Phase	Duration (min/day)	Intensity (% of HR max)	Frequency (days/wk)
1	Starter	10	60	3
2	Starter	10	60	3
3	Starter	12	60	3
4	Starter	12	70	3
5	Starter	15	70	3
6	Starter	15	70	3
7	Slow progression	20	70	3
8	Slow progression	20	70	3
9	Slow progression	25	70	3
10	Slow progression	25	70	3
11	Slow progression	30	70	3
12	Slow progression	30	70	3
13	Slow progression	35	70	3
14	Slow progression	35	70	3
15	Slow progression	40	70	3
16	Slow progression	40	70	3
17	Slow progression	40	75	3
18	Slow progression	40	75	3
19	Slow progression	40	75	3
20	Slow progression	40	75	3–4
21	Slow progression	40	75	3–4
22	Slow progression	40	75	3–4
23	Maintenance	30	75	3–4
24	Maintenance	30	75	3–4
25	Maintenance	30	75	3–4
26	Maintenance	30	75	3–4

plied to any mode of exercise. During the progression phase of the exercise program, an individual may find this type of training enjoyable because the exercise intensity does not increase. If injuries are not a problem, there is no reason why the duration of the training cannot be extended to 40 to 60 minutes/session. An advantage of continuous training is that risk of injury is lower than in more intensive training.

Interval Training

Interval training means undertaking repeated bouts or intervals of relatively intense exercise. The duration of the intervals can be varied, but a 1- to 5-minute duration is common. Each interval is followed by a rest period, which should be equal to, or slightly greater than, the interval duration. For example, if you are running 400-meter

Table 4.4

Sample Cardiorespiratory Exercise Program Designed for People in the Average or Good Fitness Category

General guidelines:
1. Begin each session with a warm-up.
2. Don't progress to the next level until you feel comfortable with your current level of exercise.
3. Monitor your heart rate during each training session.
4. End each session with a cool-down.
5. Be aware of aches and pains. If you are injury prone, choose an activity mode that is low impact, and limit your exercise duration to 20 to 30 minutes per day.

Week No.	Phase	Duration (min/day)	Intensity (% of HR max)	Frequency (days/wk)
1	Starter	10	70	3
2	Starter	15	70	3
3	Starter	15	70	3
4	Starter	20	70	3
5	Slow progression	25	70	3
6	Slow progression	25	75	3
7	Slow progression	25	75	3
8	Slow progression	30	75	3
9	Slow progression	30	75	3
10	Slow progression	35	75	3
11	Slow progression	35	75	3
12	Slow progression	40	75	3
13	Slow progression	40	75	3
14	Slow progression	40	75	3
15	Slow progression	40	80	3
16	Slow progression	40	80	3–4
17	Slow progression	40	80	3–4
18	Slow progression	40	80	3–4
19	Maintenance	30	80	3–4
20	Maintenance	30	80	3–4
21	Maintenance	30	80	3–4
22	Maintenance	30	80	3–4

intervals on a track, and it takes you approximately 90 seconds to complete each run, your rest period between efforts should be at least 90 seconds.

Interval training is a common training technique among athletes who have first established a base of endurance training and wish to attain much higher fitness levels in order to be more competitive in a particular sport. With correct spacing of exercise and rest periods, more work can be accomplished with interval training than with long, slow distance training. A major advantage of interval training is the variety of workouts it allows, which may reduce the tedium associated with other forms of training.

Fartlek Training

Fartlek is a Swedish word meaning "speed play," and it refers to a popular form of training for long-distance runners. **Fartlek training** is much like interval training, but it is not as rigid in its work-to-rest interval ratios. It consists of free-form running done out on trails, roads, golf

Table 4.5

Sample Cardiorespiratory Exercise Program Designed for People in the Excellent Fitness Category

General guidelines:
1. Begin each session with a warm-up.
2. Don't progress to the next level until you feel comfortable with your current level of exercise.
3. Monitor your heart rate during each training session.
4. End each session with a cool-down.
5. Be aware of aches and pains. If you are injury prone, choose an activity mode that is low impact, and limit your exercise duration to 20 to 30 minutes per day.

Week No.	Phase	Duration (min/day)	Intensity (% of HR max)	Frequency (days/wk)
1	Starter	15	75	3
2	Starter	20	75	3
3	Slow progression	25	75	3
4	Slow progression	30	75	3
5	Slow progression	35	75	3
6	Slow progression	40	75	3
7	Slow progression	40	75	3–4
8	Slow progression	40	75	3–4
9	Slow progression	40	80	3–4
10	Slow progression	40	80	3–4
11	Slow progression	40	80	3–4
12	Slow progression	40	80–85	3–4
13	Slow progression	40	80–85	3–4
14	Slow progression	40	80–85	3–4
15	Maintenance	30	80–85	3–4
16	Maintenance	30	80–85	3–4
17	Maintenance	30	80–85	3–4
18	Maintenance	30	80–85	3–4

courses, and the like. An advantage of fartlek training is that these workouts provide variety and reduce the possibility of boredom.

Aerobic Exercise Training: How the Body Adapts

How does the body adapt to aerobic exercise training? Endurance exercise training induces changes in the cardiovascular and respiratory system, skeletal muscles and the energy producing systems, VO$_2$ max, flexibility, and body composition, in response to regular aerobic training. A brief overview of each of these adaptations follows.

Cardiovascular System

Several adaptations occur in the cardiovascular system as a result of endurance training (15). First, although endurance training does not alter maximal heart rate, this type of training results in a decrease in heart rate during submaximal exer-

fartlek training *Fartlek* is a Swedish word meaning "speed play," and it refers to a popular form of training for long-distance runners. It is much like interval training, but it is not as rigid in its work-to-rest interval ratios. It consists of "free-form" running done out on trails, roads, golf courses, and so on.

cise compared to before training. This reduction in heart rate results because the stroke volume at submaximal loads is increased with training. Further, endurance exercise results in an increase in maximal stroke volume (SV) and a corresponding increase in maximal cardiac output (because maximal cardiac output = maximal HR × maximal SV). An increased maximal cardiac output results in an increased oxygen delivery to the exercising muscles and improved exercise tolerance.

Respiratory System

Some fitness proponents report that exercise improves lung function by expanding the volume of the lungs and increasing the efficiency of oxygen and carbon dioxide exchange. Unfortunately, there is no scientific evidence to support this belief. However, although endurance training does not alter the structure or function of the respiratory system, it does increase respiratory muscle endurance (16, 17). That is, the diaphragm and other key muscles of respiration can work harder and longer without fatigue. This improvement in respiratory muscle endurance may reduce the sensation of breathlessness during exercise and eliminate the pain in the side (often called a *stitch* in the side) that is sometimes associated with exercise.

Skeletal Muscles and Energy-Producing Systems

Endurance training increases the muscles' capacity for aerobic energy production. The practical result of an improvement in muscle aerobic capacity is an improved ability to use fat as an energy source and an increase in muscular endurance (15). Note that these changes occur only in those muscles used during the training activity. For example, endurance training using a stationary exercise cycle results in an improvement in muscular endurance in leg muscles, but has little effect on arm muscles. Finally, although endurance exercise training improves muscle tone, this type of exercise training does not result in large increases in muscle size or muscular strength.

VO_2 Max

Recall that VO_2 max is considered by many exercise physiologists to be the best single measure of cardiorespiratory fitness. Therefore, im-

provement in VO_2 max is an important physiological adaptation that occurs in response to endurance training. In general, 12 to 15 weeks of endurance exercise results in a 10% to 30% improvement in VO_2 max (15). This improvement is due to a combination of improved aerobic capacity in skeletal muscles and increased maximal cardiac output. The net result is an increased oxygen delivery and utilization by skeletal muscles during exercise. Therefore, an increase in VO_2 max translates to improved muscular endurance and less fatigue during routine daily activities.

How much VO_2 max increases after an endurance training program is dependent on several factors: fitness status at the beginning of the training program, intensity of the training program, and nutritional status during the training program. In general, people who start exercise programs with high VO_2 max values improve less than those with low initial VO_2 max values. For example, a person entering an endurance training program with a high VO_2 max may reach only a 5% improvement over a 12-week period, whereas an individual with a low VO_2 max may improve as much as 30% (see Figure 4.12). The explanation for this is that a physiological ceiling or limit for improvement in VO_2 max exists. Those people who enter fitness programs with relatively high VO_2 max values are probably closer to their limits than people who enter programs with low values.

FIGURE 4.12 The relationship between initial fitness levels and improvements in VO_2 max after a 12-week training period.

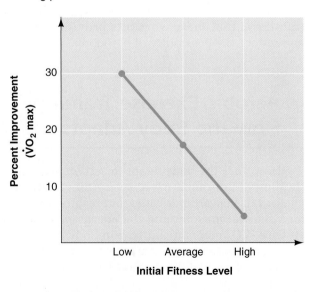

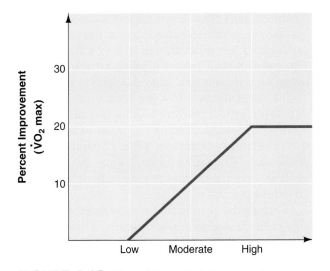

FIGURE 4.13 The relationship between training intensity and improvements in VO$_2$ max following a 12-week training period.

the intensity does not result in further improvement in fitness. In fact, training at extremely high intensities may increase the risk of injury and illness.

Finally, failure to maintain proper nutritional habits during an endurance training program will impair your improvements in VO$_2$ max. Proper nutrition means a diet that provides all of the necessary nutrients for good health. In Chapter 7 we will discuss how to construct the proper diet for health and fitness.

Flexibility

Most endurance training programs do not improve flexibility. In fact, several months of endurance training may reduce the range of motion at some joints due to muscle and tendon shortening. Therefore, to prevent a loss of flexibility, stretching exercises should always be a part of an endurance training program (see Chapter 6).

Body Composition

Endurance training generally results in a reduction in the percent of body fat (15). However, a loss of body fat in response to endurance training is not guaranteed. Whether or not an individual loses body fat as a result of exercise training is a result of many factors, including diet and the amount of exercise performed. More will be said about this in Chapter 8.

The magnitude of the exercise-induced increase in VO$_2$ max is directly related to the intensity of the training program (12). High-intensity training programs result in greater VO$_2$ max gains than low-intensity and short-duration programs (see Figure 4.13). Notice that a plateau exists in the relationship between training intensity and improvement in VO$_2$ max. Therefore, once a high-intensity of training is reached, increasing

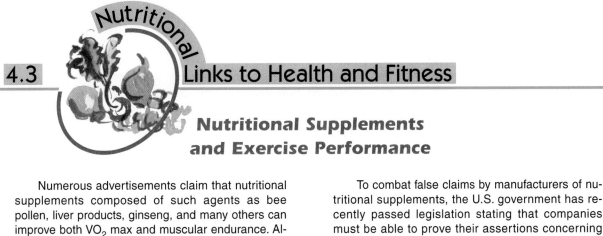

Nutritional Links to Health and Fitness

4.3

Nutritional Supplements and Exercise Performance

Numerous advertisements claim that nutritional supplements composed of such agents as bee pollen, liver products, ginseng, and many others can improve both VO$_2$ max and muscular endurance. Although some agents, such as caffeine (18) and carbohydrates (19), have been shown to be beneficial to exercise performance, most of these claims have no foundation in scientific research (20).

To combat false claims by manufacturers of nutritional supplements, the U.S. government has recently passed legislation stating that companies must be able to prove their assertions concerning the health and performance benefits of both drugs and nutritional supplements. Hopefully, this law will reduce the number of false advertisements in this area.

Summary: Endurance Training Adaptations

To summarize, endurance exercise training results in improvements in maximal cardiac output, respiratory system muscle endurance, skeletal muscle endurance, and VO_2 max. Further, endurance exercise can assist in the loss of body fat. Finally, endurance training does not improve flexibility and may even reduce flexibility if regular stretching exercises are not performed.

Motivation to Maintain Cardiorespiratory Fitness

Every year, millions of people make the decision to start an exercise routine. Unfortunately, over half those who begin a cardiorespiratory fitness program quit within the first 6 months (11). Although there are many reasons for this high dropout rate, a lack of time is commonly cited as a major one. Although finding time for exercise in a busy schedule is difficult, it is not impossible. The key is to schedule a regular time for exercise and stick with it. A small investment in time to exercise can reap large improvements in fitness and health. Think about the time required to improve cardiorespiratory fitness in the following way. There are 168 hours in every week. All you need is three, 30-minute workouts per week to improve cardiorespiratory fitness. Including the associated warm-ups, cool-downs, and showers, this is about 3 hours per week, which is less than 2% of the total week. This leaves you with 165 hours per week to accomplish all of the other things that you need to do. The bottom line is, with proper time management, anyone can find time to exercise.

In order for you to keep the commitment to develop cardiorespiratory fitness, exercise must be fun. Therefore, choose a training technique that you enjoy. Further, your chosen exercise mode should be convenient. Failure to meet both of these criteria increases your risk of becoming an exercise dropout.

One of the things that makes exercise enjoyable is the interaction with friends. Therefore, exercising with a partner is an excellent idea because it makes physical activity more fun and helps maintain your sense of commitment to a regular exercise routine. In choosing an exercise partner, choose someone that you enjoy interacting with and someone who is a good exercise role model.

Keeping a record of your training program is helpful in several ways. It assists you in keeping track of your training progress and serves as a motivating factor when you begin to notice improvements in your fitness level.

Finally, it is normal to experience some discomfort and soreness associated with your first several exercise sessions. Don't let this discourage you. In a short time, the soreness will fade and the discomfort associated with exercise will begin to disappear. As your fitness level improves, you will start to feel better and look better. Although reaching and maintaining a reasonable level of cardiorespiratory fitness will always require time and effort, the rewards will be well worth the labor.

Summary

1. Benefits of cardiorespiratory fitness include a lower risk of disease, feeling better, increased capacity to perform everyday tasks, and improved self-esteem.

2. Adenosine triphosphate is required for muscular contraction and can be produced in muscles by two systems: anaerobic (without oxygen) and aerobic (with oxygen).

3. The energy to perform many types of exercise comes from both anaerobic and aerobic sources. In general, anaerobic energy production dominates in short-term exercise, whereas aerobic energy production dominates during prolonged exercise.

4. The term *cardiorespiratory system* refers to the cooperative work of the circulatory and respiratory systems. The primary function of the circulatory system is to transport blood carrying oxygen and nutrients to body tissues. The principal function of the respiratory system is to load oxygen into and remove carbon dioxide from the blood.

5. The maximum capacity to transport and utilize oxygen during exercise is called VO_2 max; VO_2 max is considered by many exercise physiologists to be the most valid measurement of cardiorespiratory fitness.

6. Cardiac output, systolic blood pressure, and heart rate increase as a function of exercise intensity. Breathing (ventilation) also increases in proportion to exercise intensity.

7. The basis for prescribing exercise to improve cardiorespiratory fitness is knowledge of the individual's initial fitness and health status.

8. Three primary elements comprise the exercise prescription: warm-up, workout (primary conditioning period), and cool-down.

9. The purpose of a warm-up is to slowly elevate heart rate, muscle blood flow, and body temperature.

10. The components of the workout are the mode, frequency, intensity, and duration of exercise.

11. In general, the mode of exercise to be used to obtain increased cardiorespiratory endurance is one that uses a large muscle mass in a slow, rhythmical pattern for 20 to 60 minutes.

12. The target heart rate is the range of exercise heart rates that lie between 70% and 90% of maximal heart rate.

13. The recommended frequency of exercise to improve cardiorespiratory fitness is three to five times per week.

14. The purpose of a cool-down is to slowly decrease the pulse rate and return blood back to the upper body. The activity used during the training phase should be continued during the cool-down, but the intensity gradually decreased.

15. Establishing both short-term and long-term fitness goals is essential before beginning a fitness program.

16. Regardless of your initial fitness level, the exercise prescription to improve cardiorespiratory fitness has three phases: the starter phase, the slow progression phase, and the maintenance phase.

17. Common endurance training techniques to improve cardiorespiratory fitness include cross training; long, slow distance training; interval training; and fartlek training.

18. Aerobic exercise training results in an improvement in cardiorespiratory fitness (VO_2 max) and muscular endurance and can result in a reduction in percent body fat.

19. Maintaining a regular exercise routine requires proper time management and the choice of physical activities that you enjoy.

Study Questions

1. Discuss the two energy pathways used to produce muscle ATP during exercise.

2. Which energy pathway (aerobic or anaerobic) is predominantly responsible for production of ATP during the following activities: 100 meter dash, 800-meter run, 10,000-meter run, tennis, football, and weight lifting?

3. What is meant by the term *cardiorespiratory system*? List the major functions of the circulatory and respiratory systems.

4. Why is the heart called "two pumps in one"?

5. Define the following terms:

adenosine triphosphate (ATP)

cross training

hypertension

target heart rate

6. Graph the changes in heart rate, blood pressure, cardiac output, and ventilation as a function of exercise intensity.

7. Define VO_2 max.

8. Discuss the relationship between exercise intensity and lactic acid production in muscles. Define the anaerobic threshold. What is the practical significance of the anaerobic threshold for exercise?

9. What physiological changes occur as a result of endurance training?

10. Will endurance training alone result in improvement in all of the components of health-related physical fitness? Why or why not?

11. What information is necessary to develop an individualized exercise prescription?

12. What is the purpose of a warm-up prior to exercise?

13. List the criteria that must be met to obtain improvement in aerobic capacity.

14. What effect does mode of training have on obtaining increased aerobic capacity?

15. What is the range of frequency of exercise needed to improve aerobic capacity?

16. Define training threshold and give the range of intensities that are considered necessary to elicit an increase in VO_2 max.

17. What training techniques are generally used in exercise programs for improving cardiorespiratory fitness?

Suggested Reading

Cooper, K. *The aerobics program for total well-being.* M. Evans, New York, 1982.

Neiman, David C. *Fitness and sports medicine: An introduction.* 3rd ed. Bull Publishing, Palo Alto, CA, 1995.

Pollock, M. L., and J. H. Wilmore. *Exercise in health and disease.* 3rd ed. W. B. Saunders, Philadelphia, 1998.

Powers, S., and E. Howley. *Exercise physiology: Theory and application to fitness and performance.* 3rd ed. Wm. C. Brown, Dubuque, IA, 1997.

Suggested Readings on the World Wide Web

Sympatico: Healthyway (http://www.ns.sympatico.ca/healthyway/) Numerous articles, book reviews, and links to nutrition, fitness, and wellness topics.

Gatorade Sports Science Institute (http://www.gssiweb.com/library/) Many articles relating to fluid replacement during exercise. Sign up to be on a mailing list for new articles.

Marathoning: Start to Finish (http://www.teamoregon.com/publications/ marathon/) Guides to exercise in heat and cold, training for racing, ergogenic aids, and sports nutrition.

Fitness Tests: Explained (http://arnie.pec.BrockU.CA/~hsac/tests/tests.html) Tests for aerobic power, anaerobic power, flexibility, and body composition.

Fitness Files (http://www2.webpoint.com/augusta_fitness/) Fitness fundamentals, flexibility and contraindicated exercises, exercise nutrition, and treating exercise injuries.

The Running Page (http://sunsite.unc.edu/drears/running/running. html) Contains information about racing, running clubs, places to run, running related products, magazines, treating running injuries, etc.

Fitness and Sports Medicine (http://www.meriter.com/living/library/sports/ index.htm) Injury prevention and treatment, weight training, flexibility, exercise prescriptions, and more.

Health Net (http://www.health-net.com/) Weight training, low back disorders, exercise programming, heart health, nutrition, mind and body, sports medicine, managing stress, wellness, men's health, women's health, diabetes, and arthritis.

References

1. Cooper, K. H. *Aerobics.* Bantam Books, New York, 1968.

2. Wilmore, J. H. Body composition in sport and exercise: Directions for future research. *Medicine and Science in Sports and Exercise* 15:21–31, 1983.

3. Slattery, M. L. How much physical activity do we need to maintain health and prevent disease? Different diseases—different mechanisms. *Research Quarterly for Exercise and Sport* 67:209–212, 1996.

4. Bouchard, C., R. J. Shephard, T. Stevens, J. R. Sutton, and B. D. McPherson. *Exercise, fitness, and health.* Human Kinetics, Champaign, IL, 1990.

5. Stephens, T. Physical activity and mental health in the United States and Canada: Evidence from four population surveys. *Preventive Medicine* 17:35–47, 1988.

6. Neiman, David C. *Fitness and sports medicine: An introduction.* 3rd ed. Bull Publishing, Palo Alto, CA, 1995.

7. Kaplan, N. M. *Clinical hypertension.* 5th ed. Williams and Wilkins, Baltimore, MD, 1994.

8. U.S. Department of Health and Human Services. *Healthy people 2000: National health promotion and disease prevention objectives.* U.S. Government Printing Office, Washington, D.C., 1992.

9. Brooks, G. Anaerobic threshold: Review of the concept and directions for future research. *Medicine and Science in Sports and Exercise* 17:22–23, 1985.

9a. American College of Sports Medicine. *Guidelines for graded exercise testing prescription.* 5th ed. Lea & Febiger, Philadelphia, PA, 1995.

10. Wenger, H. A., and G. J. Bell. The interactions of intensity, frequency and duration of exercise training in altering cardiorespiratory fitness. *Sports Medicine* 3:346–356, 1986.

11. Dishman, R. K. Exercise adherence research: Future directions. *American Journal of Health Promotion* 3(1):52–56, 1988.

12. Hickson, R. C., et al. Reduced training intensities and loss of aerobic power, endurance, and cardiac growth. *Journal of Applied Physiology* 58:492, 1985.

13. Hickson, R. C., et al. Reduced training duration effects on aerobic power, endurance, and cardiac growth. *Journal of Applied Physiology* 53:255, 1982.

14. Hickson, R. C., and M. A. Rosenkoetter. Reduced training frequencies and maintenance of aerobic power. *Medicine and Science in Sports and Exercise* 13:13, 1982.

15. Powers, S. K. and E. T. Howley. *Exercise physiology: Theory and application to fitness and performance.* Brown and Benchmark, Dubuque, IA, 1997.

16. Powers, S., D. Criswell, F.-K. Lieu, S. Dodd, and H. Silverman. Exercise-induced cellular alterations in the diaphragm. *American Journal of Physiology* 263:R1093–R1098, 1992.

17. Powers, S., S. Grinton, J. Lawler, D. Criswell, and S. Dodd. High intensity exercise training–induced metabolic alterations in respiratory muscles. *Respiration Physiology* 89:169–177, 1992.

18. Dodd, S. L., R. A. Herb, and S. K. Powers. Caffeine and sports performance: An update. *Sports Medicine* 15(1):14–23, 1993.

19. Sherman, W. M. Carbohydrate feedings before and after exercise. In *Perspectives in exercise science and sports medicine. Vol.4. Ergogenics—Enhancement of performance in exercise and sport.* Lamb, D. R., and M. R. Williams, eds. Brown and Benchmark, Dubuque, IA, 1991.

20. Williams, M. H. *Ergogenic aids in sports.* Human Kinetics, Champaign, IL, 1983.

21. Harris, R. C., K. Soderlund, and E. Hultman. Elevation of creatine in resting and exercised muscle of normal subjects by creatine supplementation. *Clinical Science* 83:367–374, 1992.

22. Volek, J. S. Creatine supplementation and its possible role in improving physical performance. *ACSM's Health and Fitness Journal* 1(4): 23–29, 1997.

Developing Your Personal Exercise Prescription

NAME _____ DATE _____

Using Tables 4.3 through 4.5 as models, develop your personal exercise prescription based on your current fitness level and goals. Record the appropriate information in the spaces provided below. Monitor your fitness levels periodically and adjust your prescription accordingly.

Week No.	Phase	Duration (min/day)	Intensity (% of HR max)	Frequency (days/wk)	Exercise Mode	Comments
1						
2						
3						
4						
5						
6						
7						
8						
9						
10						
11						
12						
13						
14						
15						
16						

Cardiorespiratory Training Log

(Note: Make additional copies as needed)

NAME _____ DATE _____

In the spaces below keep a record of your exercise training program. Exercise heart rate can be recorded as the range of heart rates measured at various times during the training session. Use the comments section to record any useful information concerning your exercise bout such as weather conditions, time of day, how you felt, etc.

Date	Activity	Warm-Up Duration	Exercise Duration	Cool-Down Duration	Exercise Heart Rate	Comments

Date	Activity	Warm-Up Duration	Exercise Duration	Cool-Down Duration	Exercise Heart Rate	Comments

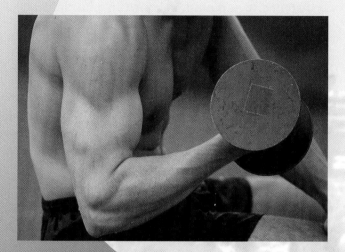

Improving Muscular Strength and Endurance

After studying this chapter, you should be able to

1 Explain the benefits of developing muscular strength and endurance.

2 Describe how muscles contract.

3 Distinguish between the various types of muscle fibers.

4 Classify the types of muscular contractions.

5 Identify the major changes that occur in skeletal muscles in response to strength training.

6 List the factors that determine muscle strength and endurance.

7 Outline the general principles used in designing a strength and endurance program.

8 Distinguish between the various types of training programs for improving strength and endurance.

9 Design a program for improving strength and endurance.

Lifting weights or performing other types of resistance exercises to build muscular strength and endurance is commonly referred to as weight training or strength training. This chapter discusses the principles and techniques employed in strength training programs. We begin with a brief overview of the benefits associated with developing muscular strength and endurance.

Benefits of Muscular Strength and Endurance

Regular strength training promotes numerous health benefits. For example, we know that the incidence of low-back pain, a common problem in both men and women, can be reduced with the appropriate strengthening exercises for the lower back and abdominal muscles (1). Further, recent studies demonstrate that muscle-strengthening exercises may reduce the occurrence of joint and/or muscle injuries that may occur during physical activity (2, 3). In addition, strength training can postpone the decreases in muscle strength experienced by sedentary older individuals (4), as well as contribute to the prevention of the bone wasting disease osteoporosis (5).

Another positive aspect of strength training is the improvement in personal appearance and self-esteem associated with increased muscular tone and strength (6). Also, increased muscular strength has many practical benefits in daily activities, such as an improved ability to carry heavy boxes, perform routine yard work, or do housework.

One of the most important benefits of strength training is that increasing muscle size results in an elevation in resting energy expenditure. Resting energy expenditure (called *resting metabolic rate*) is the total amount of energy that the body requires to perform all of the necessary functions associated with maintaining life. For example, resting metabolic rate includes the energy required to drive the heart and respiratory muscles as well as the energy needed to build and maintain body tissues. How does strength training influence resting metabolic rate? One of the primary results of strength training is an increase in muscle mass. Because muscle tissue requires energy even at rest, muscular enlargement promotes an increase in resting energy expenditure. It can be estimated that an increase of 1 pound of muscle elevates resting metabolism by approximately 2% to 3%. Further, this increase can be magnified with larger gains in muscle. For instance, a 5-pound increase in muscle mass would result in a 10% to 15% increase in resting metabolic rate. Changes in resting metabolic rate of this magnitude can play an important role in assisting in weight loss or maintaining a desirable body composition throughout life. Therefore, strength training is a key component of any physical fitness program.

Physiological Basis for Developing Strength and Endurance

The human body contains approximately 600 skeletal muscles, the primary function of which is to provide force for bodily movement. The body and its parts move when the appropriate muscles shorten and apply force to the bones. Skeletal muscles also assist in maintaining posture and regulating body temperature during cold exposure (for example, by causing heat production through the mechanism of shivering in cold weather). Because all fitness activities require the use of skeletal muscles, some appreciation of their structure and function is essential for anyone entering a physical fitness program.

Before we discuss how muscles work, let's revisit the definitions of muscular strength and endurance. Recall that muscular strength is defined as the ability of a muscle to generate maximal force (Chapter 1). In simple terms, muscular strength is the amount of weight that an individual can lift during one maximal effort. In contrast, muscular endurance is defined as the ability of a muscle to generate force over and over again. In general, increasing muscular strength by exercise training will increase muscular endurance as well. However, training aimed at improving muscular endurance does not always result in significant improvements in muscular strength. Muscular strength and endurance are related, but they are not the same thing. Techniques to improve both muscular strength and muscular endurance will be discussed later in this chapter.

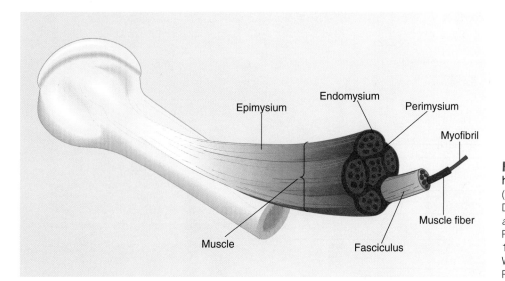

FIGURE 5.1 Design of human skeletal muscle. (Source: Wilmore, J. H., and D. L. Costill. *Physiology of sport and exercise.* Human Kinetics Publishers, Champaign, IL, 1994. Copyright 1994 by Jack H. Wilmore and David L. Costill. Reprinted by permission.)

Muscle Structure and Contraction

Muscle Structure Skeletal muscle is a collection of long thin cells called *fibers*. These fibers are surrounded by a dense layer of connective tissue called *fascia* that holds the individual fibers together and separates muscle from surrounding tissues (Figure 5.1).

Muscles are attached to bone by connective tissues known as *tendons*. Muscular contraction causes the tendons to pull on the bones, thereby causing movement. Most of the muscles involved in movement are illustrated in Figure 5.2.

Muscle Contraction Muscle contraction is regulated by signals coming from motor nerves. Motor nerves originate in the spinal cord and send nerve fibers to individual muscles throughout the body. The motor nerve and individual muscle fiber make contact at the neuromuscular junction (where the nerve and muscle fiber meet). The relationship between the motor nerve and skeletal muscle fibers is illustrated in Figure 5.3. Note that each motor nerve branches and then connects with numerous individual muscle fibers. The motor nerve and all of the muscle fibers it controls is called a **motor unit**.

A muscle contraction begins when a message to contract (called a *nerve impulse*) reaches the neuromuscular junction (Figure 5.3). The arrival of the nerve impulse triggers the contraction process by permitting the interaction of contractile proteins in muscle.

Because the nerve impulse initiates the contractile process, it is logical that the removal of the nerve signal from the muscle would "turn off" the contractile process. Indeed, when a motor nerve ceases to send signals to a muscle, the contraction stops. Occasionally, however, an uncontrolled muscular contraction occurs, resulting in a muscle cramp. The cause and prevention of muscle cramps are discussed in Nutritional Links to Health and Fitness 5.1.

Types of Muscle Contractions

Muscle contractions are classified into two major categories: isotonic and isometric. **Isotonic** (also called **dynamic**) contractions are those that result in movement of a body part. Most exercise or sports skills utilize isotonic contractions. For example, lifting a dumbbell (Figure 5.4) involves movement of a body part and is therefore classi-

motor unit A motor nerve and each of the muscle fibers that it innervates.

isotonic Refers to muscle contractions in which there is movement of a body part. Most exercise or sports skills use isotonic contractions.

dynamic Means "movement"; in reference to muscle contractions, dynamic is synonymous with isotonic contraction.

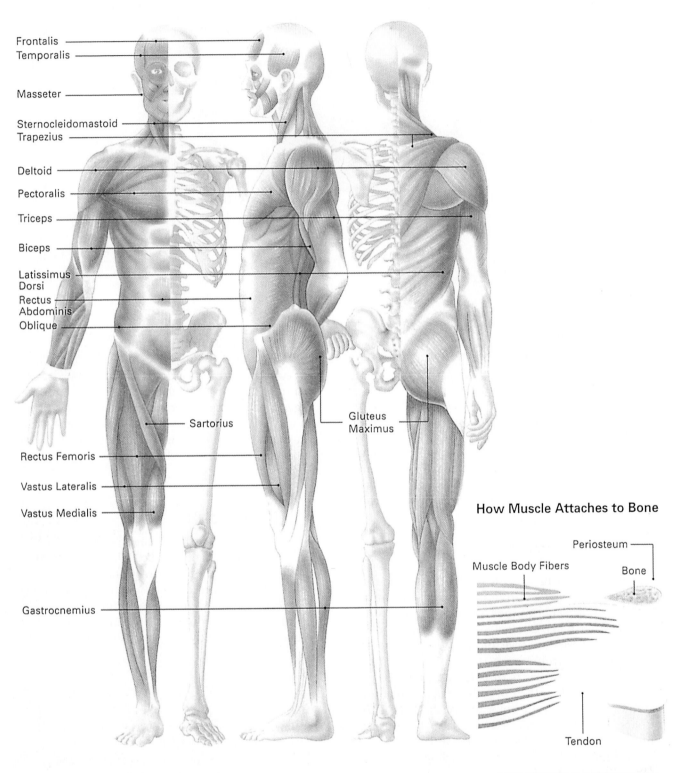

Frontalis
Temporalis
Masseter
Sternocleidomastoid
Trapezius
Deltoid
Pectoralis
Triceps
Biceps
Latissimus Dorsi
Rectus Abdominis
Oblique
Sartorius
Rectus Femoris
Vastus Lateralis
Vastus Medialis
Gastrocnemius
Gluteus Maximus

How Muscle Attaches to Bone

Muscle Body Fibers
Periosteum
Bone
Tendon

THE MUSCULAR SYSTEM

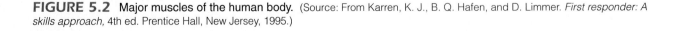

FIGURE 5.2 Major muscles of the human body. (Source: From Karren, K. J., B. Q. Hafen, and D. Limmer. *First responder: A skills approach,* 4th ed. Prentice Hall, New Jersey, 1995.)

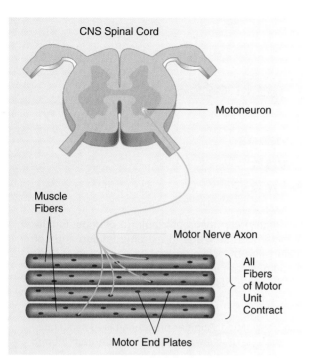

FIGURE 5.3 The concept of a motor unit. A motor nerve from the central nervous system is shown innervating several muscle fibers. With one impulse from the motor nerve, all fibers contract. (Source: Fox, Bowers, and Foss. *The physiological basis of physical education and athletics*. Brown and Benchmark, Madison, WI, 1997.)

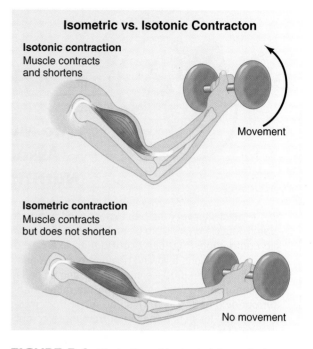

FIGURE 5.4 Illustration of isotonic (also called *dynamic*) and isometric contractions. (Source: Powers, S., and E. Howley. *Exercise physiology: Theory and application to fitness and performance*. Brown and Benchmark, Madison, WI, 1997.)

fied as an isotonic contraction. An **isometric** (also called **static**) contraction requires the development of muscular tension but results in no movement of body parts. A classic example of isometric contraction shows an individual exerting force against an iron bar mounted on the wall of a building; the muscle is developing tension but the wall is not moving and therefore neither is the body part. Isometric contractions occur commonly in the postural muscles of the body during sitting or standing; for instance, they are responsible for holding the head upright.

Note that isotonic contractions can be further subdivided into concentric, eccentric, and isokinetic contractions. **Concentric contractions** are isotonic muscle contractions that result in muscle shortening. The upward movement of the arm in Figure 5.5 is an example of a concentric contraction. In contrast, **eccentric contractions** (also called *negative contractions*) are defined as contractions in which the muscle exerts force while it lengthens. An eccentric contraction occurs when, for example, an individual resists the pull of a weight during the lowering phase of weight lifting (Figure 5.5). Here, the muscle is developing

tension, but the force developed is not great enough to prevent the weight from being lowered.

Isokinetic muscle contractions are concentric or eccentric contractions performed at a constant speed. That is, the speed of muscle shortening or lengthening is regulated at a fixed, controlled rate. This is generally accomplished by a weight-lifting machine that controls the rate of muscle shortening.

isometric Refers to muscle contractions in which muscular tension is developed but no movement of body parts takes place.

static Stationary; in reference to muscle contractions, static is synonymous with isometric contraction.

concentric contractions Isotonic muscle contractions that result in muscle shortening.

eccentric contractions Isotonic contractions in which the muscle exerts force while the muscle lengthens (also called *negative contractions*).

isokinetic A muscle contraction that is a subtype of isotonic contraction; isokinetic contractions are concentric or eccentric isotonic contractions performed at a constant speed.

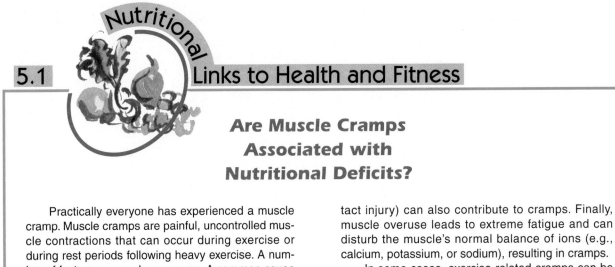

5.1   Nutritional Links to Health and Fitness

Are Muscle Cramps Associated with Nutritional Deficits?

Practically everyone has experienced a muscle cramp. Muscle cramps are painful, uncontrolled muscle contractions that can occur during exercise or during rest periods following heavy exercise. A number of factors can produce cramps. A common cause is a chemical imbalance between the muscle and surrounding body fluids. This can result from water and mineral loss via sweating or from more complicated problems such as kidney disorders. Irritation or damage to the motor nerve (such as a football con-

tact injury) can also contribute to cramps. Finally, muscle overuse leads to extreme fatigue and can disturb the muscle's normal balance of ions (e.g., calcium, potassium, or sodium), resulting in cramps.

In some cases, exercise-related cramps can be avoided by drinking water or "athletic drinks" during or after exercise to replace water and minerals lost due to sweating. Another precaution is to avoid muscle overuse. It is always better to undertrain than to overtrain.

Muscle Fiber Types

There are three types of skeletal muscle fibers: slow twitch, fast twitch, and intermediate. These fiber types differ in their speeds of contraction and in fatigue resistance (7). Most human muscles contain a mixture of all three fiber types. Before beginning a strength training program, it is helpful to have an understanding of each.

Slow-Twitch Fibers   As the name implies, **slow-twitch fibers** contract slowly and produce small amounts of force; however, these fibers are highly resistant to fatigue. Slow-twitch fibers, which are red in appearance, have the capacity to produce large quantities of ATP aerobically, making them ideally suited for a low-intensity prolonged exercise like walking or slow jogging. Further, because of their resistance to fatigue, most postural muscles are composed primarily of slow-twitch fibers.

Fast-Twitch Fibers   **Fast-twitch fibers** contract rapidly and generate great amounts of force but fatigue quickly. These fibers are white and have a low aerobic capacity, but they are well equipped to produce ATP anaerobically. With their ability to shorten rapidly and produce large amounts of force, fast-twitch fibers are used dur-

FIGURE 5.5   Illustration of concentric and eccentric contractions. (Source: Adapted from Powers, S., and E. Howley. *Exercise physiology: Theory and application to fitness and performance.* Brown and Benchmark, Madison, WI, 1997.)

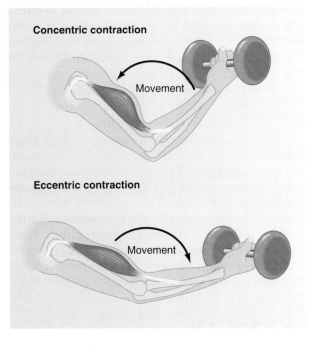

Table 5.1

Properties of Human Skeletal Muscle Fiber Types

Property	Fiber Type		
	Slow-twitch	Intermediate	Fast-twitch
Contraction speed	Slow	Intermediate	Fast
Resistance to fatigue	High	Intermediate	Low
Predominant energy system	Aerobic	Combination aerobic and anaerobic	Anaerobic
Force generation	Low	Intermediate	High

ing activities requiring rapid or forceful movement, such as jumping, sprinting, and weight lifting.

Intermediate Fibers **Intermediate fibers,** although more red in color, possess a combination of the characteristics of fast- and slow-twitch fibers. They contract rapidly, produce great force, and are fatigue resistant due to a well-developed aerobic capacity. Intermediate fibers contract

more quickly and produce more force than slow-twitch fibers but contract more slowly and produce less force than fast-twitch fibers. They are more fatigue resistant than fast-twitch fibers but less fatigue resistant than slow-twitch fibers. Table 5.1 summarizes the properties of all three fiber types.

Recruitment of Muscle Fibers during Exercise

Many types of exercise use only a small fraction of the muscle fibers available in a muscle group. For example, walking at a slow speed may use less than 30% of the muscle fibers in the legs. More intense types of exercise, however, require more force. In order for a muscle group to generate more force, a greater number of muscle fibers must be called into play. The process of involving more muscle fibers to produce increased muscu-

FIGURE 5.6 The relationship between exercise intensity and muscle–fiber type recruitment. (Source: Adapted from Powers, S., and E. Howley. *Exercise physiology: Theory and application to fitness and performance.* Brown and Benchmark, Madison, WI, 1997.)

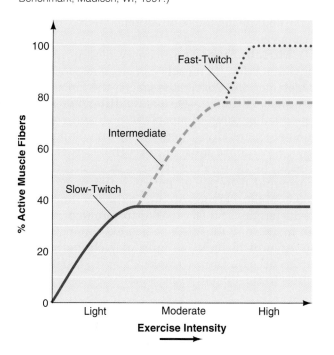

slow-twitch fibers Muscle fibers that contract slowly and are highly resistant to fatigue. Red in appearance, they have the capacity to produce large quantities of ATP aerobically, making them ideally suited for low-intensity, prolonged exercise like walking or slow jogging.

fast-twitch fibers Muscle fibers that contract rapidly but fatigue quickly. These fibers are white and have a low aerobic capacity, but they are well equipped to produce ATP anaerobically.

intermediate fibers Muscle fibers that possess a combination of the characteristics of fast- and slow-twitch fibers. They contract rapidly and are fatigue resistant due to a well-developed aerobic capacity.

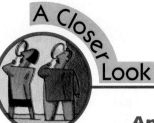

Anabolic Steroid Use Increases Muscle Size but Has Serious Side Effects

The abuse of **anabolic steroids** (primarily the hormone testosterone, which is important in muscle growth) has mushroomed over the past several decades. The fierce competition in body building and sports in which strength and power are necessary for success has driven both men and women to risk serious health consequences in order to develop large muscles.

In order for steroids to increase muscle mass, it is necessary to take large doses, which also carry several added health risks. A partial list of the side effects caused by abusing steroids includes liver cancer, increased blood pressure, increased levels of "bad" cholesterol, and prostate cancer. Prolonged use and high doses of steroids can be lethal.

---

lar force is called fiber **recruitment**. Figure 5.6 illustrates the order of recruitment of muscle fibers as the intensity of exercise increases. Note that during low-intensity exercise, only slow-twitch fibers are used. As the exercise intensity increases, progressive recruitment of fibers occurs, from slow-twitch to intermediate fibers and finally to fast-twitch fibers. High-intensity activities like weight training recruit large numbers of fast-twitch fibers.

Genetics and Fiber Type

People vary in the percentage of slow-twitch, intermediate, and fast-twitch fibers their muscles contain. Research by exercise scientists has shown that a relationship exists between muscle fiber type and success in athletics. For example, champion endurance athletes, such as marathon runners, have a predominance of slow-twitch fibers. This is logical, because endurance sports require muscles with high fatigue resistance. In contrast, elite sprinters, such as 100-meter dash runners, possess a predominance of fast-twitch fibers. The average non-athlete generally has an equal number of all three fiber types.

Although endurance exercise training has been shown to cause some fiber type conversion, the number and percentage of skeletal muscle fiber types is primarily determined by genetics. Because of the interrelationship between genetics, fiber type, and athletic success, some re-

searchers have jokingly suggested that if you want to be a champion athlete, you must pick your parents wisely!

Factors that Determine Muscular Strength

Two primary physiological factors determine the amount of force that a muscle can generate: the size of the muscle and the number of fibers recruited during the contraction.

Muscle Size The primary determinant of how much force a muscle can generate is its size. The larger the muscle, the greater the force it can produce. Although there is no difference in the chemical makeup of muscle in men and women, men are generally stronger than women because men have more muscle mass (i.e., larger muscles). The larger muscle mass in men is due to hormonal differences between the sexes; men have higher levels of the male sex hormone testosterone. The fact that testosterone promotes an increase in muscle size has led some athletes to attempt to improve muscular strength with drugs (see A Closer Look 5.1 and Nutritional Links to Health and Fitness 5.2).

Muscle Fiber Recruitment We have seen that muscle fiber recruitment influences the production of muscle force. The more muscle fibers

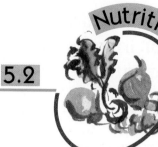

5.2

Nutritional Links to Health and Fitness

HMB: An Alternative to Steroids?

Beta-hydroxy-beta-methylbutyrate, HMB, is the latest craze to replace anabolic steroids in the quest by some athletes to find a substance to build muscle and improve exercise/athletic performance. HMB is a compound derived from the breakdown of the essential amino acid leucine. Although some evidence exists that shows HMB increases muscle mass in animals, there is little evidence to suggest that it increases muscle mass in humans.

One study performed by Nissen et al. (20) suggests that HMB, combined with weight lifting, produced increases in muscle mass (2.6 lbs) and strength (18%) greater than in control subjects over a 3-week period. Their data indicated that the HMB worked by decreasing muscle breakdown during weight lifting. These were impressive changes in such a short period of time! However, the true effectiveness of a substance such as HMB will be known

only when other controlled studies are performed to substantiate these claims. It is much too early to determine whether HMB does indeed have an anabolic effect on muscle or whether it is simply a placebo effect.

The placebo effect is the phenomenon whereby people who think they are receiving a substance that will enhance exercise performance work harder and, therefore, do make significant improvements. This increase would, of course, be due to the increased volume of training and not due to any direct effect of the substance.

As with any dietary supplement, it is unwise to waste money and take health risks if the purported benefits of the supplement are unsubstantiated. Wait until a substantial body of evidence is available concerning any dietary supplement before even considering its use.

that are stimulated to shorten, the greater the muscle force generation, because the force generated by individual fibers is additive.

Muscle fiber recruitment is regulated voluntarily through the nervous system. That is, we determine how many muscle fibers to recruit by voluntarily making a decision about how much effort to put into a particular movement. For instance, when we choose to make a minimal effort in lifting an object, we recruit only a few motor units, and the muscle develops limited force. However, if we make a decision to exert our maximal effort in lifting a heavy object, many muscle fibers are recruited and great force is generated (Figure 5.7).

FIGURE 5.7 The relationship between motor unit recruitment and muscular force production.

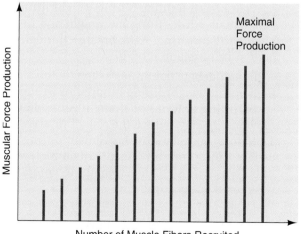

recruitment The process of involving more muscle fibers to produce increased muscular force.

anabolic steroids Hormones produced by the body which enhance muscle growth. Usually refers to the synthetic form of the hormone testosterone.

Guiding Principles for Designing a Strength and Endurance Program

In Chapter 3 we discussed the general principles of the development of training programs to improve physical fitness. Before we discuss the specifics of how to develop a strength training program, let's discuss several principles that should be considered in developing a muscular strength and endurance training program.

Progressive Resistance Exercise

The concept of **progressive resistance exercise** (PRE) is an application of the overload principle applied to strength and endurance exercise programs. Even though the two terms can be used interchangeably, PRE is preferred when discussing weight training. Progressive resistance exercise means that as strength and endurance are increased, the load against which the muscle works must be periodically elevated for strength and endurance gains to be realized.

Principle of Specificity

The principle of **specificity of training** means that development of muscular strength and endurance is specific to the muscle group that is exercised and the training intensity. First, the muscles that are trained will be the only muscles improving in strength and endurance. For example, if an individual has low-back pain and wishes to improve the strength of the supporting musculature of the lower back, it would be of no benefit to strengthen the arm muscles. The specific muscles involved with movement of the lower back should be the ones trained. Second, the training intensity determines whether the muscular adaptation is primarily an increase in strength or endurance. High-intensity training (i.e., lifting heavy weights four to six times) results in an increase in both muscular strength and size with only limited improvements in muscular endurance. Conversely, high-repetition, low-intensity training (i.e., lifting light weights 15 times or more) promotes an increase in muscular endurance, with only limited improvements in muscular size and strength.

Designing a Training Program for Increasing Muscle Strength

There are numerous approaches to the design of weight-training programs. Any program that adheres to the basic principles described earlier will result in an improvement in strength and endurance. However, the type of weight training program that you develop for yourself depends on your goals and the types of equipment available to you. Next, we discuss several other considerations in the development of a weight training program.

Safety Concerns

Before we discuss the specifics of how to develop a weight training program, the need for safety should be emphasized. Although weight training can be performed safely, some important guidelines should be followed:

1. When using free weights (like barbells), have spotters (helpers) assist you in the performance of exercises. They can help you if you are unable to complete a lift. Many weight machines reduce the need for spotters.

2. Be sure that the collars on the end of the bars of free weights are tightly secured to prevent the weights from falling off. Dropping weight plates on toes and feet can result in serious injuries. Again, many weight machines reduce the potential risk of dropping weights.

3. Warm up properly before doing any weight-lifting exercise.

4. Do not hold your breath during weight lifting. A recommended breathing pattern to prevent breath holding during weight lifting is to exhale while lifting the weight and inhale while lowering. Also, breathe through both your nose and mouth.

5. Although debate continues as to whether high-speed weight lifting is superior to slow-speed lifting in terms of strength gains, slow movements may reduce the risk of injury. Therefore, because slow movement during weight lifting certainly results in an increase in both muscle size and strength, it would be wise to take this approach.

6. Use light weights in the beginning so that the proper maneuver can be followed with each

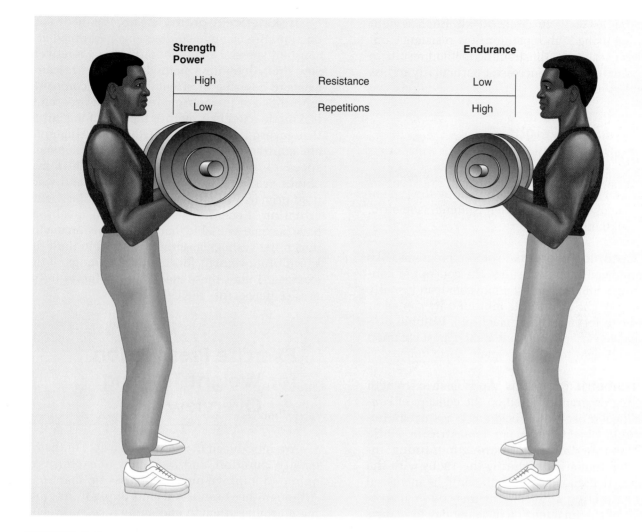

FIGURE 5.8 The strength–endurance continuum. Strength is achieved by using low repetitions/high weight, and endurance is achieved by using high repetitions/low weight.

exercise. This is particularly true when lifting free weights.

Training to Improve Strength versus Training to Improve Endurance

Weight training programs specifically designed to improve strength and programs designed to improve muscular endurance differ mainly in the number of repetitions (i.e., the number of lifts performed) and the amount of resistance (8, 9). Note in Figure 5.8 that a weight training program using low repetitions and high resistance results in the greatest strength gains, whereas a weight training program using high repetitions and low resistance results in the great-

est improvement in muscular endurance. However, it is important to appreciate that while low-repetition/high-resistance training appears to be the optimal training method to increase strength, this type of training improves muscular en-

progressive resistance exercise (PRE) The application of the overload principle applied to strength and endurance exercise programs. Even though the overload principle and PRE can be used interchangeably, PRE is preferred when discussing weight training.

specificity of training The development of muscular strength and endurance, as well as cardiorespiratory endurance, is specific to the muscle group that is exercised and the training intensity.

durance as well. In contrast, although weight training using high repetition/low resistance improves endurance, this training method results in only small strength increases, particularly in less fit individuals.

Types of Weight Training Programs

Weight training programs can be divided into three general categories classified by the type of muscle contraction involved: isotonic, isometric, and isokinetic.

Isotonic Programs Isotonic programs, like isotonic contractions, utilize the concept of contracting a muscle against a movable load (usually a free weight or weights mounted by cables or chains to form a weight machine). Isotonic programs are very popular and are the most common type of weight training program in use today.

Isometric Programs An isometric strength training program is based on the concept of contracting a muscle at a fixed angle against an immovable object, using an isometric or static contraction. Interest in strength training increased dramatically during the 1950s with the finding that maximal strength could be increased by contracting a muscle for 6 seconds at two-thirds of maximal tension once per day for 5 days per week! Although subsequent studies suggested that these claims were exaggerated (10), it is generally agreed that isometric training can increase muscular strength and endurance.

Two important aspects of isometric training make it different from isotonic training. First, in isometric training, the development of strength and endurance is specific to the joint angle at which the muscle group is trained (11). Therefore, if isometric techniques are used, isometric contractions at several different joint angles are needed to gain strength and endurance throughout a full range of motion. In contrast, because isotonic contractions generally involve the full range of joint motion, strength is developed over the full movement pattern. Second, the static nature of isometric muscle contractions can lead to breath holding (called a **valsalva maneuver**), which can reduce blood flow to the brain and cause dizziness and fainting. In an individual at high risk for coronary disease, the maneuver could be extremely dangerous and should always be avoided. Remember: Continue to breathe during any type of isometric or isotonic contraction!

Isokinetic Programs Again, isokinetic contractions are isotonic contractions performed at a constant speed. Isokinetic training is a relatively new strength training method, so limited research exists to describe its strength benefits compared with those of isometric and isotonic programs. Isokinetic exercises require the use of machines that govern the speed of movement during muscle contraction (*isokinetic* refers to constant speed of movement). The first isokinetic machines available were very expensive and were used primarily in clinical settings for injury rehabilitation. Recently, less expensive machines have become available that utilize a piston device (much like a shock absorber on a car) to limit the speed of movement throughout the range of the exercise. Today, these machines are found in fitness centers across the United States.

Exercise Prescription for Weight Training: An Overview

We introduced the general concepts of the intensity, duration, and frequency of exercise required to improve physical fitness in Chapter 3. Although these same concepts apply to improving muscular strength and endurance via weight training, the terminology used to monitor the intensity and duration of weight training is unique. For example, the intensity of weight training is measured not by heart rate but by the number of "repetition maximums." Similarly, the duration of weight training is monitored not by time but by the number of sets performed. Let's discuss these two concepts briefly.

The intensity of exercise in both isotonic and isokinetic weight training programs is measured by the concept of the **repetition maximum (RM)**. The RM is the maximal load that a muscle group can lift a specified number of times before tiring. For example, 6 RM is the maximal load that can be lifted six times. Therefore, the amount of weight lifted is greater when performing a low number of RMs than a high number of RMs; that is, the weight lifted while performing 4 RMs is greater than the weight lifted while performing 15 RMs.

The number of repetitions (reps) performed consecutively without resting is called a **set**. In the example of 6 RM, 1 set = 6 reps. Because the amount of rest required between sets will vary

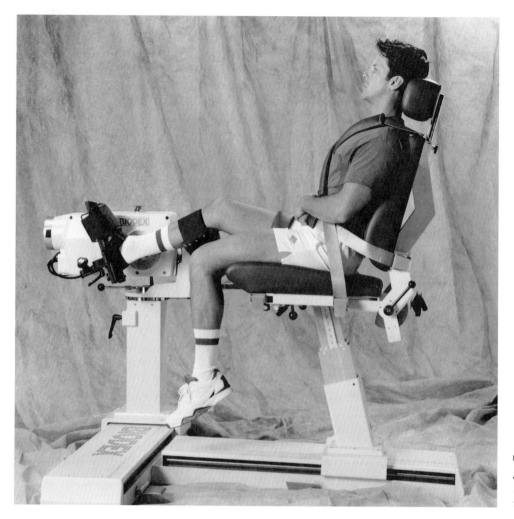

A commercially available isokinetic weight training device.

among individuals depending on how fit they are, the duration of weight training is measured by the number of sets performed, not by time.

Although disagreement exists as to the optimum number of reps and sets required to improve strength and endurance, some general guidelines can be provided. To improve strength, 3 sets of 6 reps for each exercise are generally recommended. The concept of progressive resistance applied to a strength training program involves increasing the amount of weight to be lifted a specific number of reps. For example, suppose that 3 sets of 6 RMs were selected as your exercise prescription for increasing strength. As the training progresses and you become stronger, the amount of weight lifted must be increased. A good rule of thumb is that once 8 reps can be performed, the load should be increased to a level at which 6 reps are again maximal. Figure 5.9 illustrates the relationship between strength improvement and various combinations of reps and sets. Note that in each strength training pro-

gram, 6 reps result in the greatest strength improvement. A key point in Figure 5.9 is that programs involving 3 sets result in the greatest strength gains. This is because the third set requires the greatest effort and thus is the greatest overload for the muscle.

To improve muscular endurance, 4 to 6 sets of 18 to 20 reps for each exercise are recom-

valsalva maneuver Breath holding during an intense muscle contraction that can reduce blood flow to the brain and cause dizziness and fainting.

repetition maximum (RM) The measure of the intensity of exercise in both isotonic and isokinetic weight training programs. The RM is the maximal load that a muscle group can lift a specified number of times before tiring. For example, 6 RM is the maximal load that can be lifted six times.

set The number of repetitions performed consecutively without resting.

mended. Note that endurance could be improved by either increasing the number of reps progressively while maintaining the same load, or increasing the amount of weight while maintaining the same number of reps. The advantage of the latter program is that it would also improve muscular strength.

What role does frequency play in the development of strength? Most research suggests that 2 to 3 days of exercise per week is optimal for strength gains (12). However, once the desired level of strength has been gained, studies have shown that one high-intensity training session per week is sufficient to maintain the new level of strength. Finally, although limited research exists regarding the optimal frequency of training to improve muscular endurance, 3 to 5 days per week seem adequate (13).

Starting and Maintaining a Weight Training Program

You should begin your weight training program with both short- and long-term goals. Identifying goals is an important means of maintaining

FIGURE 5.9 Strength gains from a resistance training program consisting of various sets and repetitions. All programs were performed 3 days per week for 12 weeks. Note that the greatest strength gains (+30% improvement) were obtained using three sets of 6 reps per set. (Source: Adapted from Fox, Bowers, and Foss. *Fox's Physiological Basis of Exercise and Sports.* WCB-McGraw Hill, Boston, 1998)

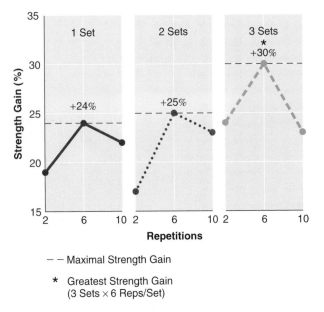

− − Maximal Strength Gain

* Greatest Strength Gain (3 Sets × 6 Reps/Set)

interest and enthusiasm for weight training. A key point is to establish realistic short-term goals that can be reached in the first several weeks of training. Reaching these goals provides the motivation needed to continue training.

Developing an Individualized Exercise Prescription

The exercise prescription for strength training has three stages: the starter phase, the slow progression phase, and the maintenance phase.

Starter Phase The primary objective of the starter phase is to build strength gradually without developing undue muscular soreness or injury. This can be accomplished by starting your weight training program slowly—beginning with light weights, a high number of repetitions, and only 2 sets per exercise. The recommended frequency of training during this phase is twice per week. The duration of this phase varies from 1 to 3 weeks, depending on your initial strength fitness level. A sedentary person might spend 3 weeks in the starter phase, whereas a relatively well-trained person may only spend 1 to 2 weeks.

Slow Progression Phase This phase may last 4 to 20 weeks depending on your initial strength level and your long-term strength goal. The transition from the starter phase to the slow progression phase involves three changes in the exercise prescription: increasing the frequency of training from 2 to 3 days per week; an increase in the amount of weight lifted and a decrease in the number of repetitions; and an increase in the number of sets performed from 2 to 3 sets.

The objective of the slow progression phase is to gradually increase muscular strength until you reach your desired level. After reaching your strength goal, your long-term objective becomes to maintain this level of strength by entering the maintenance phase of the strength training exercise prescription.

Maintenance Phase After reaching your strength goals, the problem now becomes, how do I maintain this strength level? The bad news is that maintaining strength will require a lifelong weight training effort. Strength is lost if you do not continue to exercise. The good news is that the effort required to maintain muscular strength is less than the initial effort needed to gain strength. Research has shown that as little as one workout per week is required to maintain

Table 5.2

Guidelines and Precautions to Follow Prior to Beginning a Strength Training Program

Warm up before beginning a workout. This involves 5 to 10 minutes of movement (calisthenics), using all major muscle groups.

Start slowly. The first several training sessions should involve limited exercises and light weight!

Use the proper lifting technique, as shown in the Isotonic Strength Training Exercises in this chapter. Improper technique can lead to injury.

Follow all safety rules (see section on safety guidelines).

Always lift through the full range of motion. This not only develops strength throughout the full range of motion but also assists in maintaining flexibility.

strength. A sample exercise prescription incorporating all three training phases follows.

Sample Exercise Prescription for Weight Training

Getting Started. Similar to training to improve cardiorespiratory fitness, the exercise prescription to improve muscular strength must be tailored to the individual. Before starting a program, keep in mind the guidelines and precautions presented in Table 5.2.

Details of the Prescription. Table 5.3 illustrates the stages of a suggested strength training exercise prescription. As mentioned earlier, the duration of both the starter and slow progression phases will vary depending on your initial strength fitness level. When the strength goals of the program are reached, the maintenance phase begins. This period utilizes the same routine as used during the progression phase but may be done only once per week.

Sample Strength Training Exercises. The isotonic strength training program contains 12 exercises that are designed to provide a whole body workout. Although specific machines are used in the following examples, barbells may be used for performing similar exercises. However, it is important to remember that safety and proper lifting technique are especially important when using barbells. Before beginning a program using barbells, it is a good idea to get advice from someone experienced with their use.

Follow the exercise routines provided in Exercises 5.1 through 5.12 and develop your program using the guidelines provided in Table 5.3. This selection of exercises is designed to provide a comprehensive strength training program that focuses on the major muscle groups. Although many more exercises can be performed, some exercises use the same muscle groups as the exercises covered here. Be aware of which muscle groups are involved in an exercise in order to avoid overtraining any one muscle group (see Figure 5.2). Note that it is not necessary to perform all 12 exercises in one workout session; you can perform half of the exercises on one day and the remaining exercises on an alternate day.

Table 5.3

Suggested Isotonic Strength Training Routine to Be Included in a Basic Fitness Program
The duration of the starter and slow progression phase will depend on your initial strength level.

Week No.	Phase	Frequency	Sets	Reps	Weight
1–3	Starter	2/week	2	15	15 RM
4–20	Slow progression	2–3/week	3	6	6 RM
20+	Maintenance	1–2/week	3	6	6 RM

Isotonic Strength Training Exercises

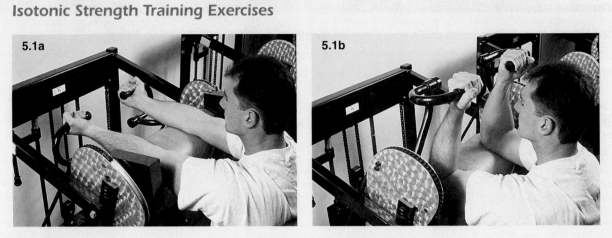

Biceps Curl

Purpose: To strengthen the muscles in the front of the upper arm, which cause flexion at the elbow.
Movement: Holding the grips with palms up and arms extended, curl up as far as possible and slowly return to the starting position.

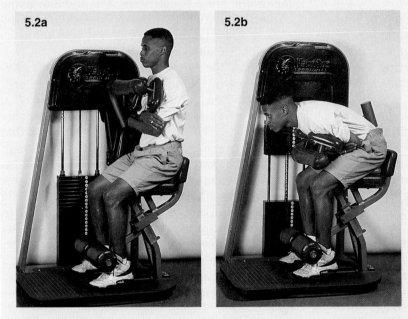

Abdominal Curl

Purpose: To strengthen the abdominal muscles.
Movement: Place hands on the abdomen and curl forward, bringing the chest toward the knees. Slowly return to the upright position.

Isotonic Strength Training Exercises

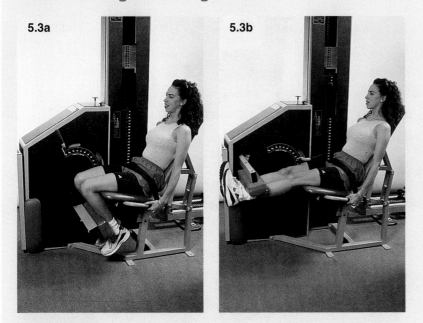

5.3a **5.3b**

Leg Extension

Purpose: To strengthen the muscles in the front of the upper leg.
Movement: Sitting in an upright position, grasp the handles on the side of the machine. Extend the legs until they are completely straight and slowly return to the starting position.

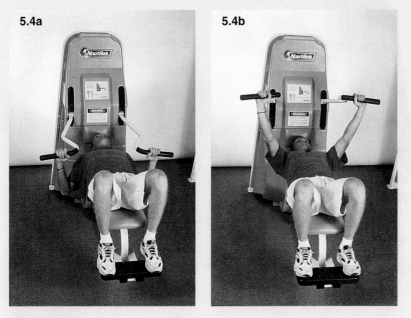

5.4a **5.4b**

Bench Press

Purpose: To strengthen the muscles in the chest, front of the shoulders, and back of the upper arm.
Movement: Lie down on the bench with the bench press bar above the chest and feet flat on the floor. Grasp the bar handles and press upward until the arms are completely extended. Return slowly to the original position. **Caution:** Do not arch your back while performing this exercise.

Isotonic Strength Training Exercises

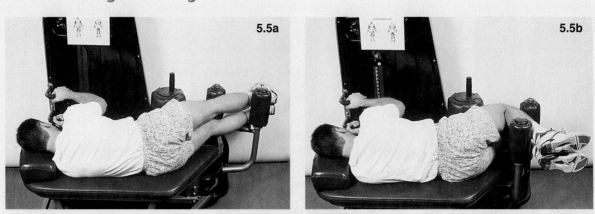

Leg Curl

Purpose: To strengthen the muscles on the back of the upper leg and the buttocks.
Movement: Lying face down, place the back of the feet under the padded bar. Curl up to at least a 90° angle and slowly return to the original position.

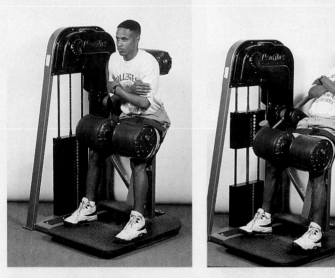

Lower Back Extension

Purpose: To strengthen the muscles of the lower back and buttocks.
Movement: Position the thighs and upper back against the padded bars. Buckle the strap around the thighs. Slowly press backward against the padded bar until the back is fully extended. Slowly return to the original position.

Isotonic Strength Training Exercises

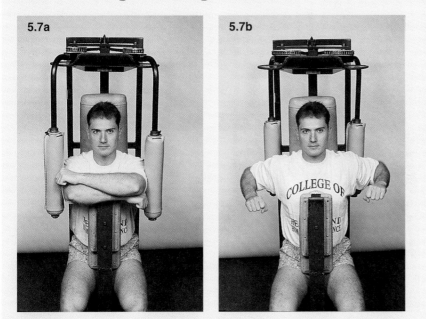

Upper Back

Purpose: To strengthen the muscles of the upper back.
Movement: Sit in the machine with elbows bent and resting against the padded bars. Press back as far as possible, drawing the shoulder blades together. Slowly return to the original position.

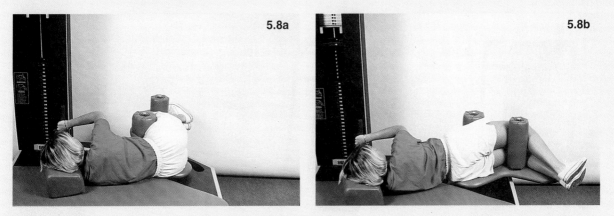

Hip and Back

Purpose: To strengthen the muscles of the hip and lower back.
Movement: Lying face up, grasp the handles at both sides for stability. Place the back of the knees against the padded bars. Alternately press the legs downward until fully extended. Slowly return to the original position and alternate legs.

Isotonic Strength Training Exercises

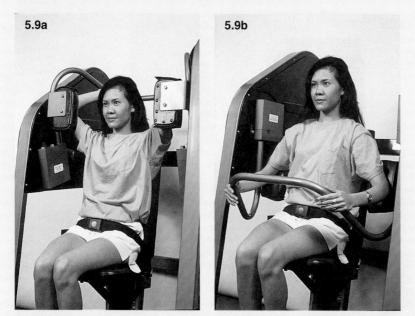

5.9a 5.9b

Pullover

Purpose: To strengthen the muscles of the chest, shoulder, and side of the trunk.

Movement: Sit with elbows against the padded end of the movement arm and grasp the bar behind your head. Press forward and downward with the arms, pulling the bar overhead down to the abdomen. Slowly return to the original position.

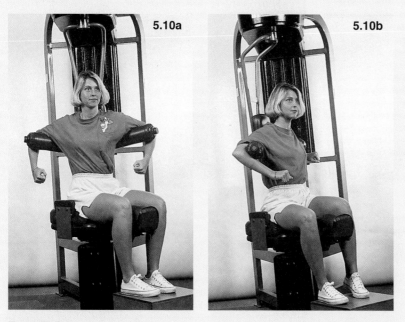

5.10a 5.10b

Torso Twist

Purpose: To strengthen the muscles on the sides of the abdomen.
Movement: Sitting upright with the elbows behind the padded bars, twist the torso as far as possible to one side. Slowly return to the original position and repeat to the other side.

Isotonic Strength Training Exercises

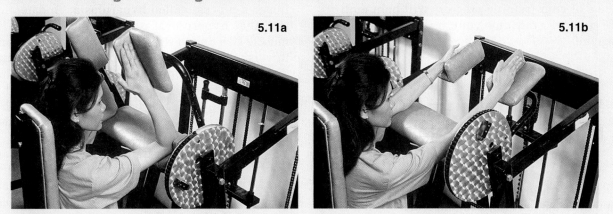

Triceps Extension

Purpose: To strengthen the muscles on the back of the upper arm.
Movement: Sit upright with elbows bent. With the little-finger side of the hand against the pad, fully extend the arms and slowly return to the original position.

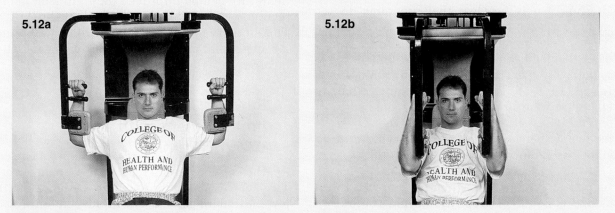

Chest Press

Purpose: To strengthen the muscles of the chest and shoulder.
Movement: With the arms up to your side, hands against the pads, and elbows bent at 90°, press the arms forward as far as possible, leading with the elbows. Slowly return to the original position.

Use Laboratory 5.1 to keep a record of your training progress. Remember: Maintenance and review of your training progress will help motivate you to continue your strength training program!

Strength Training: How the Body Adapts

What physiological changes occur as a result of strength training? How quickly can muscular strength be gained? Do men and women differ in their response to weight training programs? Let's address each of these questions separately.

Physiological Changes Due to Weight Training

It should now be clear that programs designed to improve muscular strength can do so only by increasing muscular size and/or by increasing the number of muscle fibers recruited. In fact, both these factors are altered by strength training (14, 15). Research has shown that strength training programs increase muscular strength by first altering fiber recruitment patterns due to changes in the nervous system and then by increasing muscle size (Figure 5.10).

How do muscles increase in size? Muscle size is increased primarily through an increase in fiber size, called **hypertrophy** (15). However, re-

cent research has shown that strength training can also promote the formation of new muscle fibers, a process called **hyperplasia**. To date, the role that hyperplasia plays in the increase in muscle size due to strength training remains controversial. Regardless, the increase in muscle size due to strength training depends on diet (see Nutritional Links to Health and Fitness 5.3), the muscle fiber type (fast fibers may hypertrophy more than slow fibers), blood levels of testosterone, and the type of training program.

Although strength training does not result in significant improvements in cardiorespiratory fitness (17), a regular weight training program can provide positive changes in both body composition and flexibility. For most men and women, rigorous weight training results in an increase in muscle mass and a loss of body fat, the end result being a decrease in the percent of body fat.

If weight training exercises are performed over the full range of motion possible at a joint, flexibility can be improved (8, 9). In fact, many regular weight lifters have excellent flexibility. Therefore, the notion of weightlifters becoming muscle-bound and losing flexibility is generally incorrect.

Rate of Strength Improvement with Weight Training

How rapid does strength improvement occur? The answer depends on your initial strength level. Strength gains occur rapidly in untrained

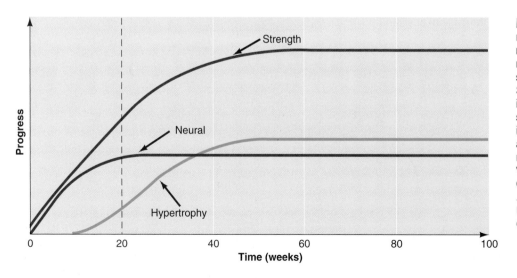

FIGURE 5.10 The relative roles of the nervous system and muscular adaptation in strength development. Strength training increases muscular strength first by changes in the nervous system and then by increasing muscle size. (Source: Wilmore, J. H., and D. L. Costill. *Physiology of sport and exercise*. Human Kinetics Publishers, Champaign, IL, 1994.)

people, whereas gains are more gradual in individuals with relatively higher strength levels (see Figure 5.11). Indeed, an exciting point about weight training for a novice lifter is that strength gains occur very quickly (18). These rapid strength gains provide motivation to continue a regular weight training program.

Gender Differences in Response to Weight Training

In terms of absolute strength, men tend to be stronger than women because men generally have a greater muscle mass. The difference is greater in the upper body where men are approximately 50% stronger than women; men are only 30% stronger than women in the lower body.

Do men and women differ in their responses to weight training programs? The answer is "no" (19). On a percentage basis, women gain strength as rapidly as men during the first 12 weeks of a strength training program (see Figure 5.12). However, as a result of long-term weight training, men generally exhibit a greater increase in muscle size than do women. This occurs because men have 20 to 30 times more testosterone (male sex hormone that builds muscles) than do women.

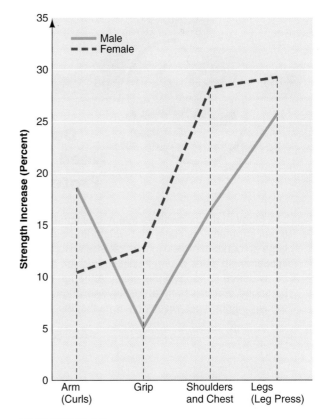

FIGURE 5.12 In relation to beginning strength levels, the increase in strength for women is equal to or greater than that seen in men for most muscle groups. (Source: Wilmore, J. Body composition and strength development. *Journal of Physical Education Research* 46(1):38–40, 1975.)

FIGURE 5.11 Time course of strength improvement in novice weight lifters versus moderately well-trained weight lifters. The rate of improvement and the total percent strength improvement is greater in the novice compared with the moderately trained weight lifter. This occurs because the moderately trained weight lifter began the weight training program with higher initial strength levels.

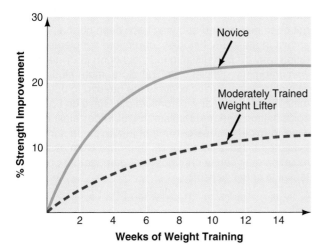

Motivation to Maintain Strength Fitness

The problems associated with starting and maintaining a weight training program are similar to those associated with cardiorespiratory training. You must find time to train regularly, so good time management is critical.

Another key feature of any successful exercise program is that training must be fun. Making weight training fun involves several elements. First, find an enjoyable place to work out. Locate a facility that contains the type of weights that

hypertrophy An increase in muscle fiber size.

hyperplasia An increase in the number of muscle fibers.

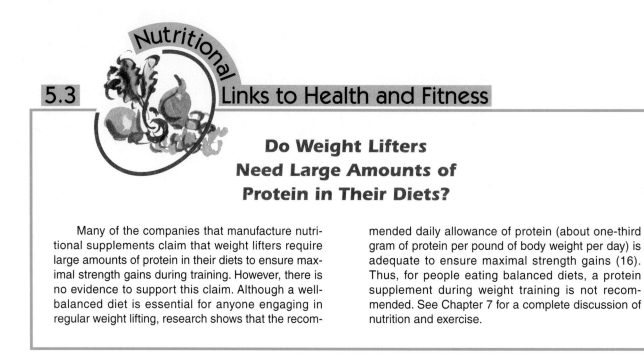

5.3 Nutritional Links to Health and Fitness

Do Weight Lifters Need Large Amounts of Protein in Their Diets?

Many of the companies that manufacture nutritional supplements claim that weight lifters require large amounts of protein in their diets to ensure maximal strength gains during training. However, there is no evidence to support this claim. Although a well-balanced diet is essential for anyone engaging in regular weight lifting, research shows that the recommended daily allowance of protein (about one-third gram of protein per pound of body weight per day) is adequate to ensure maximal strength gains (16). Thus, for people eating balanced diets, a protein supplement during weight training is not recommended. See Chapter 7 for a complete discussion of nutrition and exercise.

5.4 Nutritional Links to Health and Fitness

Chromium Picolinate: Does It Alter Body Composition?

Chromium is an essential nutrient that is present in many foods. However, chromium is poorly absorbed and exercise increases its excretion. The nutrient is important since it helps to make insulin effective in regulating metabolism. Thus, the rationale for supplementation is that chromium may be beneficial in the regulation of glucose, fat, and protein metabolism. Chromium picolinate (supplemental form of chromium for best absorption) is touted as improving glucose tolerance, reduce serum triglycerides, and increase glucose and amino acids uptake into skeletal muscle. It is thought that improvements in glucose and fat metabolism could reduce hunger and decrease caloric intake. In addition, chromium could increase muscle mass by increasing amino acid uptake in muscle for protein synthesis.

Studies have shown that supplementation in animals that are chromium deficient is beneficial. However, studies using chromium supplementation in individuals on a normal diet suggest that chromium has no beneficial effect on body fat or lean muscle mass (21, 22). There are, however, relatively few studies that have investigated this supplement. In most studies, chromium levels in the tissues have not been determined and may have been normal. As shown in the animal studies, chromium supplementation may be beneficial in individuals on poor diets with chromium deficiencies. Therefore, more studies with stringent scientific controls are needed to determine the effects, if any, chromium may have on body composition and metabolism. It would certainly be wise to avoid excess chromium intake since some evidence exists that suggests that chromium accumulation may cause chromosomal damage (i.e., potential to cause cancer).

you want to use and also provides a pleasant and motivating environment. Second, develop an enjoyable weight training routine (exercise prescription). Designing a training routine that is too hard may be good for improving strength but does not increase your desire to train. Therefore, design a program that is challenging, but fun. Further, weight training is more enjoyable if you have a regular training partner. Select a friend who is highly motivated to exercise and has strength abilities similar to yours.

Although the benefits of weight training are numerous, recent studies have shown that improved appearance, elevated self-esteem, and the overall feeling of well-being that result from regular weight training are the most important factors in motivating people to continue to train regularly. Looking your best and feeling good about yourself are excellent reasons to maintain a regular weight training program.

Summary

1. The importance of training to improve strength and endurance is evident from the fact that strength training can reduce low-back pain, reduce the incidence of exercise-related injuries, decrease the incidence of osteoporosis, and aid in maintenance of functional capacity, which normally decreases with age.

2. Muscular strength is defined as the ability of a muscle to generate maximal force (see Chapter 1). In simple terms, this refers to the amount of weight that an individual can lift during one maximal effort. In contrast, muscular endurance is defined as the ability of a muscle to generate force over and over again. In general, increasing muscular strength by exercise training will increase muscular endurance as well. In contrast, training aimed at improving muscular endurance does not always result in significant improvements in muscular strength.

3. Skeletal muscle is composed of a collection of long thin cells (fibers). Muscles are attached to bone by thick connective tissue (tendons). Therefore, muscle contraction results in the tendons pulling on bone, thereby causing movement.

4. Muscle contraction is regulated by signals coming from motor nerves. Motor nerves originate in the spinal cord and send nerve fibers to individual muscles throughout the body. The motor nerve and all of the muscle fibers it controls is called a *motor unit.*

5. Isotonic or dynamic contractions are contractions that result in movement of a body part. Isometric contractions involve the development of force but result in no movement of body parts. Concentric contractions are isotonic muscle contractions involving mus-

cle shortening. In contrast, eccentric contractions (negative contractions) are defined as isotonic contractions in which the muscle exerts force while the muscle lengthens.

6. Human skeletal muscle can be classified into three major fiber types: slow twitch, fast twitch, and intermediate fibers. Slow-twitch fibers shorten slowly but are highly fatigue resistant. Fast-twitch fibers shorten rapidly but fatigue rapidly. Intermediate fibers possess a combination of the characteristics of fast- and slow-twitch fibers.

7. The process of involving more muscle fibers to produce increased muscular force is called *fiber recruitment.*

8. The percentage of slow-, intermediate-, and fast-twitch fibers varies among individuals. Research by sports scientists has shown that a relationship exists between muscle fiber type and success in athletics. For example, champion endurance athletes (e.g., marathon runners) have a high percentage of slow-twitch fibers.

9. There are two primary physiological factors that determine the amount of force that can be generated by a muscle: the size of the muscle and the neural influences (i.e., number of fibers recruited).

10. Muscle size is increased primarily because of an increase in fiber size (hypertrophy). Further, recent research has shown that strength training can also promote the formation of new muscle fibers (hyperplasia).

11. The overload principle states that a muscle will increase in strength and/or endurance only when it works against a workload that is greater than normal.

12. The concept of progressive resistance exer-

cise (PRE) is the application of the overload principle to strength and endurance exercise programs.

13. A weight training program using low repetitions/high resistance results in the greatest strength gains, whereas a weight training program using high repetitions/low resistance results in the greatest improvement in muscular endurance.

14. Isotonic programs, like an isotonic contraction, utilize the concept of contracting a muscle against a movable load (usually a free weight or weights mounted by cables or chains to form a weight machine). An iso-

metric strength training program is based on the concept of contracting a muscle(s) at a fixed angle against an immovable object (isometric or static contraction). Isokinetic exercises require the use of machines that govern the speed of movement during muscle contraction throughout the range of motion.

15. To begin a strength training program, divide the program into 3 phases: initial phase—2 to 3 weeks/2 workouts per week/2 sets/15 RM; progression phase—20 weeks/2 to 3 workouts per week/3 sets/6 RM; maintenance phase—continues for life/1 workout per week/3 sets/6 RM.

Study Questions

1. Define the following terms:

   anabolic steroid

   hyperplasia

   hypertrophy

   motor unit

   progressive resistance exercise

   static contraction

   valsalva maneuver

2. List at least three reasons why training for strength and endurance is important.

3. Discuss the cause and prevention of muscle cramps.

4. List and discuss the characteristics of slow-twitch, fast-twitch, and intermediate skeletal muscle fibers.

5. Discuss the pattern of muscle fiber recruitment with increasing intensities of contraction.

6. Discuss the role of genetics in determining muscle fiber type.

7. What factors determine muscle strength?

8. What are the consequences of steroid abuse?

9. What physiological changes occur as a result of strength training?

10. Compare and contrast the overload principle and progressive resistance exercise.

11. Discuss the concept of specificity of training.

12. Compare and contrast the differences in training to increase strength versus training to increase endurance.

13. Define the concept of repetition maximum.

14. List the phases of a strength and endurance training program and discuss how they differ.

15. Distinguish between *concentric* and *eccentric*.

16. Describe each of the following types of muscle contraction: isokinetic, isometric, and isotonic.

Suggested Reading

Blair, S. N., and J. C. Connelly. How much physical activity should we do: The case for moderate amounts and intensities of physical activity. *Research Quarterly for Exercise and Sport* 67: 193–205, 1996.

Bouchard, C., R. Shephard, T. Stephens, J. Sutton, and B. McPherson, eds., *Exercise, fitness, and health: A consensus of current knowledge.* Human Kinetics, Champaign, IL, 1990.

Fleck, S. J., and W. J. Kraemer. *Designing resistance training programs.* Human Kinetics, Champaign, IL, 1997.

Haskell, W. L. Physical activity, sport and health: Toward the next century. *Research Quarterly for Exercise and Sport* 67: S37–S47, 1996.

Komi, P. *Strength and power in sport.* Blackwell Publishers, Oxford, 1992.

Powers, S., and E. Howley. *Exercise physiology: Theory and application to fitness and performance.* 2nd ed. Brown and Benchmark, Dubuque, IA, 1997.

Stoecker, B. J. Chromium. In: E. E. Ziegler, & L. J. Filer, Jr., eds., *Present knowledge in nutrition* 7th ed. ILSI Press, Washington, DC, 1996.

Stone, M., and H. O'Bryant. *Weight training: A scientific approach.* Bellweather Press, Minneapolis, MN, 1987.

Suggested Readings on the World Wide Web

Sympatico: Healthyway
(http://www.ns.sympatico.ca/healthyway/)
Numerous articles, book reviews, and links to nutrition, fitness, and wellness topics.

Fitness Tests: Explained
(http://arnie.pec.BrockU.CA/~hsac/tests/tests.html)
Tests for aerobic power, anaerobic power, flexibility, and body composition.

Fitness Files
(http://www2.webpoint.com/augusta_fitness/)
Fitness fundamentals, flexibility and contraindi-

cated exercises, exercise nutrition, and treating exercise injuries.

Fitness and Sports Medicine
(http://www.meriter.com/living/library/sports/index.html)
Injury prevention and treatment, weight training, flexibility, exercise prescriptions, and more.

Muscle Physiology
(http://www-neuromus.ucsd.edu/)
In-depth discussions of how muscle works and recent research articles from a world-renowned muscle physiology lab.

Weight Training: FAQ's
(ftp://ftp.cray.com/pub/misc.fitness/misc.fitness.faq.html)
Frequently asked questions about weight training.

Health Net
(http://www.health-net.com/)
Weight training, low back disorders, exercise programming, heart health, nutrition, mind and body, sports medicine, managing stress, wellness, men's health, women's health, diabetes, and arthritis.

References

1. Plowman, S. A. Physical activity, physical fitness, and low back pain. In: J. O. Holloszy, ed. *Exercise and Sports Sciences Reviews.* Vol 20. Williams and Wilkins, Baltimore, MD, 1992.

2. Stone, M. H. Muscle conditioning and muscle injuries. *Medicine and Science in Sports and Exercise.* 22:457–462, 1990.

3. Kibler, W. B., T. J. Chandler, and E. S. Stracener. Musculoskeletal adaptations and injuries due to overtraining. In: J. O. Holloszy, ed. *Exercise and sports sciences reviews,* Vol. 20. Williams and Wilkins, Baltimore, MD, 1992.

4. Larsson, L. Physical training effects on muscle morphology in sedentary males at different ages. *Medicine and Science in Sports and Exercise* 14:203–206, 1982.

5. Snow-Harter, C., and R. Marcus. Exercise, bone mineral density, and osteoporosis. In: J. O. Holloszy, ed. *Exercise and Sports Sciences Reviews.* Vol.19. Williams and Wilkins, Baltimore, MD, 1991.

6. Stephens, T. Physical activity and mental health in the United States and Canada: Evidence from four population surveys. *Preventive Medicine* 17:35–47, 1988.

7. Roy, R. R., K. M. Baldwin, and V. R. Edgerton. The plasticity of skeletal muscle: Effects of neuromuscular activity. In: J. O. Holloszy, ed. *Exercise and Sports Sciences Reviews.* Vol. 19. Williams and Wilkins, Baltimore, MD, 1991.

8. Stone, M., and H. O'Bryant. *Weight training: A scientific approach.* Burgess Publishing, Minneapolis, MN, 1987.

9. Fleck, S. J., and W. J. Kraemer. *Designing resistance training programs.* Human Kinetics, Champaign, IL. 1997.

10. Duchateau, J., and K. Hainaut. Isometric or dynamic training: Differentiated effects on mechanical properties of human muscle. *Journal of Applied Physiology* 56:296, 1984.

11. Kitai, T. A. Specificity of joint angle in isometric training. *European Journal of Applied Physiology* 58:744, 1989.

12. Braith, R. W., J. E. Graves, and M. L. Pollock. Comparison of two versus three days per week of variable resistance training during 10 and 18 week programs. *International Journal of Sports Medicine* 10:450–459, 1989.

13. Clarke, D. H. Adaptations in strength and muscular endurance resulting from exercise. In: J. H. Wilmore, ed. *Exercise and Sports Sciences Reviews.* Vol 1. Academic Press, New York, 1973.

14. Hakkinen K. Neuromuscular and hormonal adaptations in athletes to strength training in two years. *Journal of Applied Physiology* 65:2406, 1988.

15. Tesch, P. A. Skeletal muscle adaptations consequent to long-term heavy resistance exercise. *Medicine and Science in Sports and Exercise.* 20:S132, 1988.

16. Drunin, J. V. G. A. Protein requirements and physical activity. In: J. Parizkova and V. A. Rogozkin, eds. *Nutrition, Physical Fitness and Health.* University Park Press, Baltimore, MD, 1978.

17. Hickson, R. C. Strength training effects on aerobic power and short-term endurance. *Medicine and Science in Sports and Exercise* 12:336, 1980.

18. Sale, D. G. Neural adaptation to resistance training. *Medicine and Science in Sports and Exercise* 20:135, 1988.

19. Wilmore, J. H. Alterations in strength, body composition and anthropometric measurements consequent to a 10-week weight training program. *Medicine and Science in Sports and Exercise* 6:133, 1974.

20. Nissen, S. L., et al. The effect of the leucine metabolite beta-hydroxy-beta-methylbutyrate on muscle metabolism during resistance-exercise training. *Journal of Applied Physiology* 81:2095–2104, 1996.

21. Clancy, S. P., P. M. Clarkson, M. E. DeCheke, et al. Effects of chromium picolinate supplementation on body composition, strength, and urinary chromium loss in football players. *International Journal of Sport Nutrition* 4:142–153, 1994.

22. Hallmark, M. A., T. H. Reynolds, C. A. DeSouza, et al. Effects of chromium and resistive training on muscle strength and body composition. *Medicine and Science in Sports and Exercise* 28: 139–144, 1996.

Strength Training Log

NAME _____ DATE _____

The purpose of this log is to provide a record of progress in building strength in the upper and lower body.

Directions

Record the date, number of sets, reps and the weight for each of the exercises listed in the left column.

St/RP/Wt = Sets, Reps, and Weight

Example: 2/6/80 = 2 sets of 6 reps each with 80 lbs.

Date							
Exercise	St/Rp/Wt	St/Rp/Wt	St/Rp/Wt	St/Rp/Wt	St/Rp/Wt	St/Rp/Wt	St/Rp/Wt
Biceps curl							
Abdominal curl							
Leg extension							
Bench press							
Leg curl							
Lower back extension							
Upper back							
Hip and back							
Pullover							
Torso twist							
Triceps extension							
Chest press							

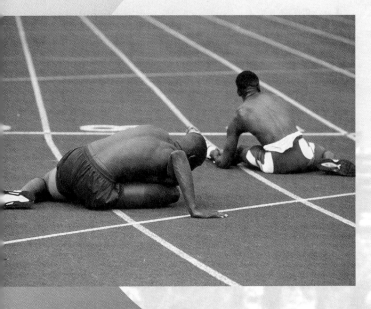

6

Improving
Flexibility

After studying this chapter, you should be able to

1 Discuss the value of flexibility.

2 Identify the structural and physiological limits to flexibility.

3 Discuss the stretch reflex.

4 Describe the three categories of stretching techniques.

5 Design a flexibility exercise program.

Flexibility is defined as the ability to move joints freely through their full range of motion. The full range of motion is determined by the physical makeup of the joint. That is, the shape of the bones play a part, as well as the composition and arrangement of muscles and tendons around the joint. For example, the elbow (a hinge-type joint) is limited in movement due to the bony makeup of the joint. However, even in hinge-type joints, connective tissue (soft tissues around the joint) also provides a major limitation to the range of joint movement (1).

Although flexibility varies between individuals because of differences in body structure, it is important to appreciate that flexibility is not a fixed property. The range of motion of most joints can be increased with proper training techniques or can decline with disuse. This chapter introduces exercises designed to improve flexibility.

Benefits of Flexibility

The many benefits of increased flexibility include: increased joint mobility, resistance to muscle injury, prevention of low-back problems, efficient body movement, and good posture, which results in improved personal appearance (2–4). Although all of these flexibility benefits are important, a key reason to improve flexibility is its role in the prevention of low-back problems. For example, most low-back pain is due to misalignment of the vertebral column and pelvic girdle caused by a lack of flexibility and/or weak muscles (4). Low-back pain is a significant problem—more than one billion dollars is lost by U.S. business yearly due to reduced productivity by workers suffering from low-back problems (5).

Physiological Basis for Developing Flexibility

The limits to flexibility are determined by the way the joint is constructed as well as by the associated muscles and tendons. Let's discuss these factors in more detail.

Structural Limitations to Movement

There are five primary factors that contribute to the limits of movement: bone; muscle; connective tissue within the joint capsule (the joint capsule is composed of **ligaments,** which hold bones together, and **cartilage,** which cushions the ends of bones); **tendons,** which connect muscle to bones and connective tissue surrounding joints; and skin. Exercise aimed at improving flexibility does not change the structure of bone, but it alters the soft tissues (i.e., muscle, joint connective tissue, and tendons) that contribute to flexibility. Table 6.1 illustrates the contribution of the various soft tissues to joint flexibility. Note that the structures associated with the joint capsule, muscles, and tendons provide most of the body's resistance to movement. Therefore, exercises aimed at improving flexibility must alter one of these three factors in order to increase the range of motion around a joint. Stretching the ligaments in the joint capsule may lead to a loose joint that would be highly susceptible to injury. However, muscle and tendon are soft tissues that can lengthen over time with stretching exercises. Stretching exercises increase the range of motion in the joint by reducing the resistance to movement offered by tight muscles and tendons.

Stretching and the Stretch Reflex

Before we examine specific exercises to improve flexibility, it is useful to discuss a key physiological response to stretching exercises. Muscles contain special receptors that are sensi-

Table 6.1

Contribution of the Soft-Tissue Structures to Limiting Joint Movement

Structure	Resistance to Flexibility (% of total)
Joint capsule	47
Muscle	41
Tendon	10
Skin	2

tive to stretch. These stretch receptors are called *muscle spindles* and are responsible for the **stretch reflex** that occurs when a doctor taps you on the knee with a rubber hammer. The stretch reflex occurs because rapid stretching of muscle spindles results in a "reflex" contraction of the muscle. This type of reflex contraction is counterproductive to stretching exercises because the muscle is shortening instead of lengthening. However, the stretch reflex can be avoided when muscles and tendons are stretched very slowly. In fact, if a muscle stretch is held for several seconds, the muscle spindles allow the muscle being stretched to further relax and permit an even greater stretch (6). Therefore, stretching exercises are most effective when they avoid promoting a stretch reflex.

Designing a Flexibility Training Program

Three kinds of stretching techniques are commonly used to increase flexibility: ballistic, static, and proprioceptive neuromuscular facilitation (7, 8). However, because ballistic stretching promotes the stretch reflex and increases the risk of injury to muscles and tendons, only the static and proprioceptive neuromuscular facilitation methods are recommended. A brief discussion of each of these stretching techniques follows.

Static Stretching

Static stretching is extremely effective for improving flexibility and has gained popularity over the last decade (8). Static stretching slowly lengthens a muscle to a point at which further movement is limited (slight discomfort is felt) and requires holding this position for a fixed period of time. The optimal amount of time to hold the stretch for maximal improvement in flexibility is unknown. However, most investigators agree that holding the stretch position for 20 to 30 seconds (repeated three to four times) results in an improvement in flexibility. Compared with ballistic stretching, the risk of injury associated with static stretching is minimal. Another benefit of static stretching is that, when performed during the cool-down period, it may reduce the muscle stiffness associated with some exercise routines (9).

Proprioceptive Neuromuscular Facilitation

A relatively new technique for improving flexibility, **proprioceptive neuromuscular facilitation (PNF)** combines stretching with alternating contracting and relaxing of muscles. There are two common types of PNF stretching: contract-relax (CR) stretching and contract-relax/antagonist contract (CRAC) stretching. The CR stretch technique calls for first contracting the muscle to be stretched. Then, after relaxing the muscle, the muscle is slowly stretched. The CRAC method calls for the same contract-relax routine but adds to this the contraction of the **antagonist** muscle, the muscle on the opposite side of the joint. The purpose of contracting the antagonist muscle is to promote a reflex relaxation of the muscle to be stretched.

How do PNF techniques compare with ballistic and static stretching? First, PNF has been shown to be safer and more effective in promoting flexibility than ballistic stretching (7). Further, studies have shown PNF programs to be equal to, or in some cases superior to, static stretching for improving flexibility (10). However, one disadvantage of PNF stretching is that some stretches require a partner.

ligaments Connective tissue within the joint capsule which holds bones together.

cartilage A tough, connective tissue that forms a pad on the end of bones in certain joints, such as the elbow, knee, and ankle. Cartilage acts as a shock absorber to cushion the weight of one bone on another and to provide protection from the friction due to joint movement.

tendons Connective tissue that connects muscles to bones.

stretch reflex Involuntary contraction of muscle that occurs due to rapid stretching of a muscle.

static stretching Stretching that slowly lengthens a muscle to a point where further movement is limited.

proprioceptive neuromuscular facilitation (PNF) Combines stretching with alternating contracting and relaxing of muscles to improve flexibility. There are two common types of PNF stretching. One is called contract-relax (C-R) stretching, while the second is called contract-relax/antagonist contract (CRAC) stretching.

antagonist The muscle on the opposite side of the joint.

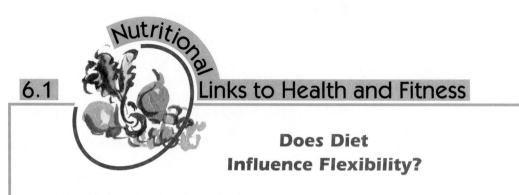

6.1 Nutritional Links to Health and Fitness

Does Diet Influence Flexibility?

Although there is no evidence that large doses of any nutrient will improve flexibility, it is well known that a vitamin C dietary deficiency can influence the range of joint motion. Vitamin C plays an important role in the synthesis of connective tissue (such as cartilage and collagen) and in maintaining bone strength. Because cartilage and collagen are key connective tissues associated with joint structure, changes in their quantity alter joint stability. Failure to consume adequate amounts of vitamin C (recommended daily allowance is 60 mg/day) can result in scurvy, which in extreme cases can result in unstable (loose) joints. An increased range of joint motion due to scurvy can lead to injury. Vitamin C deficiencies can be avoided by consuming citrus fruits, tomatoes, green salads, and green peppers. See Chapter 7 for additional details on nutrition and fitness.

FIGURE 6.1 Example of a partner-assisted PNF stretch. **(A)** Contract the calf muscles against resistance provided by partner. **(B)** Unassisted, contract shin muscles to flex the ankle. **(C)** Partner provides assistance in stretching calf muscles while contraction of shin muscles continues.

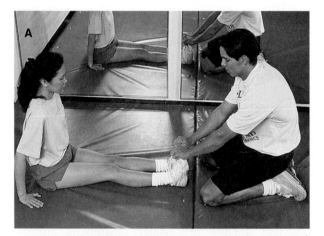

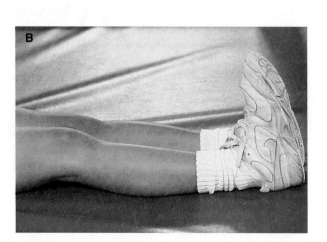

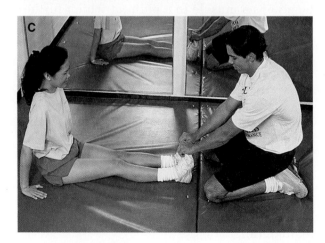

The following steps illustrate how a CRAC procedure can be done with a partner (see Figure 6.1):

1. The assistant moves the limb in the direction necessary to stretch the desired muscle to the point of tightness (mild discomfort is felt). The muscle being stretched is now briefly contracted isometrically for 3 to 5 seconds and relaxed.

2. The subject then pushes the limb in the opposite direction of the stretch, contracting the antagonist muscles. The assistant resists the contraction, and an isometric contraction occurs at this angle.

3. The isometric contraction is then held for approximately 5 seconds. The muscle is now relaxed, and the assistant slowly increases the stretch of the desired muscle.

4. The isometric contraction is then repeated for another 5 seconds, and the muscle is relaxed again. The assistant again stretches the muscle to a point of mild discomfort. This cycle is repeated three to five times.

Figure 6.2 shows how some PNF stretches can be done without a partner.

Exercise Prescription for Improving Flexibility

For safety reasons, all flexibility programs should consist of either PNF or static stretching exercises. The frequency and duration of a stretching exercise prescription should be 2 to 5 days per week for 10 to 30 minutes each day. The first week of a stretching regimen is considered the starter phase. The first week should consist of one stretching session, with one session added per week during the first 4 weeks of the slow progression phase of the program. Initially, the duration of each training session should be approximately 5 minutes, increasing gradually to approximately 20 to 30 minutes following 6 to 12 weeks of stretching during the slow progression

FIGURE 6.2 Examples of how PNF stretches may be done without a partner. Can you think of other creative ways to self-assist with PNF stretches?

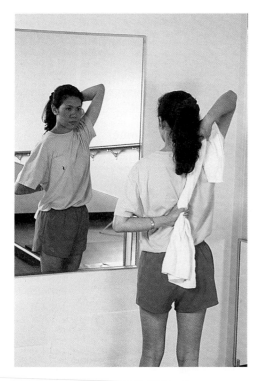
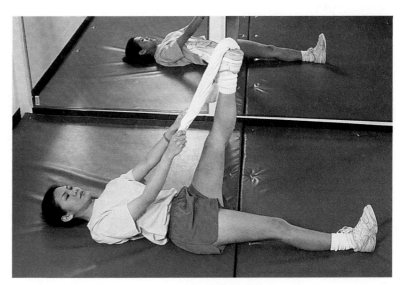

phase. The physiological rationale for increasing the duration of stretching is that each stretch position is held for progressively longer durations as the program continues. For example, begin by holding each stretched position for 15 seconds, then add 5 seconds each week up to 30 seconds. Start by performing each of the exercises once (1 rep) and progress to 4 reps.

What about the intensity of stretching? In general, a limb should not be stretched beyond a position of mild discomfort. The intensity of stretching is altered by simply increasing the range of motion during the stretch. That is, your range of motion will gradually increase as your flexibility improves during the training program. Table 6.2 illustrates a sample exercise prescription for a flexibility program.

To improve overall flexibility, all major muscle groups should be stretched. Exercises 6.1 through 6.12 illustrate the proper method of performing 12 different stretching exercises. Integrate these exercises into the program outlined in Table 6.2.

These exercises are designed to be used in a regular program of stretching to increase flexibility. Exercises are presented which use the major joints and muscle groups of the body in which range of motion tends to decrease with age and disuse. The exercises include both static and PNF movements and may require a partner.

How to Avoid Hazardous Exercises

There are many exercises that are potentially harmful to the musculoskeletal system. Which exercises actually cause an injury depends on how they are performed. Use the following key points during an exercise session to help prevent injury.

- Avoid breathholding. Try to breath as normally as possible during the exercise.
- Avoid full flexion of the knee or neck.
- Avoid full extension of the knee, neck, or back.
- Do not stretch muscles that are already stretched such as the abdominal muscles.
- Do not stretch any joint to the point that ligaments and joint capsules are stressed.
- Use extreme precaution when using an assistant to help with passive stretches.
- Avoid extension and flexion of the spine in a forceful manner.

There are many commonly practiced exercises that may cause injuries and are, therefore, contraindicated. The illustrations starting on page 143 show some of these exercises (contraindicated exercises) and provide alternatives (substitute exercises) to accomplish the same goals.

Table 6.2

Sample Flexibility Program with Considerations for Duration of Stretch Hold, Number of Repetitions, and Frequency of Training

Week No.	Phase	Duration of Stretch Hold	Repetitions	Frequency (times/wk)
1	Starter	15 sec	1	1
2	Slow progression	20 sec	2	2
3	Slow progression	25 sec	3	3
4	Slow progression	30 sec	4	3
5	Slow progression	30 sec	4	3–4
6	Slow progression	30 sec	4	4–5
7+	Maintenance	30 sec	4	4–5

Sample Flexibility Exercises

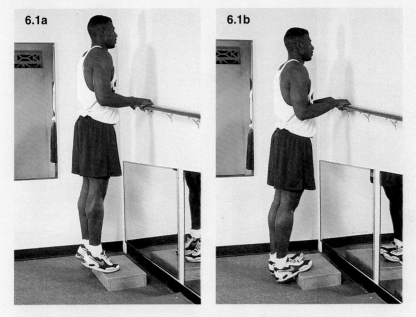

Lower Leg Stretch

Purpose: To stretch the calf muscles and the Achilles' tendon.
Position: Stand on the edge of a raised surface (e.g., a book or board) so that your heel can be lower than your toes. Have a support nearby to hold for balance.
Movement: Rise on the toes as far as possible for several seconds, then lower the heels as far as possible. Shift your body weight from one leg to the other for added stretch of the muscles.

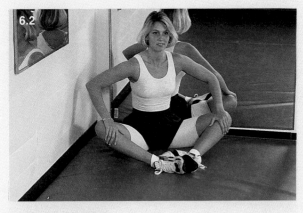

Inside Leg Stretch

Purpose: To stretch the muscle on the inside of the thighs.
Position: Sit with bottoms of the feet together. With the forearms against the knees, resist while attempting to raise the knees.
Movement: Relax and press the knees toward the floor and hold for several seconds.

Sample Flexibility Exercises

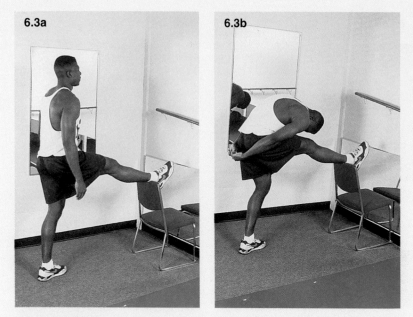

6.3a   6.3b

One-Leg Stretch

Purpose: To stretch the lower back muscles and muscles in the back of the upper leg.
Position: Stand with the heel of one foot on a support approximately knee-to-waist high. Keep both legs straight.
Movement: Press the heel down on the support for several seconds, then relax and bend forward at the waist and attempt to touch your head to your knee, and hold for several seconds. Return to the upright position and alternate legs.

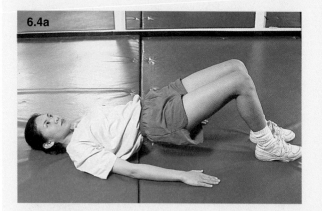
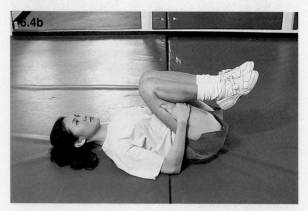

6.4a   6.4b

Lower Back Stretch

Purpose: To stretch the lower back and buttocks muscles.
Position: Lying on the floor.
Movement: First, arch your back and lift the hips off the floor, and hold for several seconds. Relax and place your hands behind the knees. Pull the knees to the chest, raise the head to meet the knees, and hold for several seconds. Repeat the sequence for the desired number of repetitions.

Sample Flexibility Exercises

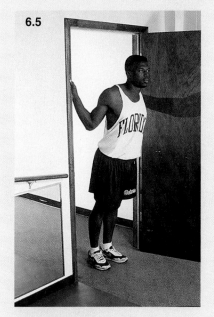

6.5

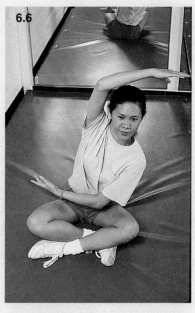

6.6

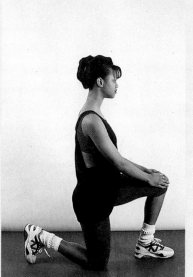

6.7

Chest Stretch

Purpose: To stretch the muscles across the chest.
Position: Stand in a doorway with hands holding it at shoulder height.
Movement: Spread your feet forward and back to maintain balance. Press forward on the doorway for several seconds. Relax and shift your weight to the forward leg so that the muscles across the chest are stretched, and hold for several seconds.

Side Stretch

Purpose: To stretch the muscles of the upper arm and side of the trunk.
Position: Sitting on the floor with legs crossed.
Movement: Stretch one arm over the head while bending at the waist in the same direction. With the opposite arm, reach across the chest as far as possible. Hold for several seconds. Do not rotate the trunk; try to stretch the muscle on the side of the trunk away from the direction of stretch.

Thigh Stretch

Purpose: To stretch the muscles in the front of the upper leg.
Position: Go down on one knee while the opposite leg is in front with the foot flat on the floor. Lift the knee off the floor and stretch the leg backward so that the knee is slightly behind the hips.
Movement: Press the hips forward and down, and hold for several seconds. Repeat on the opposite leg. On the leg in front, maintain an approximate 90° angle at the knee.

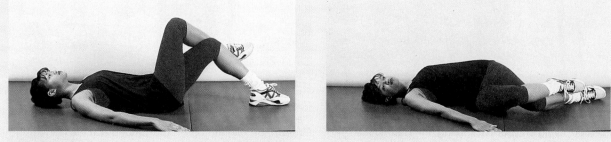

6.8a   6.8b

Spine Twister

Purpose: To stretch the muscles that rotate the trunk and thighs.
Position: Lie on your back with arms extended at shoulder level.
Movement: Cross one leg over the other while keeping arms and shoulders on the floor. Rotate the trunk to let both knees touch the floor, and hold for several seconds. Reverse the position and repeat.

Sample Flexibility Exercises

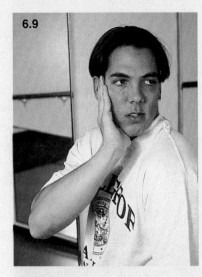

6.9

Neck Stretch

Purpose: To stretch the muscles that rotate the neck.
Position: Place the hand against the cheek with fingers toward the ear and elbow forward.
Movement: Try to turn the head and neck while resisting with the hand. Hold several seconds. Relax and turn the head in the opposite direction as far as possible, and hold for several seconds. Repeat in both directions.

6.10

Shin Stretch

Purpose: To stretch the muscles on the front of the shin.
Position: Kneel on both knees, turn to one side, and press down on the ankle.
Movement: Move the pelvis forward, and hold for several seconds. Repeat on both sides.

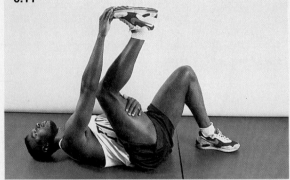

6.11

Leg Stretch

Purpose: To stretch the muscles on the back of the hip, upper leg, and lower leg.
Position: Lying on your back, bring one knee to the chest and grasp the toes with the hand on the same side. Place the opposite hand on the back of the leg just below the knee.
Movement: Pull the knee toward the chest while pushing the heel toward the ceiling and pulling toes toward the shin. Attempt to straighten the knee, and hold for several seconds. Repeat on both sides.

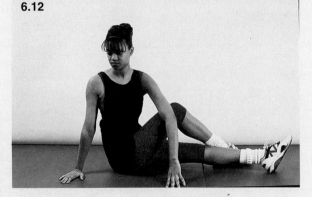

6.12

Trunk Twister

Purpose: To stretch the trunk muscles and muscles of the hip.
Position: Sit with the right leg extended and the left leg bent and crossed over the right knee, with the foot on the floor.
Movement: Place the right arm on the left side of the left leg and push against that leg while twisting the trunk to the left, and hold for several seconds. Place the left hand on the floor behind the buttocks. Reverse positions and repeat on the opposite side.

Contraindicated Exercise

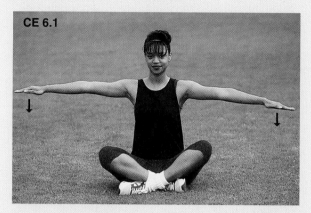

Arm Circles (Palms Down)

Purpose: To strengthen the muscles of the shoulder and upper back.
Problem: May result in irritation of the shoulder joint and, if circled forward and down, results in the use of the chest muscles instead of back muscles.

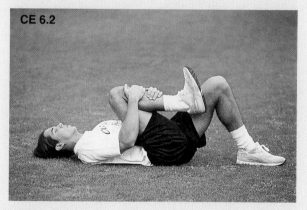

Knee Pull

Purpose: To stretch the lower back and buttocks.
Problem: Places undue stress on the knee joint.

Substitute Exercise

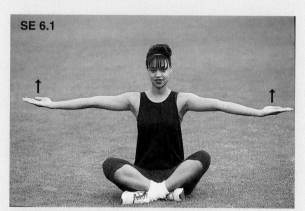

Arm Circles (Palms Up)

In a sitting position, turn the palms up and circle the arms backward.

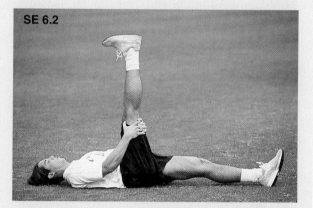

Leg Pull

Lying on your back, pull the knee to the chest by pulling on the back of your leg just below the knee joint. Then, extend the knee and point the foot to the ceiling. Continue to pull the leg toward your chest. Repeat several times with each leg.

Contraindicated Exercise

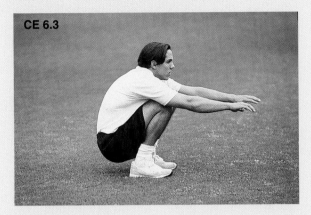

Deep Knee Bends

Purpose: To strengthen the knee extensors and flex the hip extensors.

Problem: This movement hyperflexes the knee and "opens" the joint while stretching the ligaments.

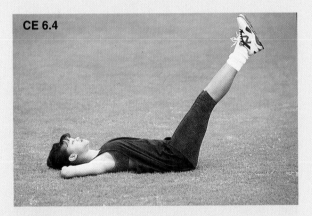

Leg Lifts

Purpose: To strengthen the abdominal muscles.

Problem: This exercise primarily recruits the hip flexor muscles and thus does not accomplish the intended purpose. These muscles are likely strong enough and do not need strengthening. In addition, this exercise produces excess compression on the vertebral disks.

Substitute Exercise

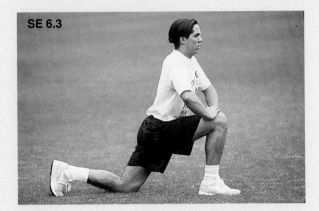

Lunges

While standing, step forward with either foot and touch the opposite knee to the floor. The front knee should be bent to a 90° angle. Repeat with the opposite leg.

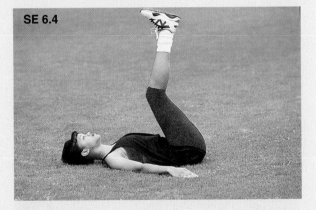

Reverse Curl

Lie on your back with knees bent, feet flat on the floor, and arms at your side. Lift your knees to your chest until your hips leave the floor. Do not let your knees go past the shoulders. Lower your legs back to the floor and repeat.

Contraindicated Exercise

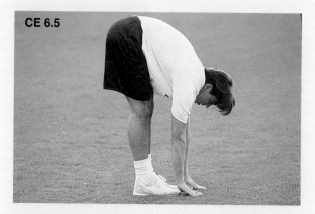

Standing Toe Touch

Purpose: To stretch the lower back, buttocks, and hamstrings.

Problem: There are two potential problems with this maneuver. First, hyperflexion of the knee could cause damage to ligaments and, second, if performed with the back flat, damage could occur to the lower back.

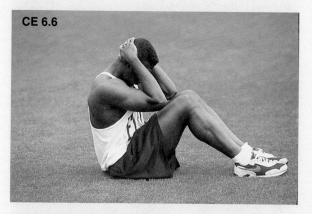

Sit-Up (Hands behind Head)

Purpose: To strengthen the abdominal muscles.

Problem: With hands behind the head, there is a tendency to jerk on the head and neck to "throw" yourself up. This could cause hyperflexion of the neck. In addition, sitting up with the back straight places undue strain on the lower back.

Substitute Exercise

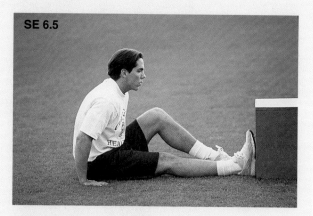

Sitting Hamstring Stretch

Sit at leg-length from a wall. With your foot on the wall and the other knee bent with the foot close to the buttocks, bend forward keeping the lower back straight. The bent knee can fall to the side.

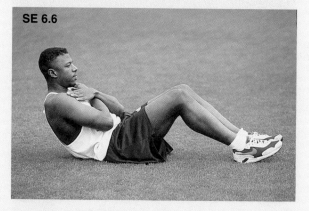

Curl Up

Keeping the knees bent while lying on your back, cross your arms over your chest so that your fingers rest on your shoulders. Curl up until the upper half of the back is off the floor and return to the starting position.

Contraindicated Exercise

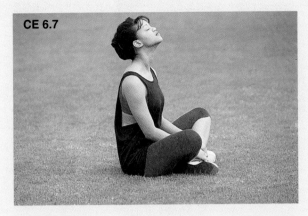

CE 6.7

Neck Circles

Purpose: To stretch the neck muscles.
Problem: Hyperextension of the neck should always be avoided. This can pinch arteries and nerves, as well as damage disks in the spine.

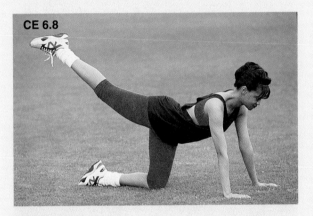

CE 6.8

Donkey Kick

Purpose: To stretch and strengthen the buttocks.
Problem: When kicking the leg back, most people hyperextend the neck and/or back.

Substitute Exercise

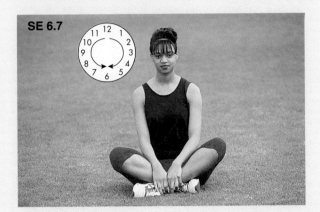

SE 6.7

Neck Stretches

In a sitting position, with your head and neck straight, move your head down to flex the neck, and return the head upright. Then, slowly turn your head from side to side as far as possible; attempt to point your chin at each shoulder.

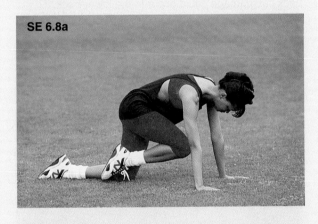

SE 6.8a

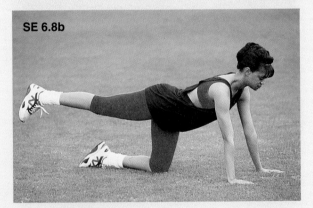

SE 6.8b

Knee-to-Nose Touch

While on your hands and knees, lift one knee to your nose and then extend your leg to horizontal. Alternate legs. Remember: Your leg should not go higher than your hips, and your neck should remain in line with your back.

Motivation to Maintain Flexibility

Maintaining flexibility requires a lifetime commitment to performing regular stretching. Similar to other types of fitness training, good time management is critical if you are going to succeed. Set aside time for 3 to 5 stretching periods per week and stick to your schedule. A key point to remember when scheduling time to perform flexibility exercises is that stretching does not require special equipment and can be performed almost anywhere. So take advantage of "windows" of free time in your day and plan stretching workouts.

You are not likely to maintain a lifetime stretching program if you do not enjoy your workouts. Therefore, how do you make stretching fun? One suggestion is to perform stretching workouts while listening to music or during a television program that you enjoy. This will allow time to pass more rapidly and will make your stretching workout more pleasant.

As in other aspects of physical fitness, establishing short-term and long-term flexibility goals are important in maintaining the motivation to stretch. Further, keeping a record of your workouts and improvements allows you to follow your flexibility progress and plan your future training schedule (see Laboratory 6.1). So, establish your stretching goals today and get started toward a lifetime of flexibility.

Summary

1. *Flexibility* is defined as the range of motion of a joint.

2. Improved flexibility results in the following benefits: increased joint mobility, resistance to muscle injury, prevention of low-back problems, efficient body movement, and improved posture and personal appearance.

3. The five structural and physiological limits to flexibility are bone, muscle, structures within the joint capsule, the tendons that connect muscle to bones and connective tissue which surround joints, and skin.

4. If muscle spindles are suddenly stretched, they respond by producing a stretch reflex. However, if the muscles and tendons are stretched slowly, the stretch reflex can be avoided.

5. Static stretches involve stretching a muscle to the limitation of movement and holding it for an extended period of time.

6. Proprioceptive neuromuscular facilitation combines stretching with alternating contracting and relaxing of muscles to improve flexibility.

Study Questions

1. Define the following terms:

   antagonist

   cartilage

   flexibility

   proprioceptive neuromuscular facilitation

2. Describe the difference in function between ligaments and tendons.

3. Compare static and ballistic stretching.

4. List three primary reasons why flexibility is important.

5. List all of the factors that limit flexibility and identify which are the major contributors.

6. Compare and contrast the two recommended methods of stretching.

7. Briefly outline the exercise prescription for improvement of flexibility.

8. Explain how a stretch reflex operates.

Suggested Reading

DeVries, H. and T. Housh. *Physiology of exercise*. 5th ed. Brown and Benchmark. Dubuque, IA, 1994.

Fox, A., S. Keteyian, and M. Foss. *The physiological basis for exercise and sports*. 6th ed. Brown and Benchmark, Dubuque, IA, 1997.

Golding, L. A. Flexiblity, stretching, and flexibility testing. *ACSM's Health and Fitness Journal* 1(2):17–20, 1997.

Hutton, R. S. Neuromuscular basis of stretching exercises. In: P. V. Komi, ed. *Strength and power in sport*. Blackwell Scientific Publications, Oxford, England, 1992.

Powers, S., and E. Howley. *Exercise physiology: Theory application to fitness and performance*. 3rd ed. Wm. C. Brown, Dubuque, IA, 1997.

Sady, S. P., M. Wortman, and D. Blanke. Flexibility training: Ballistic, static or proprioceptive neuromuscular facilitation? *Archives of Physical Medicine and Rehabilitation* 63:261–263, 1982.

Steiner, M. E. Hypermobility and knee injuries. *Physician and Sports Medicine* 15:159–168, 1987.

Wallin, D., B. Ekblom, R. Grahn, and T. Nordenberg. Improvement of muscle flexibility. A comparison between two techniques. *American Journal of Sports Medicine* 13:263–268, 1985.

Suggested Readings on the World Wide Web

Fitness Tests: Explained
(http://arnie.pec.BrockU.CA/~hsac/tests/tests.html)
Tests for aerobic power, anaerobic power, flexibility, and body composition.

Fitness Files
(http://www2.webpoint.com/augusta_fitness/)
Fitness fundamentals, flexibility and contraindicated exercises, exercise nutrition, and treating exercise injuries.

Fitness and Sports Medicine
(http://www.meriter.com/living/library/sports/index.htm)
Injury prevention and treatment, weight training, flexibility, exercise prescriptions, and more.

References

1. Johns, R., and V. Wright. Relative importance of various tissues in joint stiffness. *Journal of Applied Physiology* 17:824–828, 1962.

2. DeVries, H. Evaluation of static stretching procedures for improvement of flexibility. *Research Quarterly* 33:222–229, 1962.

3. DeVries, H., and T. Housh. *Physiology of exercise*. 5th ed. Brown and Benchmark, Dubuque, IA, 1994.

4. Plowman, S. A. Physical activity, physical fitness, and low back pain. In: J. O. Holloszy, ed. *Exercise and sports sciences reviews*. Vol. 20. Williams and Wilkins, Baltimore, MD, 1992.

5. *Back injuries: Cost, causes, cases, and prevention*. Washington D.C., Bureau of National Affairs, 1988.

6. Condon, S. M., and R. S. Hutton. Soleus muscle electromyographic activity and ankle dorsiflexion range of motion during four stretching procedures. *Journal of American Physical Therapy Association* 67:24–30, 1987.

7. Wilford, H. N., and J. F. Smith. A comparison of proprioceptive neuromuscular facilitation and static stretching techniques. *American Corrective Therapy Journal* 39(2):30, 1985.

8. Etnyre, B. R., and E. J. Lee. Chronic and acute flexibility of men and women using three different stretching techniques. *Research Quarterly for Exercise and Sport* 589:222–228, 1988.

9. Fox, A., S. Keteyian, and M. Foss. *The physiological basis for exercise and sports*. 6th ed. Brown and Benchmark, Dubuque, IA, 1997.

10. Etnyre, B. R., and E. J. Lee. Comments on proprioceptive neuromuscular facilitation stretching techniques. *Research Quarterly for Exercise and Sport* 58:184–188, 1987.

Flexibility Progression Log

NAME _____ DATE _____

The purpose of this log is to provide a record of progress in increasing flexibility in selected joints.

Directions

Record the date, sets and hold time for each of the exercises listed in the left column.

St/Hold = Sets and hold time

Example: 2/30 = 2 sets held for 30 seconds each.

Date							
Exercise	**St/Hold**	**St/Hold**	**St/Hold**	**St/Hold**	**St/Hold**	**St/Hold**	**St/Hold**
Lower leg stretch							
Inside leg stretch							
One leg stretch							
Lower back stretch							
Chest stretch							
Side stretch							
Thigh stretch							
Neck stretch							
Shin stretch							
Leg stretch							
Trunk twister							
Spine twister							

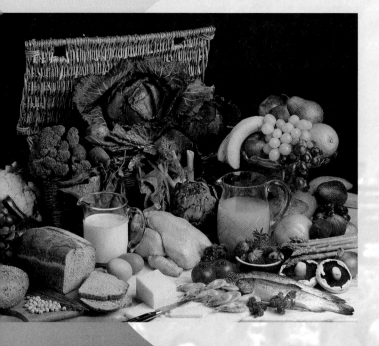

7

Nutrition, Health, and Fitness

Nutrition can be broadly defined as the study of food and the way the body uses it to produce energy and build or repair body tissues. Good nutrition means that an individual's diet supplies all of the essential foodstuffs required to maintain a healthy body. Although dietary deficiencies were a problem of the past in many industrialized countries, a primary danger associated with nutrition today is overeating.

Many diets are high in calories (see A Closer Look 7.1), sugar, fats, and sodium, and diseases linked to these dietary excesses, such as cardiovascular disease, cancer, obesity, and diabetes, are the leading killers in the United States today (1). According to the U.S. Department of Health and Human Services, over one-half of all deaths in the United States are associated with health problems linked to poor nutrition (2). Nevertheless, through diet analysis and modification, it is possible to prevent many of these nutrition-related diseases. An elementary understanding of nutrition is therefore important for everyone. This chapter outlines the fundamental concepts of good nutrition and provides guidelines for developing a healthy diet. We also discuss how exercise training can modify nutritional requirements.

Basic Nutrition

Substances contained in food that are necessary for good health are called **nutrients.** They can be divided into two categories: macronutrients and micronutrients. **Macronutrients**, which consist of carbohydrates, fats, and proteins, are necessary for building and maintaining body tissues and providing energy for daily activities. **Micronutrients** include all other substances in food such as vitamins and minerals that regulate the functions of the cells.

Macronutrients

A well-balanced diet is composed of approximately 58% carbohydrates, 30% fat, and 12% protein (Figure 7.1).

These macronutrients are called "fuel nutrients" because they are the only substances that can provide the energy necessary for bodily functions. Under normal conditions, carbohydrates and fats are the primary fuels used by the body to produce energy. The primary function of protein is to serve as the body's "building blocks" to repair tissues. However, when carbohydrate is insufficient or the body is under stress, protein can be used as a fuel.

Table 7.1 on page 154 lists the major food sources and energy content of carbohydrates, proteins, and fats. Given the importance of dietary carbohydrates, proteins, and fats to health and fitness, we will discuss these macronutrients in more detail.

Carbohydrates Carbohydrates are especially important during many types of physical activity because they are a key energy source for muscular contraction. Dietary sources of carbohydrates are breads, cereals, fruits, and vegetables. Carbohydrates can be divided into two major classes and several subclasses (Table 7.2).

7.1 A Closer Look

What is a Calorie?

A **calorie** is the unit of measure used to quantify food energy or the energy expended by the body. Technically, a calorie is the amount of energy necessary to raise the temperature of 1 gram of water 1°C. Calories contained in foods and energy expended during exercise are measured in thousands of calories, or kilocalories (kcals). By convention, the terms *calorie* and *kcal* are used interchangeably in this textbook.

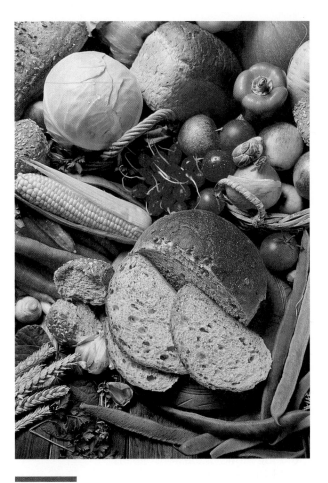

One of the main ingredients of a healthy lifestyle is a well-balanced diet.

Simple Carbohydrates Simple carbohydrates consist of one or two of the simple sugars shown in Table 7.2. **Glucose** is the most noteworthy of the simple sugars because it is the only sugar molecule that can be used by the body in its natural form. To be used for fuel, all other carbohydrates must first be converted to glucose. After a meal, glucose is stored by skeletal muscles and the liver in the form of a chain of glucose molecules called **glycogen**. The glucose remaining in the blood thereafter is often converted to fat and stored in fat cells as a future source of energy.

The body requires glucose to function normally. Indeed, the central nervous system uses glucose almost exclusively for its energy needs. If dietary intake of carbohydrates is inadequate, the body must make glucose from protein. This is undesirable because it would result in the breakdown of body protein for use as fuel. Dietary carbohydrate is not only important as a direct fuel source, but also important for its protein-sparing effect.

Other types of simple sugars include fructose, galactose, lactose, maltose, and sucrose. **Fructose**, or fruit sugar, is a naturally occurring sugar found in fruits and in honey. **Galactose** is a sugar found in the breast milk of humans and other mammals. **Lactose** (composed of galactose and glucose) and **maltose** (composed of two glucose molecules linked together) are best known as milk and malt sugar, respectively. **Sucrose** (table sugar) is composed of glucose and fructose. A key point to remember about these simple sugars is that each must be converted to glucose to be used by the body.

nutrients Substances contained in food which are necessary for good health.

macronutrients Carbohydrates, fats, and proteins, which are necessary for building and maintaining body tissues and providing energy for daily activities.

micronutrients Nutrients in food, such as vitamins and minerals, that regulate the functions of the cells.

calorie The unit of measure used to quantify food energy or the energy expended by the body. Technically, a calorie is the amount of energy necessary to raise the temperature of 1 gram of water 1°C.

carbohydrates One of the macronutrients that is especially important during many types of physical activity because they are a key energy source for muscular contraction. Dietary sources of carbohydrates are breads, cereals, fruits, and vegetables.

glucose The most noteworthy of the simple sugars because it is the only sugar molecule that can be used by the body in its natural form. All other carbohydrates must first be converted to glucose to be used for fuel.

glycogen The storage form of glucose in the liver and skeletal muscles.

fructose Also called *fruit sugar;* a naturally occurring sugar found in fruits and in honey.

galactose A simple sugar found in the breast milk of humans and other mammals.

lactose A simple sugar found in milk products; it is composed of galactose and glucose.

maltose A simple sugar found in grain products; it is composed of two glucose molecules linked together.

sucrose Also called *table sugar;* a molecule composed of glucose and fructose.

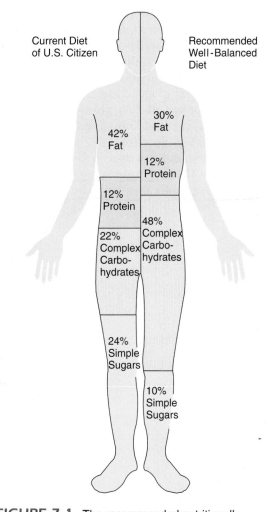

Current Diet of U.S. Citizen

Recommended Well-Balanced Diet

30% Fat

42% Fat

12% Protein

12% Protein

48% Complex Carbohydrates

22% Complex Carbohydrates

24% Simple Sugars

10% Simple Sugars

FIGURE 7.1 The recommended nutritionally balanced diet (**right**) compared with the typical U.S. diet (**left**). (Source: Donatelle, R. J., and L. G. Davis, 1996. *Access to health.* Copyright © 1996 by Allyn & Bacon.)

Complex Carbohydrates Complex carbohydrates provide both micronutrients and the glucose necessary for producing energy. They are contained in starches and fiber. **Starches** are long chains of sugars commonly found in foods such as corn, grains, potatoes, peas, and beans. Starch is stored in the body as glycogen and, as previously discussed, is used for that sudden burst of energy we often need during physical activity. **Fiber** is a stringy, nondigestible carbohydrate found in whole grains, vegetables, and fruits in its primary form, cellulose. Because fiber is nondigestible, it is not a fuel source nor does it provide micronutrients. It is, however, a key ingredient in a healthy diet.

In recent years, nutrition researchers have shown that dietary fiber provides bulk in the intestinal tract. This bulk aids in the formation and elimination of food waste products, thus reducing the time necessary for wastes to move through the digestive system and lowering the risk of colon cancer. Dietary fiber is also thought to be a factor in reducing the risk for coronary heart disease and breast cancer, and in controlling blood sugar in diabetics (3). Some types of fiber bind with cholesterol in the digestive tract and prevent its absorption into the blood, thereby reducing blood cholesterol levels.

Although a minimum of 25 grams of fiber are recommended on a daily basis, excessive amounts of fiber in the diet can cause intestinal discomfort and decreased absorption of calcium and iron into the blood (3). The following steps are recommended to increase fiber in your diet:

Table 7.1

Food Sources and Energy Content of the Macronutrients

Carbohydrate (4 calories/gram)	Protein (4 calories/gram)	Fat (9 calories/gram)
Grains	Meats	Butter
Fruits	Fish	Margarine
Vegetables	Poultry	Oils
Concentrated sweets	Eggs	Shortening
Breads	Milk	Cream
Beans/peas	Beans	
	Rice	

Table 7.2

Major Classifications of Carbohydrates and Sources of Each

Major Classifications of Carbohydrates	Subclasses of Carbohydrates	
	General Class	*Food Source*
Simple carbohydrates (simple sugars)	Fructose	Fruits and honey
	Galactose	Breast milk
	Glucose	All sugars
	Lactose	Milk sugar
	Maltose	Malt sugar
	Sucrose	Table sugar
Complex carbohydrates	Starches	Potatoes, rice, bread
	Fiber	Fruits, vegetables, bread

- Eat a variety of foods.
- Eat at least five servings of fruits and vegetables and three to six servings of whole-grain breads, cereals, and legumes per day.
- Eat less processed food.
- Eat the skins of fruits and vegetables.
- Get your fiber from foods rather than pills or powders.
- Drink plenty of liquids.

Fat Fat is an efficient storage form for energy, because each gram of fat holds more than twice the energy content of either carbohydrate or protein (see Table 7.1). Excess fat in the diet is stored in fat cells (called *adipose tissue*) located under the skin and around internal organs. Fat not only is derived from dietary sources, but also can be formed in the body from excess carbohydrate and protein in the diet. Although fat can be synthesized in the body, fat in the diet cannot be totally eliminated. Indeed, dietary fat is the only source of linoleic and linolenic acids, essential fatty acids important for normal growth and healthy skin.

Fat also gives protection to internal organs and assists in absorbing, transporting, and storing the fat-soluble vitamins A, D, E, and K. Fats are classified as simple, compound, or derived (Table 7.3). Let's discuss each of these subcategories of fat.

Simple Fats The most common of the simple fats are **triglycerides.** Triglycerides constitute approximately 95% of the fats in the diet and are the storage form of body fat. This is the form of fat that is broken down and used to produce energy to power muscle contractions during exercise.

complex carbohydrates A term that refers to carbohydrates that provide both micronutrients and the glucose necessary for producing energy. They are contained in starches and fiber.

starches Long chains of sugars commonly found in foods such as corn, grains, potatoes, peas, and beans. Starch is stored in the body as glycogen and is used for that sudden burst of energy often needed during physical activity.

fiber A stringy, nondigestible carbohydrate found in whole grains, vegetables, and fruits in its primary form, cellulose.

fat An efficient storage form for energy, because each gram of fat holds over twice the energy content of either carbohydrate or protein. Excess fat in the diet is stored in fat cells (called *adipose tissue*) located under the skin and around internal organs.

triglycerides The form of fat that is broken down and used to produce energy to power muscle contractions during exercise. Triglycerides constitute approximately 95% of the fats in the diet and are the storage form of body fat.

Table 7.3

Major Classifications of Fats and Common Examples of Each

Classification	Example
Simple fats	Triglyceride (one glycerol + three fatty acids)
Compound fats	Lipoprotein
Derived fats	Cholesterol

Fatty acids are the basic structural unit of triglycerides and are important nutritionally, not only because of their energy content, but also because they play a role in cardiovascular disease. Fatty acids are classified as either **saturated** or **unsaturated** based on their structure. Saturated fatty acids generally come from animal sources (meat and dairy products) and are solid at room temperature. However, some saturated fats, such as coconut oil, come from plant sources. Unsaturated fatty acids, which come from plants (peas, beans, grains, vegetable oils, etc.) are liquid at room temperature.

The distinction between saturated and unsaturated fatty acids has important implications for health. It is well accepted that saturated fatty acids increase blood levels of cholesterol which promote the fatty plaque build-up in the coronary arteries that can lead eventually to heart disease (see Chapter 12). Unsaturated fatty acids are generally categorized as either monounsaturated or polyunsaturated. Although polyunsaturated fatty acids were favored by nutritional researchers in the early 1980s, today the evidence suggests that polyunsaturated fatty acids may decrease beneficial cholesterol (HDL cholesterol) levels while increasing bad cholesterol (LDL cholesterol) levels (3). In contrast, because monounsaturated fatty acids seem to lower only LDL cholesterol levels, they are thought to be the least harmful of the fatty acids. Figure 7.2 illustrates the relative percentages of each of these fats in the most popular vegetable oils.

A type of unsaturated fatty acid referred to as an **omega-3 fatty acid** has recently gained widespread attention. This fatty acid is reported to lower both blood cholesterol and triglycerides and is found primarily in fresh or frozen mackerel, herring, tuna, and salmon. Note, however, that omega-3 fatty acids are not found in canned fish, because the canning process destroys the

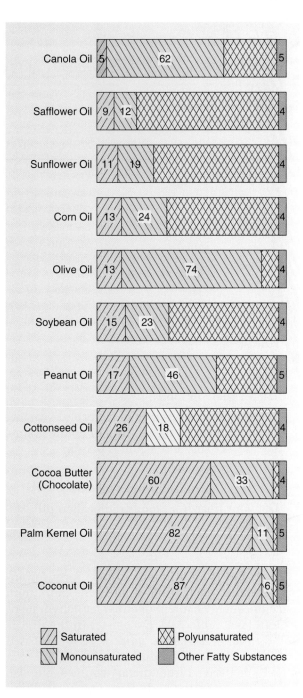

FIGURE 7.2 Percentages of saturated, polyunsaturated, and monounsaturated fats in common vegetable oils. (Source: Donatelle, R. J., and L. G. Davis, 1996. *Access to health.* Copyright © 1996. Reprinted by permission of Allyn & Bacon.)

normal structure of these molecules. Some researchers have argued that one or two servings per week of fish containing omega-3 fatty acids reduces the risk of heart disease (4). This is an exciting possibility, but more research is needed to confirm the claim.

Compound Fats For health considerations, the most important compound fats are the **lipoproteins**. These molecules are combinations of protein, triglycerides, and cholesterol. Although lipoproteins exist in several forms, the two primary types are low-density lipoproteins (LDL cholesterol) and high-density lipoproteins (HDL cholesterol). LDL cholesterol consists of a limited amount of protein and triglycerides but contains large amounts of cholesterol. It is thus associated with promoting the fatty plaque build-up in the arteries of the heart that is the primary cause of heart disease. In contrast, HDLs are primarily composed of protein with limited cholesterol and are associated with a low risk of heart disease. Because of their relationship with heart disease, HDL cholesterol is referred to as "good" cholesterol, and LDL cholesterol is referred to as "bad" cholesterol. We discuss these substances again in Chapter 12.

Derived Fats **Cholesterol** is the best example of the class of fats called **derived fats**. Although cholesterol does not contain fatty acids, it is classified as a fat because, like other fats, it is not water-soluble. Cholesterol is contained in many foods of animal sources, such as meats, shellfish, and dairy products (Table 7.4). Although a diet high in cholesterol increases your risk of heart disease, some cholesterol is essential for normal body function. Indeed, cholesterol is a constituent of cells and is used to manufacture certain types of hormones (e.g., male and female sex hormones).

Protein The primary role of dietary protein is to serve as the structural unit to build and repair body tissues. Proteins are also important for numerous other bodily functions, including the synthesis of enzymes, hormones, and antibodies. These compounds regulate body metabolism and provide protection from disease.

As mentioned earlier, proteins are not usually a major fuel source. Nevertheless, under conditions of low carbohydrate intake (e.g., dieting), proteins can be converted to glucose and used as a fuel. During periods of adequate dietary carbohydrate intake, excess proteins consumed in the diet are converted to fats and stored in adipose tissue as an energy reserve.

Table 7.4

Cholesterol Content of Common Measures of Selected Foods (in ascending order)

Food	Amount	Cholesterol (mg)
Milk, skim	1 cup	4
Mayonnaise	1 T	10
Butter	1 pat	11
Lard	1 T	12
Cottage cheese	1/2 cup	15
Milk, low fat, 2%	1 cup	22
Half and half	1/4 cup	23
Hot dog*	1	29
Ice cream, ~10% fat	1/2 cup	30
Cheese, cheddar	1 oz	30
Milk, whole*	1 cup	34
Oysters, salmon	3 oz	40
Clams, halibut, tuna	3 oz	55
Chicken, turkey	3 oz	70
Beef,* pork,* lobster	3 oz	75
Lamb, crab	3 oz	85
Shrimp	3 oz	125
Heart (beef)	3 oz	164
Egg (yolk)*	1 each	220–275
Liver (beef)	3 oz	410
Kidney	3 oz	587
Brains	3 oz	2637

*Leading contributors of cholesterol to the U.S. diet.

fatty acids The basic structural unit of triglycerides that are important nutritionally, not only because of their energy content, but also because they play a role in cardiovascular disease.

saturated A type of fatty acid that comes primarily from animal sources (meat and dairy products) and is solid at room temperature.

unsaturated A type of fatty acid that comes primarily from plant sources and is liquid at room temperature.

omega-3 fatty acid A type of unsaturated fatty acid that lowers both blood cholesterol and triglycerides and is found primarily in fresh or frozen mackerel, herring, tuna, and salmon.

lipoproteins Combinations of protein, triglycerides, and cholesterol in the blood that are important because of their role in promoting heart disease.

cholesterol A type of derived fat in the body which is necessary for cell and hormone synthesis. Can be acquired through the diet or can be made by the body.

derived fats A class of fats which does not contain fatty acids but are classified as fat because they are not soluble in water.

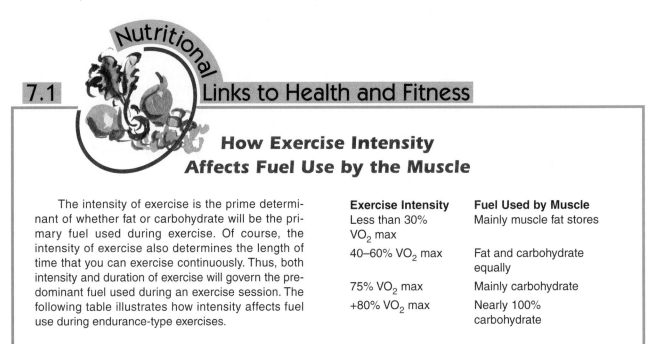

7.1 *Nutritional* Links to Health and Fitness

How Exercise Intensity Affects Fuel Use by the Muscle

The intensity of exercise is the prime determinant of whether fat or carbohydrate will be the primary fuel used during exercise. Of course, the intensity of exercise also determines the length of time that you can exercise continuously. Thus, both intensity and duration of exercise will govern the predominant fuel used during an exercise session. The following table illustrates how intensity affects fuel use during endurance-type exercises.

Exercise Intensity	Fuel Used by Muscle
Less than 30% VO_2 max	Mainly muscle fat stores
40–60% VO_2 max	Fat and carbohydrate equally
75% VO_2 max	Mainly carbohydrate
+80% VO_2 max	Nearly 100% carbohydrate

The basic structural units of proteins are called **amino acids**. Twenty different amino acids exist and can be linked end-to-end in various combinations to create different proteins with unique functions. The body can make 11 of these amino acids; because they are not needed in the diet, they are referred to as **nonessential amino acids**. The remaining nine amino acids are referred to as **essential amino acids** and cannot be manufactured by the body.

Complete proteins contain all of the essential amino acids and are found only in foods of animal origin (meats and dairy products). **Incomplete proteins** are missing one or more of the essential amino acids and can be found in numerous vegetable sources. Therefore, vegetarians must be careful to combine a variety of vegetables in their diet in order to get all of the essential amino acids (Figure 7.3).

The dietary need for protein is greatest during the adolescent years when growth is rapid. During this period, the daily recommended allowance for proteins is 1 gram of protein per kilogram of body weight (3). The recommendation decreases to 0.8 g/kg in women and 0.8 g/kg in men at the end of adolescence (see Figure 7.4). Because the average person in industrialized countries consumes more than enough protein in the diet, the nutritional problem associated with protein intake is one of excess. Protein foods from animal sources are often high in fat (and high in calories), which can lead to an increased risk of heart disease, cancer, and obesity.

FIGURE 7.3 Complementary proteins

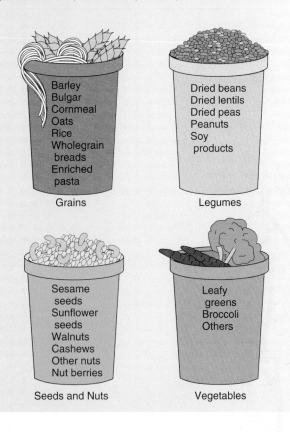

Selecting from *two* or more of these columns will help you use a process known as mutual supplementation, combining two protein-rich foods to form complementary proteins with all of the essential amino acids. These combinations make complete proteins and help us to avoid possible protein deficiencies.

Grains: Barley, Bulgar, Cornmeal, Oats, Rice, Wholegrain breads, Enriched pasta

Legumes: Dried beans, Dried lentils, Dried peas, Peanuts, Soy products

Seeds and Nuts: Sesame seeds, Sunflower seeds, Walnuts, Cashews, Other nuts, Nut berries

Vegetables: Leafy greens, Broccoli, Others

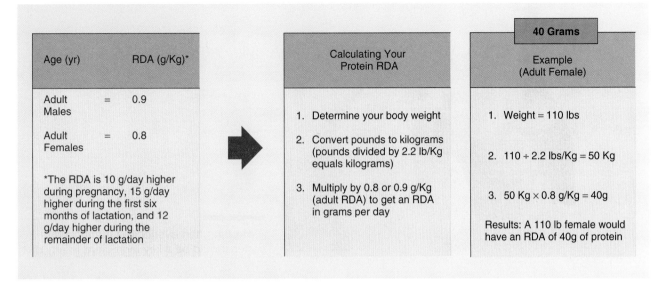

FIGURE 7.4 Estimated daily protein needs for adults. (Source: From Hales, D. R. *An Invitation to Health.* Copyright © 1994, 1992, 1989, 1986, 1983, 1980 by The Benjamin/Cummings Publishing Company, Inc. Reprinted by permission of Brooks/Cole Publishing Company, a division of International Thomson Publishing Inc., Pacific Grove, CA 93950.)

Micronutrients

The category of nutrients referred to as micronutrients consists of vitamins and minerals. Functionally, micronutrients are as important as the macronutrients and are required for sustaining life. Although they do not supply bodily energy, they are essential to the breakdown of the macronutrients.

Vitamins Vitamins are small molecules that play a key role in many bodily functions, including the regulation of growth and metabolism. They are classified according to whether they are soluble in water or fat. The class of vitamins called *water-soluble vitamins* consists of several B complex vitamins and vitamin C. Because they are soluble in body water, these vitamins can be eliminated by the kidneys. The *fat-soluble vitamins* are soluble in fat only and consist of vitamins A, D, E, and K. Because they are stored in body fat, it is possible for these vitamins to accumulate in the body to toxic levels. Table 7.5 on page 161 lists the dietary sources of both water-soluble and fat-soluble vitamins.

Most vitamins cannot be manufactured in the body and must therefore be consumed in the diet. The exceptions to this rule are vitamins A, D, and K, which can be produced by the body in small quantities. Vitamins in food can be destroyed in the process of cooking, so it is best to eat vegetables raw or steamed to retain their maximum nutritional values. Vitamins exist in almost all foods, and a balanced diet supplies all of the vitamins essential to body function.

Recent research indicates a new function for some vitamins and minerals as protectors against tissue damage (3, 5). This has important implications for individuals engaged in an exercise program. This potential new role for micronutrients will be discussed later in this chapter.

amino acids The basic structural unit of proteins. Twenty different amino acids exist and can be linked end to end in various combinations to create different proteins with unique functions.

nonessential amino acids Eleven amino acids that the body can make and are therefore not necessary in the diet.

essential amino acids Amino acids which cannot be manufactured by the body and, therefore, must be consumed in the diet.

complete proteins Contain all the essential amino acids and are found only in foods of animal origin (meats and dairy products).

incomplete proteins Proteins that are missing one or more of the essential amino acids; can be found in numerous vegetable sources.

vitamins Small molecules that play a key role in many bodily functions, including the regulation of growth and metabolism. They are classified according to whether they are soluble in water or fat.

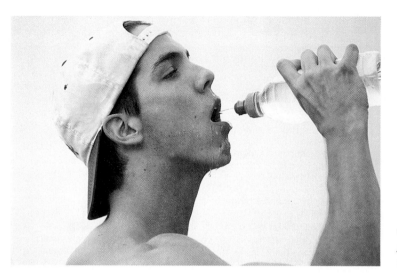

Although often overlooked nutritionally, water should be a key ingredient in any diet.

Minerals Minerals are chemical elements such as sodium and calcium required by the body for normal function. Like vitamins, minerals are contained in many foods and play important roles in regulating key body functions, such as conducting nerve impulses, muscular contraction, enzyme function, and maintenance of water balance. Minerals serve a structural function as well; calcium, phosphorus, and fluoride all are important constituents of bones and teeth.

Table 7.6 on page 163 illustrates the nutritionally important minerals and their functions. Three of the most widely recognized minerals are calcium, iron, and sodium. Calcium is important in its role in bone formation. A deficiency of calcium contributes to the development of the bone disease osteoporosis. A deficiency of dietary iron may lead to iron-deficiency anemia, which results in chronic fatigue. High sodium intake has been associated with hypertension, a major risk factor for heart disease.

Water

Approximately 60% to 70% of the body is water. Because water is involved in all vital processes in the body, it is considered to be the nutrient of greatest concern to the physically active individual. An individual performing heavy exercise in a hot, humid environment can lose 1 to 3 liters of water per hour through sweating (6).

A loss of 5% of body water causes fatigue, weakness, and the inability to concentrate. A loss of 15% can be fatal. Water is important for temperature control of the body, absorption and digestion of foods, formation of blood, and elimination of wastes. Chapter 9 provides guidelines for maintaining proper hydration during exercise training.

Water is contained in almost all foods, especially fruits and vegetables. Combining the water contained in foods and that consumed as beverages, you should consume the equivalent of 8–10 cups of water per day. This does not account for conditions that cause excess fluid loss such as excess sweating, donating blood, diarrhea, or vomiting. Figure 7.5 illustrates how the normal water balance of the body is maintained.

FIGURE 7.5 Daily water intake and output by the body. (Source: Donatelle, R. J. and Davis, L. G., 1996. *Access to health*. Copyright © 1996 by Allyn & Bacon.)

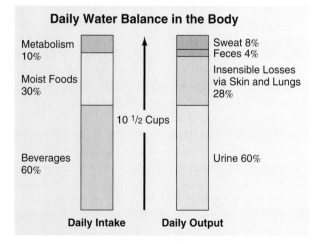

minerals Chemical elements (e.g., sodium and calcium) that are required by the body for normal functioning.

Table 7.5

Vitamins: Where You Get Them and What They Do

Vitamin	Best Sources	Main Roles	Deficiency Symptoms	Risks of Megadoses
Fat Soluble				
A	Liver; eggs; cheese; butter; fortified margarine and milk; yellow, orange, and dark-green vegetables and fruits (e.g., carrots, broccoli, spinach, cantaloupe)	Assists in the formation and maintenance of healthy skin, hair, and mucous membranes; aids in the ability to see in dim light (night vision); needed for proper bone growth, teeth development, and reproduction.	Night blindness; rough skin and mucous membranes; infection of mucous membranes; drying of the eyes; impaired growth of bones and tooth enamel	Blurred vision, loss of appetite, headaches, skin rashes, nausea, diarrhea, hair loss, menstrual irregularities, extreme fatigue, joint pain, liver damage, insomnia, abnormal bone growth, injury to brain and nervous system
D	Fortified milk; egg yolk; liver; tuna: salmon; cod-liver oil. Made on skin in sunlight.	Aids in the formation and maintenance of bones and teeth; assists in the absorption and use of calcium and phosphorus.	In children, rickets; stunted bone growth; bowed legs, malformed teeth, protruding abdomen; in adults, osteomalacia, softening of the bones leading to shortening and fractures, muscle spasms, and twitching	In infants, calcium deposits in kidneys and excessive calcium in blood; in adults, calcium deposits throughout body, deafness, nausea, loss of appetite, kidney stones, fragile bones, high blood pressure, high blood cholesterol
E	Vegetable oils; margarine; wheat germ; whole-grain cereals and bread; liver; dried beans; green leafy vegetables	Aids in the formation of red blood cells, muscles, and other tissues; protects vitamin A and essential fatty acids from oxidation.	Prolonged impairment of fat absorption	None definitely known. Reports of headache, blurred vision, extreme fatigue, muscle weakness; can destroy some vitamin K made in the gut.
K	Green leafy vegetables; cabbage; cauliflower; peas; potatoes; liver; cereals. Except in newborns, made by bacteria in human intestine.	Aids in the synthesis of substances needed for the blood to clot; helps maintain normal bone metabolism.	Hemorrhage, especially in newborn infants	Jaundice in babies; anemia in laboratory animals
Water Soluble				
Thiamin (B₁)	Pork (especially ham); liver; oysters; whole-grain and enriched cereals, pasta, and bread; wheat germ; oatmeal; peas; lima beans	Helps release energy from carbohydrates; aids in the synthesis of an important nervous system chemical.	Beriberi: mental confusion, muscular weakness, swelling of the heart, leg cramps	None known. However, because B vitamins are interdependent, excess of one may produce deficiency of others.
Riboflavin (B₂)	Liver; milk; meat; dark-green vegetables; eggs; whole-grain and enriched cereals, pasta, and bread; dried beans and peas	Helps release energy from carbohydrates, proteins, and fats; aids in the maintenance of mucous membranes.	Skin disorders, especially around nose and lips; cracks at corners of mouth; sensitivity of eyes to light	None known. See Thiamin.

(continued)

Table 7.5

Vitamins: Where You Get Them and What They Do (continued)

Vitamin	Best Sources	Main Roles	Deficiency Symptoms	Risks of Megadoses
Niacin (B_3, nicotinamide, nicotinic acid)	Liver; poultry; meat; fish; eggs; whole-grain and enriched cereals, pasta, and bread; nuts; dried peas and beans	Participates with thiamin and riboflavin in facilitating energy production in cells	Pellagra, skin disorders, diarrhea, mental confusion, irritability, mouth swelling, smooth tongue	Duodenal ulcer, abnormal liver function, elevated blood sugar, excessive uric acid in blood, possibly leading to gout
B_6 (pyridoxine)	Whole-grain (but not enriched) cereals and bread; liver; avocados; spinach; green beans; bananas; fish; poultry meats; nuts; potatoes; green leafy vegetables	Aids in the absorption and metabolism of proteins; helps the body use fats; assists in the formation of red blood cells.	Skin disorders; cracks at corners of mouth; smooth tongue; convulsions; dizziness; nausea; anemia; kidney stones	Dependency on high dose, leading to deficiency symptoms when one returns to normal amounts.
B_{12} (cobalamin)	Only in animal foods; liver; kidneys; meat; fish; eggs; milk; oysters; nutritional yeast	Aids in the formation of red blood cells; assists in the building of genetic material; helps the functioning of the nervous system.	Pernicious anemia, anemia, pale skin and mucous membranes, numbness and tingling in fingers and toes that may progress to loss of balance and weakness and pain in arms and legs	None known.
Folacin (folic acid)	Liver; kidneys; dark-green leafy vegetables; wheat germ; dried beans and peas. Stored in the body, so daily consumption is not crucial.	Acts with B_{12} in synthesizing genetic material; aids in the formation of hemoglobin in red blood cells.	Megaloblastic anemia; enlarged red blood cells, smooth tongue, diarrhea; during pregnancy, deficiency may cause loss of the fetus or fetal abnormalities. Women on oral contraceptives may need extra folacin.	Body stores it, so it is potentially hazardous. Can mask a B_2 deficiency. Diarrhea; insomnia.
C (ascorbic acid)	Citrus fruits; tomatoes; strawberries, melon; green peppers; potatoes; dark-green vegetables	Aids in the formation of collagen; helps maintain capillaries, bones, and teeth; helps protect other vitamins from oxidation; may block formation of cancer-causing nitrosamines.	Scurvy; bleeding gums; degenerating muscles; wounds that don't heal; loose teeth; brown, dry, rough skin. Early symptoms include loss of appetite, irritability, weight loss.	Dependency on high doses, possibly precipitating symptoms of scurvy when withdrawn (especially in infants if megadoses taken during pregnancy); kidney and bladder stones; diarrhea; urinary tract irritation; increased tendency for blood to clot; breakdown of red blood cells in persons with certain common genetic disorders

Source: Reprinted from *Jane Brody's Nutrition Book*, with the permission of W.W. Norton & Company, Inc. Copyright © 1981 by Jane E. Brody.

Table 7.6

Minerals: Where You Get Them and What They Do

Best Sources	Main Roles	Deficiency Symptoms	Risks of Megadoses
Macrominerals			
Calcium			
Milk and milk products; sardines; canned salmon eaten with bones; dark-green, leafy vegetables; citrus fruits; dried beans and peas	Building bones and teeth and maintaining bone strength; muscle contraction; maintaining cell membranes; blood clotting; absorption of B_2; activation of enzymes	In children: distorted bone growth (rickets); in adults: loss of bone (osteoporosis) and increased susceptibility to fractures	Drowsiness; extreme lethargy; impaired absorption of iron, zinc, and manganese; calcium deposits in tissues throughout body, mimicking cancer on X-ray
Phosphorus			
Meat; poultry; fish; eggs, dried beans and peas; milk and milk products; phosphates in processed foods, especially soft drinks	Building bones and teeth; release of energy from carbohydrates, proteins, and fats; formation of genetic material, cell membranes, and many enzymes	Weakness, loss of appetite, malaise, bone pain. Dietary shortages uncommon, but prolonged use of antacids can cause deficiency.	Distortion of calcium-to-phosphorus ratio, creating relative deficiency of calcium
Magnesium			
Green, leafy, vegetables (eaten raw); nuts (especially almonds and cashews); soybeans; seeds; whole grains	Building bones; manufacture of proteins; release of energy from muscle glycogen; conduction of nerve impulse to muscles; adjustment to cold	Muscular twitching and tremors; irregular heartbeat; insomnia; muscle weakness; leg and foot cramps; shaky hands	Disturbed nervous system function because the calcium-to-magnesium ratio is unbalanced; catharsis: hazard to persons with poor kidney function
Potassium			
Orange juice; bananas; dried fruits; meats; bran; peanut butter; dried beans and peas; potatoes; coffee; tea; cocoa	Muscle contraction; maintenance of fluid and electrolyte balance in cells; transmission of nerve impulses; release of energy from carbohydrates, proteins, and fats	Abnormal heart rhythm; muscular weakness; lethargy; kidney and lung failure	Excessive potassium in blood, causing muscular paralysis and abnormal heart rhythms.
Sulfur			
Beef; wheat germ; dried beans and peas; peanuts; clams	In every cell as part of sulfur-containing amino acids; forms bridges between molecules to create firm proteins of hair, nails, and skin.	None known in humans.	Unknown
Chlorine			
Table salt and other naturally occurring salts	Regulation of balance of body fluids and acids and bases; activation of enzyme in saliva; part of stomach acid	Disturbed acid-base balance in body fluids (very rare)	Disturbed acid-base balance

(continued)

Table 7.6

Minerals: Where You Get Them and What They Do (continued)

Trace Minerals

Iron

| Liver; kidneys; red meats; egg yolk; green, leafy vegetables; dried fruits; dried beans and peas; potatoes; black-strap molasses; enriched and whole-grain cereals | Formation of hemoglobin in blood and myoglobin in muscles, which supply oxygen to cells; part of several enzymes and proteins | Anemia, with fatigue, weakness, pallor, and shortness of breath | Toxic buildup in liver, pancreas, and heart |

Copper

| Oysters; nuts; cocoa powder; beef and pork liver; kidneys; dried beans; corn-oil margarine | Formation of red blood cells; part of several respiratory enzymes | In animals: anemia; faulty development of bone and nervous tissue; loss of elasticity in tendons and major arteries; abnormal lung development; abnormal structure and pigmentation of hair | Violent vomiting and diarrhea. Cooking acid foods in unlined copper pots can lead to toxic accumulation of copper. |

Zinc

| Meat; liver; eggs; poultry; seafood; followed by milk and whole grains | Constituent of about 100 enzymes | Delayed wound healing; diminished taste sensation; loss of appetite. In children: failure to grow and mature sexually. Prenatally: abnormal brain development | Nausea, vomiting; anemia; bleeding in stomach; premature birth and stillbirth; abdominal pain; fever. Can aggravate marginal copper deficiency. May produce atherosclerosis. |

Iodine

| Seafood; saltwater fish; seaweed; iodized salt; sea salt | Part of thyroid hormones; essential for normal reproduction | Goiter (enlarged thyroid with low hormone production). Newborns: cretinism, retarded growth, protruding abdomen, swollen features | Not known to be a problem, but could cause iodine poisoning or sensitivity reaction. |

Fluorine

| Fish; tea; most animal foods; fluoridated water; foods grown with or cooked in fluoridated water | Formation of strong, decay-resistant teeth; maintenance of bone strength | Excessive dental decay; possibly osteoporosis | Mottling of teeth and bones; in larger doses, a deadly poison |

Manganese

| Nuts; whole grains; vegetables and fruits; tea; instant coffee; cocoa powder | Functioning of central nervous system; normal bone structure; reproduction; part of important enzymes | None known in human beings. In animals: poor reproduction; retarded growth; birth defects; abnormal bone development | Masklike facial expression; blurred speech; involuntary laughing; spastic gait; hand tremors |

Guidelines for a Healthy Diet

Several national health agencies have suggested guidelines for healthy diets. Although they don't agree on all points, in essence, they do agree on the following, as suggested by the Senate Select Committee on Nutrition and Human Needs (1):

1. Maintain ideal body weight (see chapter 8).
2. Increase the consumption of complex carbohydrates to > 58% of total calories.
3. Reduce fat intake to < 30% of total calories (saturated fat to < 10%).
4. Reduce cholesterol consumption to < 300 mg/day.
5. Reduce simple sugars in the diet.
6. Reduce sodium intake to < 3000 mg/day.

The following sections provide general rules for selection of the macro- and micronutrients to meet the goals of a healthy diet. In addition, we will discuss how to critically analyze your diet using a dietary record.

Nutrients

The general rule for meeting the body's need for macronutrients is that an individual should consume approximately 58% of needed calories from carbohydrates (48% complex carbohydrates and 10% simple sugars), 30% or less in fats (approximately 10% saturated and 20% unsaturated fats), and 12% in proteins (3). Again, the daily protein requirement for adults is approximately 0.8 grams of protein per kilogram (2.2 lbs) of body weight.

To meet the need for micronutrients, the U.S. Council (7) has established guidelines concerning the quantities of each micronutrient required to meet the minimum needs of most individuals. These Recommended Dietary Allowances (RDAs) are contained in Table 7.7.

When you know the recommended daily requirements for nutrients, the key question is, "How do I choose foods to meet these goals?" Previous dietary guidelines suggested choosing foods from four basic food groups. These groups are fruits and vegetables; poultry, fish, meat, and eggs; beans, grains, and nuts; and dairy products. Although these guidelines are still generally acceptable, they do not illustrate the most desirable proportions of different foods. Government health agencies responsible for setting nutritional guidelines (7) have altered their recommendations about how we should choose foods from these groups. Figure 7.6 on page 169 illustrates these latest recommendations for a healthy diet using the "eating-right pyramid."

The use of the eating-right pyramid in forming a diet accomplishes two important goals. First, the relative proportions of foods known to promote disease are minimized. Second, "nutrient dense" foods, that is, foods high in micronutrients per calorie, are maximized. Thus, by following the pyramid approach, you are assured of getting the proper balance of macro- and micronutrients.

Until recently, nutrition labeling provided little help in choosing the right foods. Labels were required on only 60% of packaged foods, making it difficult to follow the RDA guidelines. Further, the terms used on labels were often undefined, poorly organized, and misleading. In 1994, consumer groups and major health organizations prompted the U.S. Food and Drug Administration to adopt a new set of requirements for food labeling. As illustrated in Figure 7.7 on page 170, the labeling system now enables consumers to choose foods based on current, accurate, and easy-to-understand information.

Calories

The number of calories in the diet is a key consideration for developing good eating habits. As mentioned, the problem with most U.S. diets is not the lack of nutrients, but excess caloric consumption. Therefore, monitor your total caloric intake to prevent overconsumption of food energy.

When monitoring your dietary calories, remember these two important points. First, most people consume too many calories from simple sugars. The primary simple sugar in most diets is sucrose (i.e., table sugar). The principal nutritional problem related to simple sugars is that they are not nutrient-dense. In other words, simple sugars contain many calories but few micronutrients. A second concern when determining caloric intake is the amount of fat in the diet. Fat is high in calories, often rich in cholesterol, and contains over twice as many calories as a gram of carbohydrate or protein (1 gram of fat = 9 calories; 1 gram of carbohydrate = 4 calories; and 1 gram of protein = 4 calories). Limiting fat in the diet reduces both the risk of heart disease and excess caloric intake. We will discuss how to determine the optimal caloric intake for a healthy body weight in much greater detail in Chapter 8.

Table 7.7

Recommended Dietary Allowances (Revised 1989)*

Age (years) and Gender	Reference Weight		Height		Protein	Vitamins											Minerals						
						Vitamin A	Thiamin	Riboflavin	Niacin	Vitamin B₆	Folacin	Vitamin B₁₂	Vitamin C	Vitamin D	Vitamin E	Vitamin K	Calcium	Iodine	Iron	Magnesium	Phosphorus	Selenium	Zinc
	kg	lbs	cm	in	g	RE	mg	mg	NE	mg	µg	µg	mg	µg	αTE	µg	mg	µg	mg	mg	mg	µg	mg
Infants																							
0.0–0.5	6	13	60	24	13	375	0.3	0.4	5	0.3	25	0.3	30	7.5	3	5	400	40	6	40	300	10	5
0.5–1.0	9	20	71	28	14	375	0.4	0.5	6	0.3	35	0.5	35	10	4	10	600	50	10	60	500	15	5
Children																							
1–3	13	29	90	35	16	400	0.7	0.8	9	1.0	50	0.7	40	10	6	15	800	70	10	80	800	20	10
4–6	20	44	112	44	24	500	0.9	1.1	12	1.1	75	1.0	45	10	7	20	800	90	10	120	800	20	10
7–10	28	62	132	52	28	700	1.0	1.2	13	1.4	100	1.4	45	10	7	30	800	120	10	170	800	30	10
Males																							
11–14	45	99	157	62	45	1000	1.3	1.5	17	1.7	150	2.0	50	10	10	45	1200	150	12	270	1200	40	15
15–18	66	145	176	69	59	1000	1.5	1.8	20	2.0	200	2.0	60	10	10	65	1200	150	12	400	1200	50	15
19–24	72	160	177	70	58	1000	1.5	1.7	19	2.0	200	2.0	60	10	10	70	1200	150	10	350	1200	70	15
25–50	79	174	176	70	63	1000	1.5	1.7	19	2.0	200	2.0	60	5	10	80	800	150	10	350	800	70	15
51+	77	170	173	68	63	1000	1.2	1.4	15	2.0	200	2.0	60	5	10	80	800	150	10	350	800	70	15

(continued)

Table 7.7

Recommended Dietary Allowances (Revised 1989) * (continued)

Age (years) and Gender	Reference Weight kg	lbs	Height cm	in	Protein g	Vitamins Vitamin A RE	Thiamin mg	Riboflavin mg	Niacin NE	Vitamin B6 mg	Folacin µg	Vitamin B12 µg	Vitamin C mg	Vitamin D µg	Vitamin E αTE	Vitamin K µg	Minerals Calcium mg	Iodine µg	Iron mg	Magnesium mg	Phosphorus mg	Selenium µg	Zinc mg
Females																							
11–14	46	101	157	62	46	800	1.1	1.3	15	1.4	150	2.0	50	10	8	45	1200	150	15	280	1200	45	12
15–18	55	120	163	64	44	800	1.1	1.3	15	1.5	180	2.0	60	10	8	55	1200	150	15	300	1200	50	12
19–24	58	128	164	65	46	800	1.1	1.3	15	1.6	180	2.0	60	10	8	60	1200	150	15	280	1200	55	12
25–50	63	138	163	64	50	800	1.1	1.3	15	1.6	180	2.0	60	5	8	65	800	150	15	280	800	55	12
51+	65	143	160	63	50	800	1.0	1.2	13	1.6	180	2.0	60	5	8	65	800	150	10	280	800	55	12
Pregnant/ Lactating					60	800	1.5	1.6	17	2.2	400	2.2	70	10	10	65	1200	175	30	320	1200	65	15
1st 6 mo					65	1300	1.6	1.8	20	2.1	280	2.6	95	10	12	65	1200	200	15	355	1200	75	19
2nd 6 mo					62	1200	1.6	1.7	20	2.1	260	2.6	90	10	11	65	1200	200	15	340	1200	75	16

*National Academy of Sciences, *Recommended dietary allowances.* 10th rev. ed. Washington D.C.: National Academy Press, 1989.

Definitions: mcg or µg = micrograms; 1000 mcg = 1 mg; 1000 mg = 1 gram; thiamin = vitamin B_1; riboflavin = vitamin B_2; niacin = vitamin B_3; RE (retinol equivalents) = 1 µg vitamin A from animal sources, or 6 µg of vitamin A from B-carotene (plant sources);

vitamin D: 10 µg of vitamin D (as cholecalciferol) = 400 IU (international units); vitamin E: 1 mg of d-α tocopherol = 1 α -TE (TE = tocopherol equivalent); niacin (vitamin B_3); NE (niacin equivalent) is 1 mg of niacin or 60 mg of dietary tryptophan (also referred to as mg-NE).

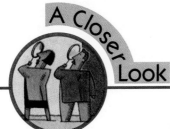

New Guidelines for Dietary Nutrients!

Recommended Dietary Allowances (also known as RDAs) are the daily amounts of the different food nutrients deemed adequate for healthy individuals by the National Academy of Sciences. To account for the differences in people's ability to absorb nutrients, the RDAs are set somewhat higher than the body's actual needs. To date, there are RDAs for protein, 11 vitamins (A, C, D, E, K, thiamin, riboflavin, niacin, B6, folic acid, and B12) and 7 minerals (calcium, iodine, iron, magnesium, phosphorus, selenium, and zinc). The Academy reviews and updates these recommendations every 5 to 10 years (see Table 7.7).

Times have changed. Since nutritional supplementation has become a popular topic of discussion in the last few years, people are now asking questions such as, "What are the minimal amounts of nutrients I need?" and "What are the maximal amounts that are safe?" Recently, the National Academy of Sciences has decided to revamp the reporting system. In August, 1997, they issued the first in a series of new guidelines (Dietary Reference Intakes—DRIs) to address these questions. DRIs were devised as multilevel recommendations that will update and eventually replace the old RDAs. The new DRIs are divided into four separate categories, each of which addresses a different nutritional issue. They are:

- **Recommended Dietary Allowance (RDA):** Unlike their predecessors, these RDAs recommend the amount of nutrient that will meet the needs of almost every healthy person in a specific age and gender group (such as 19- to 30-year-old women). Also, these RDAs are meant to reduce disease risk, not just prevent deficiency.

- **Adequate Intake (AI):** This is a value that is used when the RDA is not known because the scientific data isn't strong enough to come up with a final number, yet there is enough evidence to give a general guideline.

- **Estimated Average Requirement (EAR):** This is a value that is used for evaluating and planning the diets of large groups of people, like the army, not individuals.

- **Tolerable Upper Intake Level (UL):** This value is the maximum amount that a person can take without risking "adverse health effects." Anything above this amount might result in toxic reactions. In most cases, this number refers to total intake of the nutrient—from food, fortified foods, and nutritional supplements.

The nutrients are reported in various groups according to their functions. The following list shows the groupings and examples of the nutrients in each:

- **calcium, phosphorus, magnesium, vitamin D, and fluoride**
- **folate and other B vitamins**
- **antioxidants (e.g., vitamins C and E, selenium)**
- **macronutrients (e.g., protein, fat, carbohydrates)**
- **trace elements (e.g., iron, zinc)**
- **electrolytes and water, and**
- **other food components (e.g., fiber, phytoestrogens)**

Dietary Analysis

From the preceding discussions, it is clear that eating a balanced diet is the key to good nutrition. Now the critical question is, "How do I know if I'm eating a well-balanced diet?" The answer is to perform a dietary analysis by keeping a 3-day record of everything you eat. It is a good idea to include both weekdays and weekends in your record (two weekdays and one weekend day is generally recommended). At the end of each day, look up the nutrient content of each food (see the Appendix) and record this information in the tables provided in Laboratory 7.1. The process of analyzing your diet by hand is often time consuming and can be simplified by using computerized dietary analysis software.

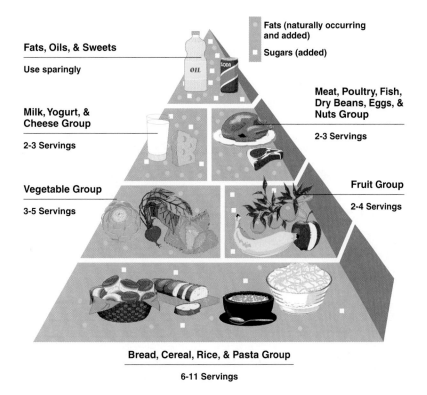

Fats, Oils, & Sweets

Use sparingly

Fats (naturally occurring and added)

Sugars (added)

Milk, Yogurt, & Cheese Group

2-3 Servings

Meat, Poultry, Fish, Dry Beans, Eggs, & Nuts Group

2-3 Servings

Vegetable Group

3-5 Servings

Fruit Group

2-4 Servings

Bread, Cereal, Rice, & Pasta Group

6-11 Servings

FIGURE 7.6 The eating right pyramid. The basic diet should consist primarily of those foods on the lower two tiers of the pyramid, with decreasing amounts of foods from the top. (Source: Donatelle, R. J., and L. G. Davis, 1996. *Access to health.* Copyright © 1996. Reprinted by permission of Allyn & Bacon.)

When you have recorded the nutritive values for each day of your 3-day record, compare your average nutrient intake with the recommended dietary allowances for your age and gender (Laboratory 7.1). These results will provide you with a good index of your dietary strengths and limitations. If you find your diet to be deficient in any macro- or micronutrient (compared with RDA values), you should modify your diet to include foods that will provide adequate amounts of the missing nutrient. In contrast, if you find your diet to be excessive in any macro- or micronutrient, modify it to reduce the values to those suggested elsewhere in this chapter.

A careful and honest dietary analysis is a critical step in modifying a poor diet and planning a well-balanced one. It is also an eye-opening experience, because most of us are not aware of the nutrient contents of common foods. After performing a 3-day dietary analysis, many people are surprised by their high fat intake. The average U.S. diet contains approximately 42% fat (% of total calories), which is well above the recommended 30% (see Figure 7.1). As mentioned earlier, a high fat intake results in an increased risk of disease and obesity.

Family and cultural influences often dictate the foods we choose.

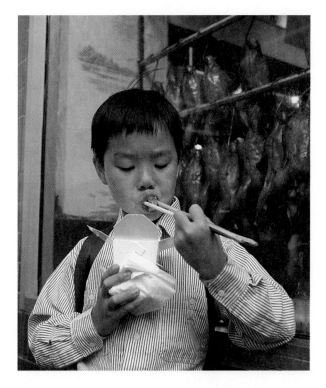

THE NEW LABEL

1 — **Nutrition labeling** is now required on nearly all foods regulated by the FDA (exceptions include spices, foods prepared in retail stores, and restaurant foods). Foods regulated by the USDA, including meat and poultry, are *not* covered. Nutritional data for fresh fruits and vegetables will be described on the shelf in booklets.

2 — **Serving size.** Now requires uniformity of serving size, based on a commonly consumed portion as determined by the FDA.

3 — **New data:** Amount of saturated fat, fiber, and cholesterol, plus calories from fat. Also, % Daily Value gives you the % of total daily needs of each nutrient based on a 2000-calorie diet.

4 — The most critical vitamins and minerals are listed with the % of daily values of each. Optional listings are thiamin, riboflavin, and niacin.

5 — **Health claims.** These must be supported by "significant agreement" about scientific evidence (this may be tricky to judge). Claims are permitted in these well-established areas: fiber may reduce the risk of colon cancer and heart disease; low fat may reduce the risk of heart disease and cancer; low salt may reduce the risk of high blood pressure; calcium may help prevent osteoporosis. Model messages for claims will be developed by the U.S. Public Health Service.

6 — Formal definitions for such labeling terms as "low-fat" and "high-fiber" have now been developed.

1

2

Nutrition Facts

Serving size 1/2 cup (91g)
Servings Per Container 5

Amount Per Serving

Calories 58	Calories from Fat 0

3

	% **Daily Value***
Total Fat 0g	0%
Saturated Fat 0g	0%
Cholesterol 0mg	0%
Sodium 45mg	2%
Total Carbohydrate 12g	4%
Dietary Fiber 3g	12%
Sugars 3g	
Protein 3g	

Vitamin A	92%	•	Vitamin C	16%
Calcium	2%	•	Iron	5%

4

*Percent Daily Values are based on a 2,000 calorie diet. Your daily values may be higher or lower depending on your calorie needs:

	Calories	2,000	2,500
Total Fat	Less than	65g	80g
Sat fat	Less than	20g	25g
Cholesterol	Less than	300mg	300mg
Sodium	Less than	2,400mg	2,400mg
Total Carbohydrate		300g	375g
Fiber		25g	30g

Calories per gram:
Fat 9   •   Carbohydrates 4   •   Protein 4

Many factors affect cancer risk. ————— 5
Eating a diet low in fat and high in fiber may lower risk of this disease.

• GOOD SOURCE OF FIBER ————— 6
• LOWFAT

FIGURE 7.7 The food labeling system. Food labels now required by the federal government list both the total amount and % daily value of the nutrients shown on the sample label. Note that the % daily values are based on a 2000-calorie diet. (Source: Donatelle, R. J., and L. G. Davis, 1996. *Access to health.* Copyright © 1996. Reprinted by permission of Allyn & Bacon.)

Thus, in dietary analysis, the most likely deficiency you will encounter is too few micronutrients in your diet. The most likely problem of excess you may encounter is overconsumption of fat, simple sugars, and calories. Remember, by following the eating-right pyramid and counting calories, you can protect your diet against these common pitfalls.

Foods to Avoid

Now that we have outlined the macro- and micronutrients that should be included in your diet, remember that there are several foods that should be minimized in order to maintain a healthy diet. Even if you do not have the health problems that will be discussed next, determine whether close relatives have these problems. If they do, you may be a prime candidate for developing the problem later in life if you do not change your eating habits now.

First and foremost on the list of foods to avoid are those with a high fat content. Both saturated and unsaturated fats are linked to heart disease, obesity, and certain cancers. In addition, it is often overlooked that dietary fat contributes more to body fat than does protein or carbohydrate (8). Table 7.8 provides guidelines to help you cut fat intake from your diet.

Although cholesterol is a substance that the body needs to function properly, too much contributes to heart disease. Lowering blood cholesterol by dietary modifications can lower your risk of heart disease. Improvement in one's coronary heart disease risk is closely related to a decrease in dietary cholesterol, and a 1% reduction in cholesterol results in a 2% reduction in risk (see Chapter 12). The new food labeling system will help identify foods high in cholesterol; however, some unlabeled foods may surprise you with their cholesterol content. Many foods that are high in cholesterol are also high in fat. Table 7.9 on page 172 will help you determine your cholesterol/saturated fat index in order to rate the cardiovascular risks of certain foods.

Although salt (sodium chloride) is a necessary micronutrient, the body's daily requirement is small (less than 1/4 of a teaspoon). For very active people who perspire a great deal, this need may increase to over 1.5 teaspoons/day. To put this into perspective, the average diet in the United States ranges from 3 to 10 teaspoons/day! Most people are totally unaware of the amount of salt in some foods. Figure 7.8 on page 174 illustrates the "hidden" salt in an average pizza.

An excess of salt should be avoided because it is a complicating factor in people with high blood pressure. In countries where salt is not added to foods, during cooking or at the table, high blood pressure is virtually unknown. Thus, even if you don't already have high blood pressure, you should limit salt in your diet to only the minimal daily requirements (see A Closer Look 7.3).

It has been estimated that the average U.S. citizen consumes half of their dietary intake of carbohydrates in the form of simple sugars as sucrose (table sugar) and corn syrup (commercial sweetener)(3). This represents more than 80 pounds of table sugar and 45 pounds of corn syrup per person each year! Sucrose and corn syrup are used to make cakes, candies, and ice cream, as well as to sweeten beverages, cereals, and other foods. Although overconsumption of these simple sugars has been linked to health problems—from hyperactivity in children to diabetes—there is little evidence to support these claims. There are, however, several effects from overconsumption of these simple sugars which

---

Table 7.8

Guidelines for Cutting Fat from the Diet

Read food labels. Keep in mind that 30% or less of total calories should come from fat and that no more than 10% should be saturated fat.

Many foods are now fat-free or low in fat and should be chosen over high-fat foods.

For baking and sautéing, choose vegetable oils, such as olive oil, that do not raise cholesterol levels.

Choose margarines with the lowest levels of *trans-fatty acids.*

Choose only lean meats, fish, and poultry. Always remove the skin before eating, and bake or broil meats whenever possible. Meats that are the most well-done have fewer calories and are less likely to cause food poisoning. Drain off all oils from meats after cooking.

Eliminate most cold cuts from your diet (i.e., bacon, sausage, hot dogs, etc.). Beware of meat products claiming "95% fat-free," because they may still have a high fat content.

Select nonfat dairy products whenever possible. Part skim milk cheeses such as mozzarella, farmer's, lappi, and ricotta are the best choices.

Substitute other products for butter, margarine, oils, sour cream, mayonnaise, and salad dressings when cooking. Chicken broths, wine, vinegar, and low-calorie dressings make good flavorings and/or cooking ingredients.

Think of food intake as an average over a day or couple of days. A high-fat breakfast can be offset by a low-fat lunch or dinner.

Table 7.9

The Cholesterol/Saturated Fat Index: Which Foods Promote Cardiovascular Disease?

The cholesterol/saturated fat index (CSI) compares the saturated fat in foods with the amount of cholesterol. The value indicated for each food gives the relative contribution of that food to promoting cardiovascular disease. The lower the saturated fat and cholesterol, the lower the CSI. For example, fruits and vegetables have a CSI of zero (the best). A food that is high in cholesterol, but low in saturated fat, would have an intermediate CSI value. Shrimp, for example, would have a CSI of 6 with 182 mg of cholesterol but virtually no saturated fat. In contrast, lean hamburger, with approximately 95 mg of cholesterol and 6.3 grams of fat, would have a CSI of 10 and carry a greater risk for promoting cardiovascular disease. For a healthy diet, the total daily CSI should range from 22 to 50, depending on the caloric content of your diet (22 for a 1200 calorie diet; 50 for a 2800 calorie diet).

	Cholesterol (mg)	Saturated Fat (g)	CSI
Fish, shellfish, cooked (3.5 oz)			
Sole	50	3	4
Salmon	74	1.5	5
Shrimp, crab, lobster	182	0.2	6
Poultry, no skin (3.5 oz.)	84.7	1	6
Beef, pork, lamb (3.5 oz.)			
15% fat (ground round)	94.6	6.3	10
30% fat (ground beef)	88.6	11.4	18
Cheeses (3.5 oz)			
1–2% fat (low-fat, cottage cheese)	7.9	1.2	1
5–10% fat (cottage cheese)	15.1	2.8	6
32–38% fat (cheddar, cream cheese)	104.7	20.9	26
Eggs			
Whites (3)	0	0	0
Whole (1)	246	2.41	15
Fats (1/4 cup, 4 tablespoons, or 55 g)			
Most vegetable oils	0	7	8
Soft vegetable margarines	0	7.8	10
Stick margarines	0	8.5	15
Butter	124	28.7	37
Frozen desserts (1 serving)			
Frozen low-fat yogurt	*	*	2
Ice milk	13.6	2.4	6
Ice cream (10% fat)	60.6	9	13
Specialty ice cream (22% fat)	*	*	34

*Varies according to brand.

Source: Adapted with permission of Simon & Schuster Inc. from *The New American Diet* by Sonja L. Connor, M.S., R.D. and William E. Connor, M.D. Copyright © 1986 by Sonja L. Connor, M.S., R.D. and William E. Connor, M.D.

should be avoided. First, the amount of sugar in sweets adds a tremendous amount of calories to the diet. This leads to obesity, which contributes to many health problems (e.g., diabetes). In addition, calories from sweets are considered "empty" calories because they provide little of the micronutrients necessary for the body to metabolize the macronutrients. Thus, complex carbohydrates are preferred because they are "saturated" with micronutrients. Second, sugar in sweets also leads to tooth decay. Although brushing your teeth after eating sweets can prevent this problem, it will not solve the other problems of over-consumption of sugar. One way of avoiding

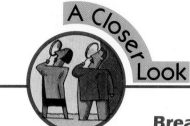

A Closer Look

7.3

Breaking the Salt Habit

Check labels on food to determine the salt content of the foods you buy. You may be surprised to find salt in many of the foods you eat. By buying foods low in salt and eliminating the use of salt as seasoning in cooking and at the table, you can easily lower your salt intake to fewer than 3000 mg/day. Use the following tips to help you eliminate salt from your diet.

- Always taste food before salting.

- Check labels of processed foods for sodium content.

- Flavor cooking water with a bay leaf instead of salt.

- Use onion or garlic powder, not onion salt or garlic salt.

- Substitute pepper, lemon, herbs, or spices as food flavorings.

- Choose fresh fruits and vegetables, rather than canned or frozen, whenever possible.

---

sucrose in the diet is to use fructose as a sweetener. Fructose is twice as sweet as sucrose, so you get equal sweetness for fewer calories.

Like table sugar, alcohol provides empty calories. In addition, chronic alcohol consumption tends to deplete the body's stores of some vitamins, which could lead to severe deficiencies. Thus, if for no other reason, alcohol consumption should be limited because of its addition of empty calories to your diet. Table 7.10 lists those foods that, because of their content of the aforementioned nutrients, should be minimized or avoided in your diet.

Your New Diet

Now that we have presented the guidelines for a healthy diet, let's put these principles into practice and illustrate how to construct a new diet. Refer to Table 7.11 on page 176 as we discuss the steps for choosing the right foods. Table 7.11 presents both a sample of a healthy diet and how each of the foods meets the guidelines that have been presented. Let's construct a 1-day diet for a college-age woman weighing 110 pounds. Thus, our projected daily caloric need, assuming light daily activities, should be approximately 1690 calories. For your use of this diet plan, adjust the quantities accordingly.

Because the diet should consist of mainly complex carbohydrates, let's start each meal with a selection of food from the lower two levels of the eating right pyramid. This will provide mainly carbohydrates, which should be >58% of the total caloric intake, or 980 calories. These calories may be spread out over the day in any proportion you choose. We will use foods from the upper two levels of the pyramid to "fill in" where certain nutrients are needed.

Breakfast. Our subject first chooses a banana, a cup of milk, yogurt, and a cup of apple juice, which provide plenty of complex carbohydrates from fruits and dairy products. The bran flakes add lots of vitamin A and iron. The grapefruit adds plenty of vitamin C.

Lunch. Our subject can't resist a slice of pizza for lunch and gets approximately one-fourth of her daily salt, fat, and cholesterol. This is not as bad as it may seem if consumed in small quantities. She also gets protein, complex carbohydrates, and some micronutrients. The lunch also consists of a turkey sandwich, which adds considerably to the salt load but also adds other needed nutrients. The carrots add considerably to the vitamin A and C totals. In addition, low-fat milk gives more of the much needed calcium.

Dinner. Any nutritional needs that are not met during the day should be met at dinner. The fish provides a low-fat source of high protein as well as calcium, which is so important for our subject. This dinner provides an excellent example of how foods such as margarine and diet cola provide so little nutrient value. The margarine provides mainly fat and calories, and the cola provides only sodium.

Special Dietary Considerations

There are several conditions that require special dietary considerations, especially as they pertain to people who lead an active lifestyle. Following is a list of nutrients that may need to be supplemented, depending on need.

Vitamins As mentioned previously, healthy people who eat a balanced diet generally do not need vitamin supplements. Some individuals, however, may not be getting proper nutrition because of poor diet or disease. Therefore, the following people may find a multivitamin supplement helpful:

- strict vegetarians
- people with chronic illnesses that depress appetite or the absorption of nutrients
- people on medications that affect appetite or digestion
- athletes engaged in a rigorous training program
- pregnant women or women who are breast-feeding infants
- individuals on prolonged low-calorie diets
- the elderly

Iron Iron is an essential component of red blood cells which carry oxygen to all our tissues for energy production. A deficiency of iron can result in a decreased oxygen transport to tissues and thus an energy crisis. Getting enough iron is a major problem for women who are menstruating, pregnant, or nursing. Indeed, only one-half of all women of child-bearing age get the necessary 15 mg of iron per day (3). Five percent suffer from iron-deficiency anemia! Although these individuals should not take iron supplements unless their physician prescribes them, they can modify their diets to assure getting the RDA of iron. To meet this requirement, the following dietary modifications should be undertaken:

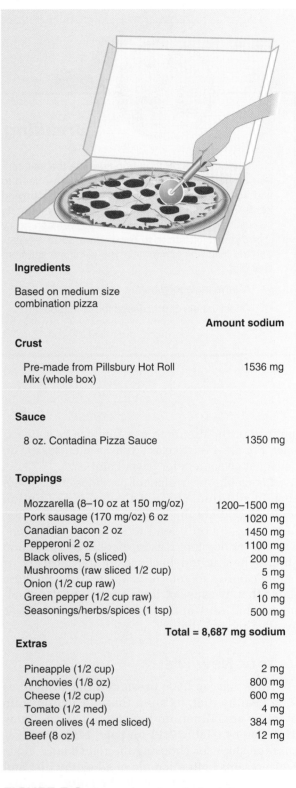

Ingredients

Based on medium size
combination pizza

	Amount sodium
Crust	
Pre-made from Pillsbury Hot Roll Mix (whole box)	1536 mg
Sauce	
8 oz. Contadina Pizza Sauce	1350 mg
Toppings	
Mozzarella (8–10 oz at 150 mg/oz)	1200–1500 mg
Pork sausage (170 mg/oz) 6 oz	1020 mg
Canadian bacon 2 oz	1450 mg
Pepperoni 2 oz	1100 mg
Black olives, 5 (sliced)	200 mg
Mushrooms (raw sliced 1/2 cup)	5 mg
Onion (1/2 cup raw)	6 mg
Green pepper (1/2 cup raw)	10 mg
Seasonings/herbs/spices (1 tsp)	500 mg
Total = 8,687 mg sodium	
Extras	
Pineapple (1/2 cup)	2 mg
Anchovies (1/8 oz)	800 mg
Cheese (1/2 cup)	600 mg
Tomato (1/2 med)	4 mg
Green olives (4 med sliced)	384 mg
Beef (8 oz)	12 mg

FIGURE 7.8 Some of our favorite foods have "hidden" salt. (Source: Donatelle, R. J., and L. G. Davis, 1993. *Access to health.* Copyright © 1993. Reprinted by permission of Allyn & Bacon.)

Table 7.10

Foods to Minimize for a Healthy Diet*

| | Ingredient | | | |
Food	Fat	Cholesterol	Salt	Sugar
Cakes, pies and cookies	X	?		X
Candy	?	?		X
Cheese	X	X		
Cooking oils	X			
Eggs	X	X		
Fish		?		
French fries	X	?	X	
Granola	X			
Ice cream	X	X		X
Potato chips	X	?	X	
Meat	X	X		
Salad dressings	X	X		
Shellfish		X		
Soft drinks				X
Whole milk	X	X		

*See Appendix for nutritional contents of various fast foods.
X indicates that this ingredient is present in above-average amounts in these foods.
? indicates ingredient may be present in excess in some foods in this category.

- Eat vegetables and carbohydrates high in iron: legumes, fresh fruits, whole-grain cereals, and broccoli.
- Also eat foods high in vitamin C; vitamin C helps iron absorption.
- Eat lean red meats high in iron at least two or three times per week.
- Eat iron-rich organ meats, such as liver, once or twice per month.
- Don't drink tea with your meals; it interferes with iron absorption.

Calcium Calcium, the most abundant mineral in the body, is essential for building bones and teeth, as well as normal nerve and muscle function. Adequate calcium is especially important for pregnant or nursing women. There is some evidence that calcium may help in the prevention of colon cancer (9).

The RDAs call for an intake of 1200 mg of calcium for both sexes from ages 11 to 24. Adequate calcium during these years may be crucial in preventing osteoporosis in later years. Osteoporosis

strikes one of every four women over the age of 60 (9). The RDA for adults over age 24 is 800 mg. This amount has been shown to maintain strong bones and prevent fractures. However, some research suggests that women at high risk of osteoporosis should consume 1000 to 1500 mg/day (3). The following tips may help in adding calcium to your diet.

- Add dairy products to your diet, but remember, choose those low in fat.
- Choose other calcium-rich alternatives, such as canned fish (packed in water), turnip and mustard greens, and broccoli.
- Eat foods rich in vitamin C to boost absorption of calcium.
- Use an acidic dressing, made with citrus juices or vinegar, to enhance calcium absorption from salad greens.
- If you can't get enough calcium in the foods you like, add a supplement. Beware, however, of those made with dolomite or bone meal; they may be contaminated with lead.

Table 7.11

Sample Diet for a College-Age Female Weighing 110 Pounds, Assuming Light Daily Activities

	kcal	Fat (g)	Sat. Fat (g)	Chol. (mg)	Sod. (mg)	CHO (g)	Pro (g)	Vit A (RE)	Vit C (mg)	Ca (mg)	Iron (mg)
Breakfast											
1/2 grapefruit	38	0.1	0.02	0	0	9.7	0.8	2	41.3	14	0.1
2/3 cup bran flakes	90	0	0	0	220	18	3	380	1.2	20	18
1 cup whole milk	150	8.2	5.1	33	120	11.4	8	65	2.3	291	0.1
1 cup lowfat yogurt	225	2.6	1.7	10	121	42	9	20	1.4	314	0.1
1 banana	105	0.6	0.2	0	1	26.7	1.2	35	10.3	7	0.4
1 cup apple juice	92	0.5	0.02	0	1	24	0.3	24	7.8	16	1.4
Lunch											
Turkey sandwich with mustard	171	3.7	0.7	9	784	25	9.4	0	0	78	2.2
1 slice pizza	327	10.3	4.6	51	643	44	17	48	14	150	2
1 cup carrots (raw)	48	0.2	0.04	0	38	11.2	1.1	1400	10.2	30	0.54
1 cup low-fat milk	102	2.6	1.6	10	123	11.7	8	38	2.4	300	0.1
Dinner											
Baked fish with mushrooms (3 oz)	112	1.9	0.3	46	83	1.6	21	2	5.5	120	1.4
Baked potato	116	0.14	0.04	0	7	27	2.3	0	10	10	0.4
2 tsp margarine	100	11.4	2.1	0	150	0	0	32	0.02	3.75	0
3 slices tomato	12	0.15	0.02	0	5	2.4	0.5	62	11	3.9	0.3
1 diet cola	1	0	0	0	63	0.2	0	0	0	0	0.1
TOTALS	1689	42	16	159	2359	255	81.6	2108	117	1358	27
RDA	1690	<30%	<10%	<300	<3000	>58%	40	1000	60	1200	15
% of RDA	100	76	90	53	79	105	204	210	196	114	175

Abbreviations: Sat. Fat, saturated fat; Chol., cholesterol; Sod., sodium; CHO, carbohydrate; Pro., protein; RE, retinol equivalents; Ca, calcium.

Nutritional Aspects of Physical Fitness

The number of myths about physical fitness and nutrition increases every year. Radio, T.V., newspaper, and magazine advertisements create a never-ending source of fallacies. Successful athletes are often viewed as experts by the public, and their endorsements of various nutritional products are an attempt to convince the public that a particular food or beverage is responsible for their success. Even though most of the claims made in commercial endorsements are not supported by research, the claims are so highly publicized that they become accepted as fact. The truth is, there are no miracle foods to improve physical fitness or exercise performance. In the paragraphs that follow, we discuss the specific needs of individuals engaging in a regular exercise program.

Carbohydrates

The increased energy expenditure during exercise creates a greater demand for fuel. Recall that the primary fuels used to provide energy for exercise are carbohydrates and fat. Because even very lean people have a large amount of energy stored as fat, lack of fat for fuel is not a problem during exercise. In contrast, the carbohydrate stores in the liver and muscles can reach critically low levels during intense or prolonged exercise (6) (Figure 7.9).

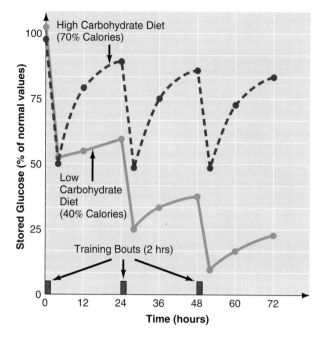

FIGURE 7.9 The importance of a high carbohydrate diet during exercise training. Stored glucose in the muscle (glycogen) is depleted with daily exercise training and a low carbohydrate diet (**solid line**). If a high carbohydrate diet is consumed (**dashed line**), glycogen levels are maintained at near normal levels. (Source: Neiman, David C. *Fitness and sports medicine: An introduction.* Bull Publishing, Palo Alto, CA, 1995. Used with permission.)

Because carbohydrates play a critical role in providing fuel during exercise, some exercise scientists have suggested that people participating in daily exercise programs should increase the complex carbohydrates in their diet from 58% to 70% of the total calories consumed (fat intake is then reduced to 18% of total caloric intake)(10). If exercise is intense, carbohydrates can be depleted from the liver and muscles, and the result is fatigue. The intensity of the exercise dictates whether carbohydrates or fat is the predominant source of energy production (6, 11).

Manufacturers of sweets have perpetrated the notion that candy can give you a quick burst of energy when needed. Does a candy bar consumed prior to exercise provide a quick burst of energy? The answer is "no." In fact, there are at least two potential problems with this type of carbohydrate consumption. First, simple sugar in the form of sweets contains only minimal amounts of the micronutrients necessary for energy production. Second, if candy is consumed prior to exercise, the resulting rapid rise in blood glucose will promote hormonal changes that reduce blood glucose levels below normal and can create a feeling of fatigue. In this case, the effect is opposite of the one intended. Increasing the percentage of complex carbohydrates in the diet and maintaining sufficient caloric intake can ensure that adequate supplies of energy from carbohydrates are stored in the muscles and the liver to meet the needs of a rigorous exercise training program.

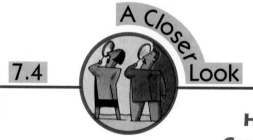

7.4 — A Closer Look

How to Control Cravings for Sweets

The following guidelines will help in your quest to control your sweet tooth.

- Know how to spot sugar. When you see terms such as *sucrose, glucose, maltose, dextrose, fructose,* or *corn syrup* on food labels, beware. These are all forms of sugar.

- If sugar or its "pseudos" are in the first three ingredients on a label, avoid the product. It has a high sugar content by weight.

- Cut back on all sugars, including honey and brown sugar as well as white sugar.

- Eat graham crackers, yogurt, fresh fruits, popcorn, and other healthy substitutes for high-sugar sweets when you have the munchies.

- Buy cereals that do not have sugars listed among their top ingredients. Shredded Wheat, Cheerios, and oatmeal are among the best choices.

- When baking, try cutting the sugar in recipes by one-fourth or more and substitute fruit juices for sweetness or use spices such as cinnamon, anise, ginger, and nutmeg for flavorings.

- If you can't resist sweets, at least eat foods that give you some nutritional value. For example, put bananas on your oatmeal rather than brown sugar; make oatmeal cookies rather than sugar cookies.

Source: Boyle, M., and G. Zyla. *Personal nutrition.* West Publishers, St. Paul, MN, 1991.

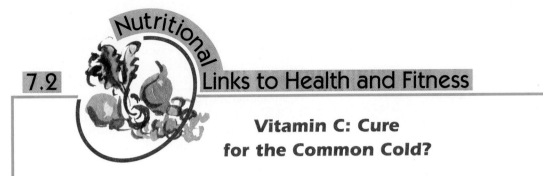

Vitamin C: Cure for the Common Cold?

Vitamin C (also called ascorbic acid), probably the best-known vitamin in the world, has been proclaimed by some individuals to prevent colds. However, to date, the studies that have examined this possibility have found that vitamin C may be beneficial in reducing the severity of cold symptoms but not in preventing or curing a cold. Vitamin C is a great stimulator of white cells in the immune system. In fact, one researcher has said, "Unless the white blood cells are saturated with ascorbic acid, they are like soldiers without bullets."

Foods that are high in vitamin C are citrus fruits, tomatoes, potatoes, greens, raw cabbage, peppers, and melon. These foods may be good food choices during a cold to decrease the symptoms and the period of sickness. Remember that no one food is ideal, and eating a wide variety of foods is a good idea.

Increased intake of vitamin C is recommended for stressful situations and periods of increased exposure to cold and flu viruses. Conditions such as fatigue, trauma, and air pollution are common stressful conditions that can lower the body's resistance. The RDA for vitamin C ranges from 30 mg/day in infants to 90 mg/day in pregnant women. Some researchers, such as Nobel Laureate Dr. Linus Pauling, have suggested that several grams per day may be necessary to be effective in combating cold viruses. The exact amount needed to be effective is not known.

In summary, although vitamin C will not prevent you from getting a cold, it is effective in reducing the severity and length of colds. Make sure your diet contains the RDA of vitamin C. If you don't get your daily allowance in your foods, use a vitamin supplement to get the necessary amount.

Protein

Another common myth among individuals involved in strength training programs is that additional amounts of protein are necessary to promote muscular growth. In fact, many body-builders consume large quantities of protein to supplement their normal dietary protein. Research has shown that the protein requirements of most body-builders is met by a normal, well-balanced diet (12, 13). Therefore, the increased caloric needs of an individual engaged in a strength training program should come from additional amounts of food from the eating right pyramid and not from simply additional protein. In this way, not only are the extra macronutrients supplied, but also the micronutrients necessary for energy production.

Vitamins

Some vitamin manufacturers have argued that megadoses of vitamins can improve exercise performance (5). This belief is based on the notion that exercise increases the need for energy and, because vitamins are necessary for the breakdown of foods for energy, an extra loading of vitamins should be helpful. There is no evidence to support this claim (14). The energy supplied for muscle contraction is not enhanced by vitamin supplements. In fact, megadoses of vitamins may interfere with the delicate balance of other micronutrients and can be toxic as well (3).

Antioxidants

Although large doses of vitamins may be counterproductive, recent research has discovered a new function for some vitamins and other micronutrients (3). These vitamins and micronutrients provide cellular protection by working as antioxidants. **Antioxidants** are chemicals that prevent a damaging form of oxygen (called *oxygen free radicals*) from causing damage to the cells. Although free radicals are constantly produced by the body, excess production of these has been implicated in cancer, lung disease, heart disease, and even the aging process (15). If cellular antioxidants can combine with the free radicals as they are produced, the free radicals become neutralized before they cause damage. Therefore, increasing the level of cellular antioxidants may be beneficial to health. Several of the micronutrients have been identified as potent antioxidants; these antioxidants are vitamins A, E, and C, beta-carotene, zinc, and selenium.

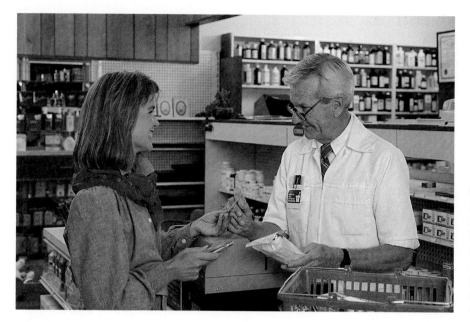

Many special considerations such as age, gender, size, and activity must be assessed in determining vitamin requirements. Consult your pharmacist or a registered dietician when considering any dietary supplementation.

Current Topics in Food Safety

There are many aspects of nutrition, such as food safety, that indicate significant effects on health. In recent years there have been increased reports of illness and death due to improperly stored and prepared foods. Let's examine some of the latest suggestions for improving food safety.

Foodborne Infections

According to the Institute of Food Technologists, approximately 80 million cases of foodborne bacterial disease occur each year. These illnesses produce nausea, vomiting, and diarrhea from 12 hours to 5 days after infection (17). The severity of the illness depends on the microorganism ingested and the victim's overall health. Indeed, they can be fatal in people with compromised immune systems or those in ill health.

One of the most common types of food poisoning is caused by the bacterium *Salmonella*. It is usually found on undercooked chicken, eggs, and processed meats. A relatively uncommon but sometimes fatal form of food poisoning is *botulism*, which is usually found with improper home-canning procedures. Use the following guidelines for preventing food poisoning:

- Clean food thoroughly. Wash all produce and raw meats and make sure cans show no sign of leaks or bulges.

- Drink only pasteurized milk.
- Don't eat raw eggs.
- Cook chicken thoroughly.
- Cook pork to an internal temperature of 170°F to kill parasites called Trichina.
- Cook all shellfish thoroughly; steaming them open may not be sufficient.
- Be wary of raw fish; it may contain parasitic roundworms. Keep fish frozen and cook until well done.
- Wash utensils, plates, cutting boards, knives, blenders, and other cooking equipment with soap and very hot water after preparing raw poultry.

Food Additives

Food additives are used to lengthen storage time, change the taste, alter the color, or make modifications that make it more appealing. They provide benefits such as preventing discoloration

antioxidants Chemicals that prevent a damaging form of oxygen (called *oxygen free radicals*) from causing destruction to the cells. Although free radicals are constantly produced by the body, excess production of these compounds has been implicated in cancer, lung disease, heart disease, and even the aging process.

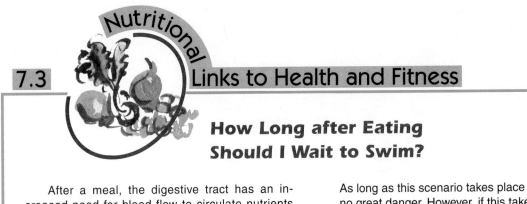

7.3 Nutritional Links to Health and Fitness

How Long after Eating Should I Wait to Swim?

After a meal, the digestive tract has an increased need for blood flow to circulate nutrients throughout the body. Likewise, exercising muscles have a great need for blood to deliver oxygen and remove waste products. Therefore, if you exercise strenuously after a meal, the muscles are in competition with the digestive tract for blood. If the exercise is strenuous and prolonged, and robs the digestive tract of blood, you may become nauseated and sick. In these cases, stop exercising or lower the intensity.

As long as this scenario takes place on land, there is no great danger. However, if this takes place in water (especially deep water), drowning may result. Thus, although playing in a shallow swimming pool after a meal may not present a great danger, swimming in deep water can be life threatening. As a rule of thumb, wait at least 2 hours after a meal before swimming in deep water. Even then, never swim alone, and make sure emergency rescue equipment is available.

and enhancing flavor, but may also pose a risk. One example is nitrites, which are found in foods such as bacon, sausages, and lunch meats. Nitrites inhibit spoilage and prevent botulism but also form cancer-causing agents (nitrosamines) in the body.

Organically Grown Foods

Each year, over one million pounds of commercial pesticides are used in the United States. Although these chemicals are necessary to save crops from disease and pests, they may also endanger human health. In recent years, many people have begun to purchase organically grown foods. **Organic** refers to foods that are grown without the use of pesticides. Organically grown foods are more expensive than foods commonly supplied by supermarkets, and many have been found to contain significant levels of pesticides. Thus, beware of foods labeled "organically grown." Check with the vendor to validate the claim!

In the near future, look for new genetics techniques in biology to spawn a new world of pest- and insecticide-free foods. These new techniques allow the combination of genetic material from various plants that are resistant to diseases and pests, producing high-yield crops that are high in quality and free of chemicals. These techniques also allow the combination of plants, which can maximize nutritional value as well.

Irradiated Foods

Irradiation is the use of radioactivity (X-rays) to kill microorganisms that grow on food. This does not make the food radioactive, but serves to prolong the useful life of the food (17). Indeed, irradiated food can be stored for years in sealed containers at room temperature without spoiling. In addition, irradiation can delay the sprouting of vegetables such as potatoes and onions and delay the ripening of fruits such as bananas, mangoes, tomatoes, pears, and avocados. This can result in significant cost savings.

Are these irradiated foods safe to eat? Currently, the best answer is a qualified "yes." All research indicates that the foods are safe, but only limited data exist (18). In addition, most studies have used very low radiation levels to irradiate foods. This raises the question, "What is a safe level of radiation for the treatment of foods?"

organic Refers to foods that are grown without pesticides.

7.4 Nutritional Links to Health and Fitness

Do Antioxidants Prevent Muscle Injury or Fatigue?

Recent research suggests that the increased muscle metabolism associated with exercise may cause an increase in free radical production (16). Several studies have shown that this increase in free radicals may contribute to fatigue, and maybe even muscle damage. The obvious question is, "Do active individuals need to increase their consumption of antioxidants?" Several preliminary studies have indicated a positive role for antioxidants, primarily vitamin E, in neutralizing exercise-produced free rad-

icals. In fact, recent reports have demonstrated a reduction in muscle fatigue following administration of antioxidants (16a). Several researchers have suggested that an additional 400 I.U. of vitamin E be consumed daily to protect against free radical damage. However, you should consult your pharmacist or nutritionist before consuming more than the RDA of fat-soluble vitamins. Remember: Fat-soluble vitamins are stored in the body and accumulation may lead to toxicity.

Animals Treated with Antibiotics and Hormones

In recent years, consumers have grown suspicious of eating meat from animals that have been treated with antibiotics to prevent infections. Concern has developed because of the possibility that eating the meat could lead to the development of antibiotic-resistant bacteria in humans. At present, a definitive answer to this issue is not available.

Another recent concern has been the use of hormones to increase production of meat and milk. Most notably, a form of growth hormone, bovine somatotropin, has been used to increase the production of milk. Some people fear that hormones may result in health problems that have not yet been determined. Many supermarkets are restricting the sale of milk produced with the aid of hormone supplements.

Summary

1. Nutrition is the study of food and its relationship to health and disease. The current primary problem in nutrition in industrialized countries is overeating.

2. A well-balanced diet is composed of approximately 55% to 60% complex carbohydrates, 25% to 30% fat, and 12% to 15% protein. These macronutrients are also called the fuel nutrients, because they are the only substances that can be used as fuel and, therefore, provide the energy (calories) necessary for bodily functions.

3. Carbohydrate is a primary fuel used by the body to provide energy. The calorie is a unit of measure of the energy value of food or the energy required for physical activity.

4. Simple carbohydrates consist of sugar (glucose, fructose, sucrose) and double sugar units (galactose, lactose, and maltose).

5. The complex carbohydrates consist of the starches and fiber. Starches are composed of chains of simple sugars. Fiber is a nondigestible but essential form of complex carbohydrates (contained in whole grains, vegetables, and fruits).

6. Fat is an efficient storage form for energy, because each gram contains over twice the energy content of either carbohydrate or protein.

Fat can be derived from dietary sources, and it can be formed from excess carbohydrate and protein consumed in the diet. Excess fat in the diet is stored as fat in the adipose tissues located under the skin and around internal organs. Fats are classified as either simple, compound, or derived. The triglycerides are the most notable of the simple fats. Fatty acids are classified as either saturated or unsaturated, depending on their chemical structures. For nutritional considerations, the most important of the compound fats are the lipoproteins. Cholesterol is the best example of the class of fats called derived fats.

7. The primary role of protein consumed in the diet is to serve as the structural unit to build and repair cells in all tissues of the body. Protein consists of amino acids made by the body (11 nonessential amino acids) and those available only through dietary sources (nine essential amino acids).

8. Vitamins serve many important functions in the body, including regulation of growth and metabolism. The class of water-soluble vitamins consists of several B-complex vitamins and vitamin C. The fat-soluble vitamins are A, D, E, and K.

9. Minerals are chemical elements contained in many foods. Like vitamins, minerals serve many important roles in regulating body functions.

10. Approximately 60% of the body is water. Water is involved in all vital processes in the body and is the nutrient of greatest concern to the physically active individual. In addition to the water contained in foods, it is recommended that an additional eight glasses of water be consumed daily.

11. The basic goals of developing good nutritional habits are to maintain ideal body weight; eat a variety of foods, following the "eating right pyramid" model; avoid consuming too much fat, saturated fat, and cholesterol; eat foods with adequate starch and fiber; avoid consuming too much simple sugar; avoid consuming too much sodium; and if you drink alcohol, do so in moderation.

12. The general rule for meeting the body's need for macronutrients is that an individual should consume approximately 55% to 60% of needed calories in carbohydrates (50% complex carbohydrates and 10% simple sugars), 25% to 30% or less in fats (approximately 10% saturated and 20% unsaturated fats), and 12% to 15% in proteins.

13. In order to have a healthy diet, several nutrients should be minimized. These are fats (especially saturated or animal fats), cholesterol, salt, sugar/corn syrup, and alcohol.

14. The intensity of exercise dictates the relative proportions of fat and carbohydrate that are consumed as fuel during exercise. In general, the lower the intensity of exercise, the more fat is used as a fuel. Conversely, the greater the intensity of exercise, the more carbohydrate is used as a fuel.

15. Antioxidants are nutrients that prevent oxygen free radicals from combining with cells and damaging them. Several micronutrients have been identified as potent antioxidants. These are vitamins E and C, beta-carotene, zinc, and selenium.

16. Food storage and preparation is key to the prevention of food poisoning. Select foods that appear clean and fresh; keep foods cold or frozen to prevent bacteria from growing; thoroughly clean fresh fruits, vegetables, and meats (especially chicken); cook all meats thoroughly, and order well-done meats when dining out.

Study Questions

1. What is the role of the carbohydrate in the diet?

2. List the major food sources of dietary carbohydrates.

3. List the various subcategories of carbohydrates.

4. Compare the three classes of fats.

5. Define *triglyceride* and discuss its use in the body.

6. Distinguish between saturated and unsaturated fatty acids.

7. What are omega-3 fatty acids?

8. Discuss the role of protein in the diet.

9. Distinguish between essential and nonessential amino acids.

10. What are the classes of vitamins, and what is the role of vitamins in body function?

11. Outline the role of minerals in body function.

12. Discuss the importance of water in the diet.

13. What proportions of carbohydrate, fat, and protein in the diet are recommended daily?

14. Discuss the "eating right pyramid" and its role in the selection of foods for the diet.

15. How many calories are contained in a gram of carbohydrate, fat, and protein, respectively?

16. Discuss the special need for carbohydrate in an individual who is engaging in an exercise training program.

17. Discuss the special need for protein for an individual who is engaging in an exercise training program.

18. What is the potential role of antioxidants in the diet?

19. Define the following:

    antioxidants

    calorie

20. Discuss the impact of the following on heart disease:

    high-density lipoproteins (HDL cholesterol)

    low-density lipoproteins (LDL cholesterol)

Suggested Reading

Butterfield, G. Ergogenic aids: Evaluating sport nutrition products. *International Journal of Sport Nutrition* 6:191–197, 1996.

Clark, N. Fluid facts: What, when, and how much to drink. *Physician and Sports Medicine* 20(11):34–36, 1992.

Connor, S., and W. Connor. *New American diet systems.* Simon and Schuster, New York, 1992.

Diplock, A. T. Safety of antioxidant vitamins and b-carotene. *American Journal of Clinical Nutrition* 62: 1510S–1516S, 1995.

Food Marketing Institute. *Trends in the United States: Consumer attitudes and the supermarket,* 1996.

Gershoff, S. N. Vitamin C (ascorbic acid): New roles, new requirements? *Nutrition Review* 51: 313–326, 1993.

Hamilton, E., E. Whitney, and F. Sizer. *Nutrition concepts and controversies.* West, St. Paul, MN, 1992.

Lee, M., J. G. Sebranek, D. G. Olson, and J. S. Dickson. Irradiation and packaging of fresh meat and poultry, *Journal of Food Protection* 59(1):62–72, 1996.

Nutrition Reviews. Dietary supplements: Recent chronology and legislation. *Nutrition Reviews* 53: 31–36, 1995.

Williams, Melvin. The gospel truth about dietary supplements. *ACSM's Health and Fitness Journal* 1(1):24–29, 1997.

Suggested Readings on the World Wide Web

Inside the USOC: Nutrition
(http://test.olympic-usa.org/inside/in_1_3_6_1.html)
Excellent information and resources concerning all aspects of sports nutrition.

The Blonz Guide
(http://www.wenet.net/blonz)
Links to many of the best nutrition, food information, food companies and health association sites on the web.

What's New: USDA Reports on Food Safety
(http://www.usda.gov/whatsnew.htm)
Reports on governmental initiatives to enhance food safety. Good information on defining the problems, potential solutions, and costs to business and consumers.

Ask the Dietician
(http://www.dietitian.com)
Sound nutritional advice on many diet related questions. Excellent "Healthy Body Calculator" for determination of body weight, diet, and exercise.

USDA Nutrient Values
(http://www.rahul.net/cgi-bin/fatfree/usda/usda.cgi)
Searchable data base of foods and nutrient contents.

USDA Food and Nutrition Information Center
(http://www.nal.usda.gov/fnic/)
Government information on food safety, general nutrition, nutrition research, dietary guidelines and the Food Guide Pyramid.

USDA Center for Nutrition Policy and Promotion
(http://www.usda.gov/fcs/cnpp.htm)
Governmental guidelines for diets and use of the Food Guide Pyramid.

USDA Food Safety Guidelines
(http://www.usda.gov/agency/fsis/pubconsu.htm)
Articles about all aspects of safety in food preparation, storage, etc.

Fast Food Finder
(http://www.olen.com/food/)
Search for desired fast food (by restaurant or food) and find nutritional information.
Fat-Free Recipe Center
(http://www.rahul.net/cgi-bin/fatfree/recipes.cgi)
Large collection of fat-free recipes.
Veggies Unite! On-line guide to vegetarianism
(http://www.vegweb.com)
Recipes, books, articles, discussions.
American Dietetic Association
(http://www.eatright.org/index.html)
Nutritional resources, FAQ's, links, and more.

Sympatico: Healthyway
(http://www.ns.sympatico.ca/healthyway/)
Numerous articles, book reviews, and links to nutrition, fitness, and wellness topics.
Gatorade Sports Science Institute
(http://www.gssiweb.com/library/)
Many articles relating to fluid replacement during exercise. Sign-up to be on a mailing list for new articles.
Nutrition for Normal People
(http://www.phys.com)
Self-analysis, articles, nutritional encyclopedia, forums, dietary calculator, and more.

References

1. Cheraskin, E., W. Ringsdorf, and J. Clark. *Diet and disease.* 3d ed. Keats Publishing, New Canaan, CT, 1995.

2. U.S. Department of Health and Human Services. *The Surgeon General's report on nutrition and health.* DHHS (PHS) Publication No. 88-50211. U.S. Government Printing Office: Washington, D.C., 1994.

3. Brown, J. E. *The science of human nutrition.* Harcourt, Brace, and Jovanovich, New York, 1990.

4. Kromhout, D., E. B. Bosschiefer, and C. Lezenne-Coulander. The inverse relation between fish consumption and 20-year mortality from coronary heart disease. *New England Journal of Medicine* 312:1205–1209, 1985.

5. Belko, A. Z. Vitamins and exercise—An update. *Medicine and Science in Sports and Exercise* 19:S191–S196, 1987.

6. Powers, S. K., and E. T. Howley. *Exercise physiology: Theory and application to fitness and performance.* Brown and Benchmark, Dubuque, IA, 1997.

7. *Recommended dietary allowances.* 10th ed. Food and Nutrition Board, National Research Council, Washington D.C., National Academy of Sciences, 1989.

8. Seeley, R. R., T. D. Stephens, and P. Tate. *Anatomy and physiology.* Mosby, St. Louis, MO, 1995.

9. Hales, D. *An invitation to health.* 6th ed. Benajmin Cummings, Redwood City, CA, 1997.

10. Nieman, David C. *Fitness and sports medicine: An introduction.* 3rd ed. Bull Publishing, Palo Alto, CA, 1995.

11. Holloszy, J. O. Muscle metabolism during exercise. *Archives of Physical Medicine and Rehabilitation* 63:231–233, 1982.

12. Lemon, P. W. R. Protein and exercise: Update 1987. *Medicine and Science in Sports and Exercise* 19:S179–S190, 1987.

13. Tarnopolsky, M. A., J. D. MacDougall, and S. A. Atkinson. Influence of protein intake and training status on nitrogen balance and lean body mass. *Journal of Applied Physiology* 64:187–193, 1988.

14. Weight, L. M., T. D. Noakes, J. Graves, P. Jacobs, and P. A. Berman. Vitamin and mineral status of trained athletes including the effects of supplementation. *American Journal of Clinical Nutrition* 47:186–192, 1988.

15. Halliwell, B., and J. M. C. Gutteridge. *Free radicals in biology and medicine.* 2d ed. Oxford University Press, Oxford, 1990.

16. Jenkins, R. R. Free radical chemistry: Relationship to exercise. *Sports Medicine* 5:156–170, 1988.

16a. Kanter, M. Free radicals and exercise: Effects of nutritional antioxidant supplementation. *Exercise and Sports Sciences Reviews* 23:375–398, 1995.

17. Donatelle, R. J. and L. G. Davis. *Access to health.* 4th ed. Prentice-Hall, Englewood Cliffs, NJ, 1996.

18. Rogan, A., and G. Glaros. Food irradiation: The process and implications for dietitians. *Journal of American Dietetic Association* 88:833–838, 1988.

Diet Analysis

NAME _____ DATE _____

The purpose of this exercise is to analyze eating habits during a 3-day period.

Directions

For a 3-day period (two weekdays and one weekend day), eat the typical foods that constitute your normal diet. At the end of each day, record on the following chart the foods eaten for that day and the amounts of the listed nutrients contained in each. Most packaged foods now have the amounts of the nutrients listed on the package. See the appendix for the listings of the nutrients contained in various foods. Total the values for each nutrient at the bottom of the chart. Transfer the total to the next chart. At the end of the 3-day period, total the daily values and divide by 3 to get the average dietary intake for each of the nutrients analyzed. Compare your average intake for each of the nutrients with those recommended at the bottom of the page for your sex and age group. Remember that this analysis is only as representative of your normal diet as the foods you eat over the 3-day period.

Write-up

In the space provided, list the strengths and weaknesses in your diet and discuss the steps that can be taken to improve it.

Daily Nutrient Intake

Name: _____   Date: _____

Foods	Amount	kcals (total)	kcals from fat	Protein (gm)	CHO (gm)	Fiber (gm)	Fat (gm)	Fat % (kcal)	Sat. Fat (gm)	Chol. (mg)	Sodium (mg)	Vit. A (I.U.)	Vit. C (mg)	Calcium (mg)	Iron (mg)	Vit. B_1 (mg)	Vit. B_2 (mg)	Niacin (mg)
Totals																		

Make additional copies of this form for additional days.

Three Day Nutrient Summary

Name: _____ Date: _____

Day	kcals Total	kcals from Fat	Protein (gm)	CHO (gm)	Fiber (gm)	Fat (gm)	Fat % (kcal)	Sat. Fat (gm)	Chol. (mg)	Sodium (mg)	Vit. A (I.U.)	Vit. C (mg)	Calcium (mg)	Iron (mg)	Vit. B$_1$ (mg)	Vit. B$_2$ (mg)	Niacin (mg)
One																	
Two																	
Three																	
Totals																	
Average																	

Recommended Dietary Allowances for Comparison

	kcals Total	kcals from Fat	Protein (gm)	CHO (gm)	Fiber (gm)	Fat (gm)	Fat % (kcal)	Sat. Fat (gm)	Chol. (mg)	Sodium (mg)	Vit. A (I.U.)	Vit. C (mg)	Calcium (mg)	Iron (mg)	Vit. B$_1$ (mg)	Vit. B$_2$ (mg)	Niacin (mg)
Men 15–18	See Below	< 30%	See Below	> 58%	~ 30%	< 30%		< 10%	< 300	3000	1000	60	1200	12	1.5	1.8	20
Men 19–24		< 30%		> 58%	~ 30%	< 30%		< 10%	< 300	3000	1000	60	1200	12	1.5	1.8	20
Men 25–50		< 30%		> 58%	~ 30%	< 30%		< 10%	< 300	3000	1000	60	1200	12	1.5	1.8	20
Men 51+		< 30%		> 58%	~ 30%	< 30%		< 10%	< 300	3000	1000	60	1200	12	1.5	1.8	20
Women 15–18		< 30%		> 58%	~ 30%	< 30%		< 10%	< 300	3000	1000	60	1200	12	1.5	1.8	20
Women 19–24		< 30%		> 58%	~ 30%	< 30%		< 10%	< 300	3000	1000	60	1200	12	1.5	1.8	20
Women 25–50		< 30%		> 58%	~ 30%	< 30%		< 10%	< 300	3000	1000	60	1200	12	1.5	1.8	20
Women 51+		< 30%		> 58%	~ 30%	< 30%		< 10%	< 300	3000	1000	60	1200	12	1.5	1.8	20
Pregnant		< 30%		> 58%	~ 30%	< 30%		< 10%	< 300	3000	1000	60	1200	12	1.5	1.8	20
Lactating		< 30%		> 58%	~ 30%	< 30%		< 10%	< 300	3000	1000	60	1200	12	1.5	1.8	20

See Chapter 8 for determination of kcal requirements.

Protein intake should be 0.8 grams/kg of body weight (0.36 grams per lb). Pregnant women should add 15 g, and lactating women should add 20 g.

All recommended allowances for macronutrients come from nutrition experts.

Reprinted with permission from "Recommended Dietary Allowances," 10th edition, 1989, by the National Academy of Sciences. Published by National Academy Press, Washington, D.C.

Construct a New Diet

NAME _____   DATE _____

The purpose of this exercise is to construct a new diet using the principles outlined in Chapter 7.

Directions

After completing Laboratory 7.1, you should have a general idea of how your diet may need modification. Follow the example given in Table 7.11 and the discussion in the text to choose foods to construct a new diet that meets the recommended dietary goals presented in this chapter. Fill in the blanks on the following chart with the requested information obtained from the Appendix or package labels. Use the totals for each column and the RDA for each nutrient (see Laboratory 7.1 or Table 7.7) to determine your percent of RDA for each nutrient.

	Kcal	Fat (g)	Sat.Fat (g)	Chol (mg)	Sod. (mg)	CHO (g)	Pro (g)	Vit A (I.U.)	Vit C (mg)	Ca (mg)	Iron (mg)
Breakfast											
Lunch											
Dinner											
Totals											
RDA	*	<30%	<10%	<300	3000	>58%	**	4000	60	1200	15
% of RDA											

* See Chapter 8 for determination of kcal requirements.

**Protein intake should be 0.8 grams/kg of body weight (0.36 grams/lb).
Pregnant women should add 15g, and lactating women should add 20g.

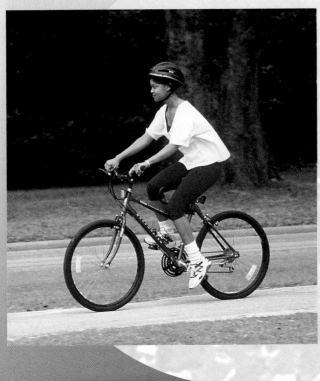

8

Exercise, Diet, and Weight Control

Millions of people in the United States believe they are too fat. This is evidenced by the fact that 30% to 40% of adult women and 20% to 25% of adult men are currently trying to lose weight (1). Interest in weight loss has opened the door to numerous commercial weight loss programs and a billion-dollar industry. Many commercial weight loss programs advertise that they are highly successful in promoting individual weight loss. Unfortunately, research demonstrates that if no other treatment is given, only 5% of individuals maintain the weight loss for 5 years after completion of the program (2).

A key element in any weight loss program is education. This chapter, therefore, provides a general overview of body fat control. Specifically, we will discuss the principles of determining an ideal body weight for health and fitness; ways to achieve loss of body fat, using a combination of diet, exercise, and behavior modification; and the principles involved in maintaining a desirable body weight throughout life.

Obesity

Obesity is a term applied to individuals with a high percentage of body fat, generally over 25% for men and over 30% for women (3–7). Obesity is a major health problem in the United States, and numerous diseases have been linked to being over-fat (see A Closer Look 8.1). Current estimates for the United States suggest that over 65 million people meet the criteria for obesity (1, 8).

What causes obesity? There is no single answer. Obesity is related to both genetic traits and characteristics of a person's lifestyle (13, 14). Studies have demonstrated that children of obese parents have a greater potential to become obese than children of non-obese parents (14). Further, adopted children with low genetic potential for obesity have a greater chance of becoming obese if their adoptive parents are obese (14).

The link between genetics and obesity is poorly understood. Researchers continue to search for specific genes that could influence body fatness. In contrast, the tie between lifestyle and obesity is well defined. Nutritional studies have demonstrated that families consuming high-fat meals have a greater risk of obesity than families who eat low-fat diets (4, 5, 13). Similarly, children raised in households where physical activity is not encouraged have a greater potential for obesity than children reared in homes where physical activity is encouraged (4, 15).

Many individuals who do not have a genetic link to obesity may gradually add fat over the years and become obese at some point in their lives. This slow increase in body fat is often called **creeping obesity** because it gradually "sneaks up" on us (9). This type of weight gain is usually attributed to poor diet (including increased food intake) and a gradual decline in

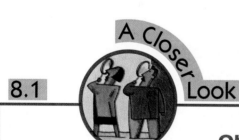

A Closer Look

8.1

Obesity and Disease

Obesity increases the risk for at least twenty-six diseases (9–11). Some of the most serious of these include heart disease, colon cancer, hypertension (high blood pressure), kidney disease, arthritis, and diabetes (10). For example, obesity increases the risk of heart attack by 60% to 80% (12,12a). Further, there is a high correlation between the onset of type II diabetes and body fatness, as over 80% of type II diabetics are obese (1). Because of the strong link between obesity and disease, the National Institutes of Health concluded that obesity may indirectly account for 15% to 20% of the deaths in the United States (11).

Obesity may also contribute to emotional concerns, particularly in adolescents and young adults who are very conscious of their body image (individual feelings toward one's body). A poor body image resulting from obesity may contribute to low self-esteem and reduce the quality of life.

physical activity (9). Figure 8.1 illustrates the process of creeping obesity over a 5-year period. In this example, the individual is gaining one-half pound of fat per month (6 pounds per year), resulting in a total weight gain of 30 pounds over 5 years.

Regional Fat Storage

Recall (Chapter 2) that much of our body fat is stored beneath the skin (Figure 8.2). The fact that people vary in their regional pattern of fat storage is well known. What factor determines where body fat is stored? The answer is genetics. We inherit specific fat storage traits that determine the regional distribution of fat. This occurs

Obesity tends to run in families

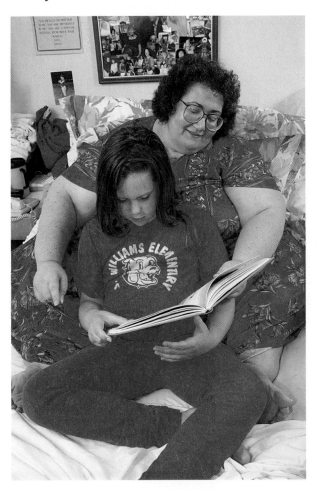

due to the fact that fat cells are unequally distributed throughout the body. For example, many men have a high number of fat cells in the upper body, which results in a predominance of fat storage within the abdominal or waist area. In contrast, most women contain a high number of fat cells in the lower body, resulting in fat storage in the waist, hips, and thighs. As we have seen, people who carry body fat primarily in the abdominal or waist area are at greater risk for development of heart disease than are those who store body fat in the hips or lower part of the body. Therefore, obtaining a desirable body weight with proper fat distribution is a primary health goal (1, 12).

Optimal Body Weight

Almost everyone has an idea about how much they should weigh for optimal physical appearance. However, a key question is, *"What is my optimal body weight for health and fitness?"* Although researchers disagree on the answer to this question, some guidelines are available. In general, optimal body fat for health and fitness in men ranges from 10% to 20%, whereas the optimal range of body fat for women is 15% to 25% (15–20) (Figure 8.3). These ranges allow for individual differences in physical activity and appearance and are associated with limited risk of the diseases linked to body fatness.

Optimal Body Weight Based on Percent Fat

In Chapter 2, we discussed the skinfold caliper technique for body fatness assessment. Now that we know how to compute percent body fat and the optimal range of body fat, how can we determine the desired range of body weight? Consider the following example of a male college stu-

obesity A term applied to individuals with a high percentage of body fat, generally over 25% for men and over 30% for women.

creeping obesity A slow increase in body fat collected over a period of several years.

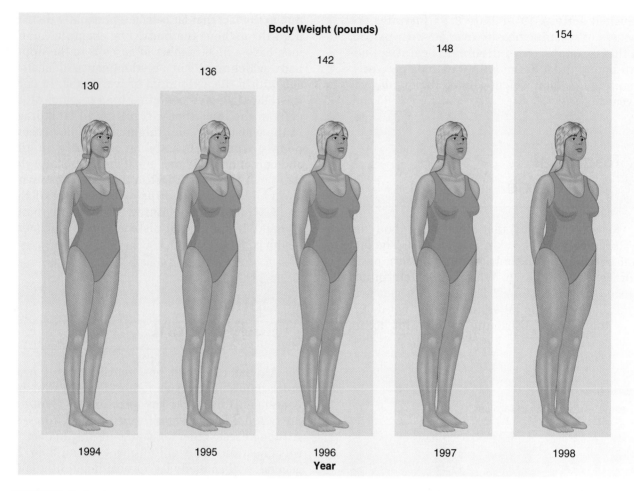

FIGURE 8.1 The concept of creeping obesity.

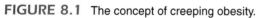
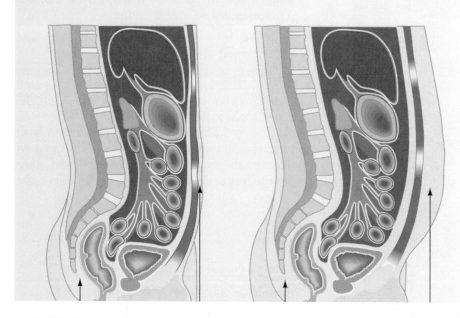

FIGURE 8.2 Much of our body fat is stored beneath
the skin.

dent who has 25% body fat and weighs 185 pounds. What is the optimal range of body weight for health and fitness in this individual? The calculations can be done in two simple steps:

Step 1. Compute fat-free weight (i.e., the amount of body weight contained in bones, organs, muscles).

100% body weight - 25% fat weight = 75% fat-free weight (75% of total body weight is fat-free)

Therefore,

75% × 185 pounds = 138.8 pounds fat-free weight

Step 2. Calculate the optimal weight (remember that optimal body fat range for men is 10% to 20%). The formula to compute optimal body weight is

Optimal weight = fat-free weight ÷ (1 − optimal % fat)

Note that optimal % fat should be expressed as a fraction. Therefore, the optimal weight range for 10% and 20% body fat would be

For 10%: Optimal weight = 138.8 ÷ (1 − 0.10) = 154.2 pounds

For 20%: Optimal weight = 138.8 ÷ (1 − 0.2) = 173.5 pounds

Hence, the optimal body weight for this individual is between 154.2 and 173.5 pounds. Laboratory 8.1 provides the opportunity to compute your optimal body weight, using both percent body fat and body mass index (introduced in Chapter 2).

Men tend to store body fat in the upper body.

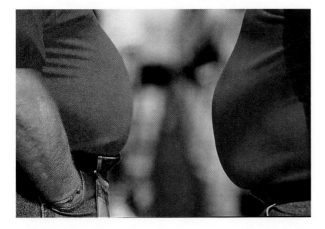

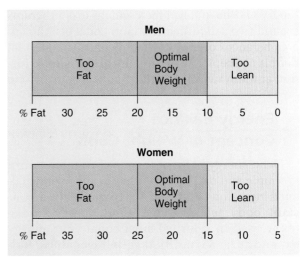

FIGURE 8.3 The concept of ideal body weight based on a desirable percent of body fat.

Physiology of Weight Control

Before we discuss how to begin a weight loss program, it is necessary to outline some key physiological concepts associated with weight loss. One of the oldest theories of weight control is called the **set point theory**. This theory centers around the concept that body weight is regulated at a set point by a weight-regulating control center within an area of the brain called the hypothalamus (4, 7). The control center has a set point, similar to the thermostat in your home, that maintains body weight at a constant level. According to the set point theory of weight loss, when we lose weight by dieting, the body will react by reducing energy expenditure and increasing appetite. As a result, we will eventually gain weight to get back to the set point body weight. Nonetheless, while the set point theory may explain some types of obesity, it probably does not explain creeping obesity or the fat gain that most of us experience around holidays due to high-calorie meals. Given this fact, many weight control researchers have discarded the set point

set point theory A theory of weight regulation that centers around the concept that body weight is controlled at a set point by a weight-regulating control center within the brain.

theory and have developed weight loss programs around two scientifically sound concepts: the energy balance concept of weight control and the fat deficit concept of weight control. Let's look further at these two concepts.

Energy Balance Concept of Weight Control

The energy balance theory of weight control is simple and can be illustrated by the energy balance equation (Figure 8.4). To maintain a constant body weight, your food energy intake (expressed in calories) must equal your energy expenditure, a condition called **isocaloric balance** (see Figure 8.4A). If you consume more calories than you expend, you gain body fat. Consuming more calories than you expend results in a **positive caloric balance** (see Figure 8.4B). Finally, if you expend more calories than you consume, you lose body fat and have a **negative caloric balance** (see Figure 8.4C).

From the energy balance equation presented in Figure 8.4, you might conclude that weight gain can be prevented by either decreasing your energy (food) intake or increasing your energy (exercise) expenditure. In practice, good weight loss programs include both a reduction in caloric intake and an increase in caloric expenditure achieved through exercise (7, 20–22).

Energy Expenditure   Estimating your daily energy expenditure is a key factor in planning a weight loss program and adjusting the energy balance equation. The daily expenditure of energy involves both the resting metabolic rate and exercise metabolic rate. Let's examine each of these individually.

Resting metabolic rate (RMR) is the amount of energy expended during all sedentary activities. That is, RMR includes the energy required to maintain necessary bodily functions (called the *basal metabolic rate*) plus the additional energy required to perform such activities as sitting, reading, typing, and digestion of food. The RMR is an important component of the energy balance equation because it represents approximately 90% of the total daily energy expenditure in sedentary individuals (23).

Exercise metabolic rate (EMR) represents the energy expenditure during any form of exercise (walking, climbing steps, weight lifting, etc.). In the sedentary individual, EMR comprises only 10% of the total daily energy expenditure. By comparison, EMR can account for 20% to 40% of

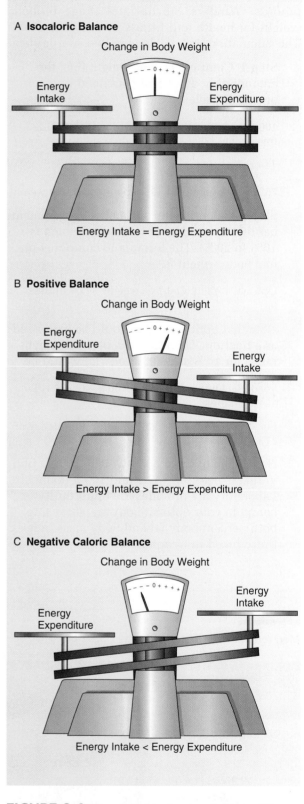

A **Isocaloric Balance**

Change in Body Weight

Energy Intake   Energy Expenditure

Energy Intake = Energy Expenditure

B **Positive Balance**

Change in Body Weight

Energy Expenditure

Energy Intake

Energy Intake > Energy Expenditure

C **Negative Caloric Balance**

Change in Body Weight

Energy Intake

Energy Expenditure

Energy Intake < Energy Expenditure

FIGURE 8.4   The concept of energy balance. **(A)** illustrates an isocaloric balance, **(B)** illustrates a positive caloric balance, and **(C)** illustrates a negative caloric balance.

Table 8.1

Estimation of Daily Caloric Expenditure Based on Body Weight and Physical Activity
To compute your estimated daily caloric expenditure, multiply your body weight in pounds by the calories per pound that corresponds to your activity level.

Activity Level	Description	Calories per Pound of Body Weight Expended during a 24-Hour Period
1	Very sedentary (restricted movement, such as a patient confined to a house)	13
2	Sedentary (most U. S. citizens, doing light work or office job)	14
3	Moderate activity (many college students, performing some daily activity and weekend recreation)	15
4	Very physically active (vigorous activity at least 3–4 times/week)	16
5	Competitive athlete (daily activity in high-energy sport)	17–18

the total daily energy expenditure in the active individual (23). For example, during heavy exercise, EMR may be 10 to 20 times greater than RMR (20). Therefore, increased daily exercise results in an increase in the EMR and is a key factor in weight control programs.

Estimating Daily Energy Expenditure

Dieting is widespread in the United States as people try to reduce body fat by decreasing energy intake. The obvious goal of dieting is to consume less energy than is expended and therefore create a negative energy balance and resulting weight loss. The first step in this process is to estimate your daily caloric expenditure. One of the simplest ways to do so is presented in Table 8.1, which provides estimates of daily caloric energy expenditure based on body weight and physical activity. For example, let's compute the estimated daily caloric expenditure for a college-age woman whose body weight is 120 pounds and who is involved in only moderate physical activity on weekends. Using Table 8.1, we locate her activity level on the left (i.e., level 3) and her estimated calories expended per pound of body weight (15 calories/pound/day) in the right-hand column. To calculate her total daily energy expenditure, we multiply her body weight by her caloric expenditure:

Daily caloric expenditure = 120 pounds × 15 calories/pound/day = 1800 calories/day

Do this same calculation for your own daily caloric expenditure. If you need to lose weight, you are now prepared to create a negative energy balance by reducing your energy intake. Note that after losing 5 pounds of body weight, you should recalculate your estimated caloric expenditure; this is necessary because the weight loss results in a lower daily energy expenditure (see Laboratory 8.2).

Fat Deficit Concept of Weight Control

The general concept that weight loss occurs due to a negative energy balance is straightforward and easy to understand. Nonetheless, recent evidence suggests that creating a fat deficit is an-

isocaloric balance Food energy intake that equals energy expenditure.

positive caloric balance Consuming more calories than are expended.

negative caloric balance Expending more calories than are consumed.

resting metabolic rate (RMR) The amount of energy expended during all sedentary activities.

exercise metabolic rate (EMR) The energy expenditure during any form of exercise.

other essential factor in weight loss that is often overlooked (24). For instance, it is now accepted that dietary fat is more easily stored as body fat than either carbohydrate or protein (24). This occurs because dietary fat is not used as a body fuel as rapidly as is carbohydrate or protein. For example, if a positive caloric balance is created by eating large amounts of carbohydrate or proteins, many of the excess calories are used to repair body tissues, replace body carbohydrate stores, or metabolize to provide body energy. In contrast, if excess calories are consumed as fat, they are more likely to be stored as body fat (24).

The importance of a low-fat diet in weight control can best be illustrated by the fact that body fat gain is a result of a continual imbalance of fat intake and fat metabolism (fat burned in the body). In other words, if you ingest more fat than you burn during the day, you gain weight (Figure 8.5A). It follows that if you consume and burn equal amounts of fat, your weight remains constant (Figure 8.5B). Finally, if you burn more fat than you consume (a fat deficit), you lose body fat and weight (Figure 8.5C). Thus, losing body fat is not as simple as creating an energy deficit; your diet must provide a caloric deficit which also results in a fat deficit. How to design a diet plan that is low in fat and calories and high in carbohydrates will be discussed shortly.

What Is a Safe Rate of Weight Loss?

Before we discuss how to design a weight loss program, we should address two general points about weight loss. First, the maximum recommended rate for weight loss is 1 to 2 pounds per week. Diets resulting in a weight loss of more than 2 pounds per week are associated with a significant loss of lean body mass (i.e., muscle and body organs). In general, a weight loss goal of 1 pound per week is a safe and reasonable goal. The negative energy balance required to lose 1 pound per week is approximately 3500 calories. Therefore, a negative energy balance of 500 calories per day would theoretically result in a loss of 1 pound of fat per week (500 calories/day × 7 days = 3500 calories).

A second general point about weight loss is that the rate of loss during the first several days of dieting will be greater than later in the dieting period. This is true because at the onset of a diet, in addition to fat loss, there is an initial reduction in body carbohydrate and water stores, which also results in some weight loss (20). Further, some lean tissue, such as muscle, may also be lost during the beginning of any diet; the caloric content of lean tissue is less than fat. Therefore, more than 1 pound will be lost during the first 3500-calorie deficit. However, as the diet continues, weight loss will occur at a slower rate. This fact should not discourage you, because subsequent weight loss will be primarily from body fat stores. Sticking with your weight plan for several weeks will result in a significant fat loss, and you will like the associated changes.

Where on the Body Does Fat Reduction Occur?

A key weight loss question is, "Where on the body do changes occur when fat is lost?" The answer is that most weight loss occurs in the body areas that contain the greatest fat storage. Figure 8.6 illustrates this point in a study of obese women who completed a 14-week weight loss program which resulted in each participant losing approximately 20 pounds of fat (25). At the

FIGURE 8.5 Importance of a low-fat diet in creating a fat deficit and promoting weight loss.

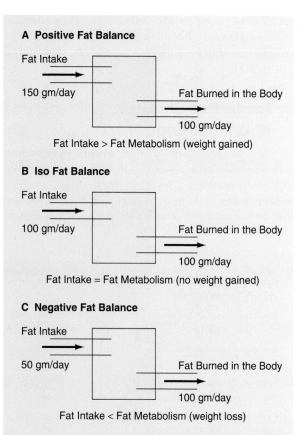

A Positive Fat Balance

Fat Intake

150 gm/day

Fat Burned in the Body

100 gm/day

Fat Intake > Fat Metabolism (weight gained)

B Iso Fat Balance

Fat Intake

100 gm/day

Fat Burned in the Body

100 gm/day

Fat Intake = Fat Metabolism (no weight gained)

C Negative Fat Balance

Fat Intake

50 gm/day

Fat Burned in the Body

100 gm/day

Fat Intake < Fat Metabolism (weight loss)

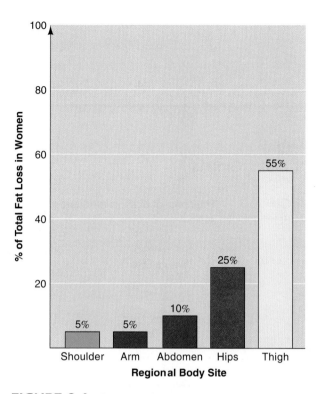

FIGURE 8.6 Fat is lost from the areas of the body that contain the greatest fat storage. (Data from King, M., and F. Katch. Changes in body density, fatfolds, and girths at 2.3 kg increments of weight loss. *Human Biology* 58:709, 1986.)

beginning of the study, regional fat storage was assessed using skinfold measurements, and it was determined that the largest percentage of fat was stored in the abdomen, hips, and thighs. At the completion of the study, regional fat storage was reassessed to determine where the fat loss occurred. Approximately 90% of the fat loss occurred in the body regions with the highest fat storage (Figure 8.6). This is good news because most people want to lose fat from those areas.

Establishing a Successful Weight Loss Program

With proper knowledge and motivation, almost anyone can design a program of weight loss. The four basic components of a comprehensive weight control program are establishment of weight loss goals; a reduced caloric diet stressing balanced nutrition, high carbohydrate intake, and low fat intake; an exercise program designed to increase caloric expenditure and maintain or increase muscle mass; and a behavior modification program aimed toward changing eating habits that contribute to weight gain.

Weight Loss Goals

The establishment of weight loss goals is a key component of any weight loss program. The first step is to decide where your percent body fat should be within the optimal range (10% to 20% for men, 15% to 25% for women). Many people who are beginning a comprehensive weight loss program choose a long-term weight loss goal that will place them in the middle of the optimal weight range (15% body fat for men, 20% body fat for women). After choosing your long-term goal, it is also useful to establish short-term weight loss goals—usually expressed in the number of pounds lost per week (see A Closer Look 8.2 and Laboratory 8.3).

Role of Diet in Weight Loss

Bookstore shelves are filled with diet books, and television and radio advertisements promote "miracle" diets. While some of these diets may promote weight loss, many do not provide balanced nutrition. When assessing new diets, a general rule of thumb is to avoid diets that promise fast and easy weight loss. If you have concerns about the safety or effectiveness of a published diet, you can contact your local branch of the American Dietetic Association for information or approach a dietitian at a hospital or college. By learning the basic nutrition principles contained in this chapter and in Chapter 7, you should be able to critically evaluate most diet plans.

Table 8.2 presents a brief summary of some of the major types of diets used in weight loss programs (20). Of these, only plan 4 is a nutritionally balanced, low-caloric diet; it is the only one recommended. Any safe and nutritionally sound diet should adhere to the following guidelines (4–7, 9, 18):

1. The diet should be low in calories but provide all the essential nutrients required by the body.

2. The diet should be low in fat (less than 30% of total calories) and high in complex carbohydrates (approximately 60% of total calories). Remember, a diet low in fat is essential to creating a fat deficit. Establishing a diet that creates a negative caloric balance with less than 30% of the total calories coming from fat will ensure that your daily fat intake is less than your daily fat metabolism.

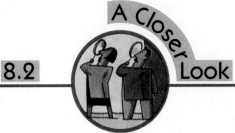

A Closer Look

8.2

Short-Term and Long-Term Weight Loss Goals

Short-term weight loss goals are designed to provide achievable weight loss targets that can be reached within a 2- to 4-week period. For example, an initial short-term weight loss goal might be to lose 2 pounds during the first 2 weeks of your weight loss program. Achievement of a short-term goal provides the motivation to establish another short-term goal and continue the weight loss program (Figure 8.7).

Long-term weight loss goals generally focus on reaching the desired percent of body fat. For instance, a long-term goal for a male college student might be to reach 15% body fat within the first year of his weight loss program. After reaching this long-term goal, his objective then becomes the maintenance of this desired body composition.

FIGURE 8.7 The concept of short-term and long-term weight loss goals.

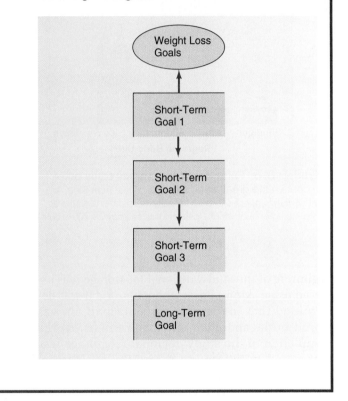

3. The diet should employ a variety of foods to appeal to your taste and to prevent hunger between meals.

4. The diet should be compatible with your lifestyle, and the foods should be obtained easily.

5. The diet should be a lifelong diet; that is, it should be one that you can follow for the remainder of your life. This type of diet greatly increases your chances of maintaining an ideal weight in the future.

6. The diet should provide foods that adhere to the principles of eating for health.

In addition to these diet guidelines, here are some helpful reminders from Chapter 7 for planning a successful balanced diet:

1. Avoid high-calorie, low-nutrient foods such as those high in sugar (e.g., candy bars, cookies). Instead, select low-calorie, nutrient-dense foods such as fruits, vegetables, and whole-grain breads.

2. Reduce the amount of fat in your diet. High-fat foods are high in calories. For example, eat less butter and choose meats that are low in fat, like lean cuts of beef, chicken, and fish. Avoid fried foods; broil, bake, or micro-

wave your food. If you must use oil in your cooking, use monosaturated oils such as olive or peanut oil.

3. Although milk-exchange products are excellent sources of protein, these products may be high in calories unless the fat has been removed. Use nonfat or low-fat milk, low-fat cottage cheese, and similar products.

4. Eat more fruits, vegetables, and whole grains. Select fresh fruits when possible and avoid fruits that are canned in heavy syrup.

5. Limit salt intake. Use herbs and other seasonings as substitutes for salt.

6. Drink fewer alcoholic beverages. Alcoholic beverages are low in nutrients and high in calories.

7. Eat three meals per day, and do not snack in between.

Remember that a negative energy balance of 500 calories/day will result in a weight loss of approximately 1 pound per week. The key to maintaining a caloric deficit of 500 calories/day is careful planning of meals and accurate calorie counting.

Exercise and Weight Loss

Exercise plays a key role in weight loss for several reasons (see ref. 22 for a review). First, increased physical activity will elevate your daily

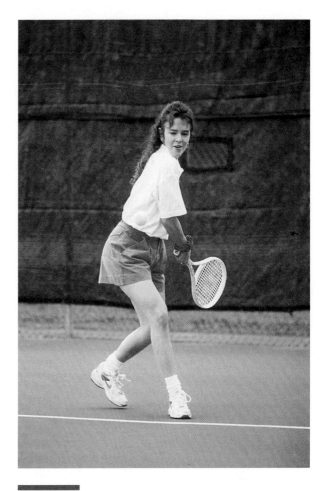

Exercise is a key component of any weight loss program.

Table 8.2

Examples of Weight Loss Diets

Type of Diet	Description/Comments	Recommendation
Nutritionally unbalanced	Low carbohydrate diet (high fat or protein intake), not safe for long time periods	Not recommended (see 8.1 Nutritional Links to Health and Fitness)
Nutritionally balanced	Low-calorie liquid diet, monotonous and unsatisfying	Not recommended
Nutritionally unbalanced	Very low-calorie liquid diet (protein/carbohydrate mixture: 300–600 calories/day); not safe for long time periods	Not recommended
Nutritionally balanced	Balanced low-calorie diet (caloric deficit of 500–1000 calories per day); diet is high in carbohydrates (approximately 60% of total calorie intake) and low in fat (less than 30% of total calories)	Recommended

caloric expenditure and therefore assist you in creating a negative energy balance. Second, regular cardiorespiratory exercise training results in an improved ability of skeletal muscles to burn fat as energy. Third, regular resistance exercise (such as weight training) can reduce the loss of muscle that occurs during a diet. This is important because your primary goal in dieting is not to lose muscle mass but to promote fat loss. Finally, increasing your muscle mass by weight training results in an increased resting metabolic rate which further aids in weight loss (26).

What type of exercise should be performed to assist in weight loss? A sound recommendation is that both cardiorespiratory training (i.e., running, cycling, swimming, etc.) and strength training be performed while dieting. The combination of these two types of training will maintain cardiorespiratory fitness and reduce the loss of muscle.

How much exercise must be performed during a weight loss program? In general, exercise sessions designed to promote weight loss should be in excess of 250 calories. Further, it is recommended that the negative caloric balance should be shared equally by exercise and diet. For instance, if an individual wishes to achieve a 500-calorie/day deficit, this should be done by

increasing energy expenditure (exercise) by 250 calories/day and by decreasing caloric intake by 250 calories.

Although intensity of exercise is an important factor in improving cardiorespiratory fitness, it is the total amount of energy expended and fat burned that is important in weight loss. Some authors have argued that low-intensity prolonged exercise is better than short-term high-intensity exercise (i.e., sprinting 50 yards) in burning fat calories and promoting weight loss (27, 28). However, recent evidence clearly demonstrates that both high- and low-intensity exercise can promote fat loss (see ref. 20 for a review). Nonetheless, for the sedentary or obese individual, low-intensity exercise is the proper choice because it can be performed for longer time periods and this type of training results in an increase in the ability of skeletal muscle to metabolize fat as an energy source (20, 29). A brief discussion of the energy cost of various activities follows.

Table 8.3 contains an estimation of the caloric cost of several types of physical activities. To compute your caloric expenditure (per minute) during an activity, simply multiply your body weight in kilograms (2.2 pounds = 1 kilogram) by the values in the right-hand column of Table 8.3 and by the exercise time. For example, suppose a

Table 8.3

Energy Costs for Selected Sporting Activities

	Cal/min./kg	Cal/min.*	METS
Archery (American Round)	0.0412	2.8	2.3
Bowling (with three other bowlers)	0.0471	3.2	2.7
Golf (playing in a foursome)	0.0559	3.8	3.2
Walking (17-min. mile on a grass surface)	0.0794	5.4	4.5
Cycling (6.4-min. mile)	0.0985	6.7	5.6
Canoeing (15-min. mile)	0.1029	7.0	5.8
Swimming (50-yd./min.)	0.1333	9.1	7.6
Running (10-min. mile)	0.1471	10.0	8.0
Cycling (5-min. mile)	0.1559	10.6	8.5
Handball (singles)	0.1603	10.9	9.1
Skipping rope (80 turns/min.)	0.1655	11.3	9.5
Running (8-min. mile)	0.1856	12.6	10.0
Running (6-min. mile)	0.2350	16.0	12.8

*These are values for a 150-lb (68kg) person.

Source: From Getchell, B., 1992. *Physical fitness: A way of life.* Copyright © 1992. Reprinted with permission from Allyn & Bacon.

8.1 Nutritional Links to Health and Fitness

Low-Carbohydrate Diets: Are They Safe and Effective?

Many different types of low-carbohydrate diets have been popularized over the years. Names of some low-carbohydrate diets include the Zone diet, Atkins New Diet Revolution, Calories Don't Count, Scarsdale Diet, and the Mayo Diet. New ones continue to be introduced but essentially they are the same diet.

Any diet low in carbohydrate will promote responses similar to low calorie diets. Each of the low-carbohydrate diets mentioned above have enjoyed a surge of popularity due to the initial weight loss that occurs. The sales pitch is that "you never feel hungry" and that "you will lose weight fast."

Both claims are true, but misleading. Loss of appetite occurs with any low-calorie diet. Further, low-carbohydrate diets result in a loss of body water. This loss of body water explains the rapid weight loss observed with these diets; however, the water is rapidly regained as soon as a normal diet is resumed (34).

Are low-carbohydrate diets safe? The answer is no! Many physiological hazards accompany low carbohydrate diets. For example, these diets have been associated with high blood cholesterol, hypoglycemia, mineral imbalances, and other metabolic disorders. In short, these diets can be very dangerous and are never recommended by knowledgeable practitioners.

70-kilogram (kg) individual plays 20 minutes of racquetball. How many calories did he or she expend during the time of play? The total estimated caloric expenditure is computed as follows:

Caloric expenditure = 70 kg × 0.178 calories/kg/min × 20 min = 249 calories

Exercise and Appetite

A common question is, "Does exercise increase appetite?" Although the high-intensity training programs used by many athletes may increase appetite, it is generally believed that when a moderate exercise program is introduced to a sedentary or obese population, appetite does not increase (30). In fact, moderate exercise training may diminish appetite (30).

Behavior Modification

Research demonstrates that behavior modification plays a key role in both achieving short-term weight loss and maintaining weight loss over the years (4–7). **Behavior modification** is a technique used in psychological therapy to promote desirable changes in behavior. The rationale behind it is that many behaviors are learned. For

example, attending movies at the theater elicits, in many people, a response of eating popcorn and candy. Because these types of responses are learned, they can also be eliminated (unlearned). In regard to weight control, behavior modification is used primarily to reduce or (ideally) eliminate social or environmental stimuli that promote overeating.

The first step in a diet-related behavior modification program is to identify those social or environmental factors that promote overeating. This can be done by keeping a written record of daily activities for 1 or 2 weeks to identify factors associated with consumption of high-calorie meals. In recording your daily eating habits, consider the following (9):

1. *Activities.* What activities are associated with eating? You may find a correlation between specific types of activities, such as watching TV and snacks.

behavior modification A technique used in psychological therapy to promote desirable changes in behavior.

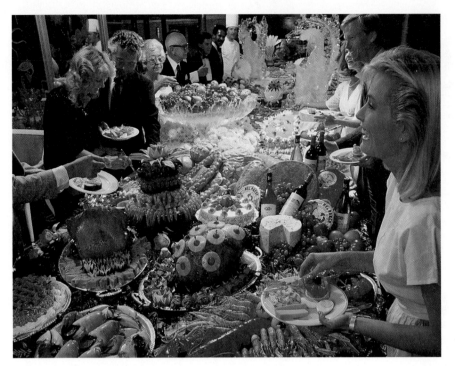

Avoid parties or social gatherings that encourage overeating.

2. *Emotional behavior before or during eating.* What emotions are associated with eating? For instance, do you overeat when you are depressed or under stress? (*Overeating* is defined as the consumption of high-calorie meals that leads to a positive calorie balance).

3. *Location of meals.* Where do you eat? Are specific rooms associated with snacks?

4. *Time of day and level of hunger.* Do you eat at specific times of the day? When you eat, are you always hungry?

5. *People involved.* With whom do you eat? Are specific people associated with periods of overeating?

After identifying the factors that influence your eating behavior, start a program aimed at correcting those behaviors that contribute to weight gain. The following weight control techniques have been used successfully for many years. Although it is not essential to use each of them, adhering to many will make weight control easier (9).

1. *Make a personal commitment to losing weight.* This is the first step toward behavior modification and weight loss. The establishment of realistic short-term and long-term weight loss goals assists in maintaining a lifelong commitment to weight control.

2. *Develop healthy low-calorie eating patterns.* Avoid eating when you are not hungry. Learn to eat slowly and only while sitting at the table. Finally, keep food quantities to the minimum amount within your calorie guidelines.

3. *Avoid social settings where overeating is encouraged.* If you go to parties where high-calorie foods are served, don't go to these functions hungry. Eat a low-calorie meal before going.

4. *Avoid snacking.* If snacks must be eaten, eat low-calorie foods such as carrots or celery.

5. *Engage in daily exercise.* Regular exercise that uses large-muscle groups can play an important role in increasing your daily caloric expenditure and can therefore assist in weight control.

6. *Reward yourself for successful weight loss with nonfood rewards.* Rewards or positive feedback are an important part of behavior modification. For example, after reaching part of your weight loss goal, reward yourself by doing something you like to do (going to the beach, going hiking, or buying a new CD.)

7. *Think positively.* Avoid negative thinking about how difficult weight loss is going to be. Positive thinking promotes confidence and maintains the enthusiasm necessary for a lifetime of successful weight control.

Lifetime Weight Control

The good news about weight loss is that any-body with the proper motivation can lose body fat. The bad news is that there is no simple way of losing body fat and keeping the fat off forever. Weight control over the course of a lifetime is only accomplished by the proper combination of diet, exercise, and behavior modification. The key factors in long-term weight control are a positive attitude toward weight control, regular exercise, and a personal commitment to maintaining a desired body composition.

Similar to many other facets of personal or professional life, weight control will have its ups and downs. Be prepared for occasional setbacks. For instance, gaining weight during holiday periods is common and experienced by everyone at some time. When this type of weight gain occurs, avoid self-criticism, quickly reestablish your personal commitment to a short-term weight loss goal, and develop a new diet and exercise plan to lose the undesired fat. Remember, any amount of weight gain can be lost by applying the principles discussed in this chapter.

Finally, the importance of family and friends in lifetime weight control cannot be overemphasized. Their encouragement and support can assist you in maintaining good eating habits, as well as provide the needed support to sustain a lifetime commitment to exercise. It is much easier to lose weight if your close associates are trying to help you achieve your goals rather than tempting you to eat improperly. Therefore, surround yourself with friends that will support you in your weight control goals.

Weight Loss Myths

Numerous weight loss myths cause confusion among people who are attempting to lose weight. Several common ones are discussed next.

Diet Pills

There are a number of over-the-counter diet pills on the market. Most contain caffeine or other mild stimulants. Unfortunately, none has been scientifically shown to assist in achieving a safe and permanent weight loss. A 1989 study of individuals using commercially available diet pills reported that fewer than 3% lost weight and maintained this weight loss longer than 12 months (2).

Spot Reduction

The notion that exercise applied to a specific region of the body will result in fat loss in that region is called **spot reduction**. Will performing sit-ups, for example, result in a reduction in abdominal fat? Unfortunately, the answer is "no." To date, there is no scientific evidence to show that exercise promotes fat loss in local regions of the body (31). As we have seen, the evidence suggests that when a caloric deficit exists, fat loss will occur from the largest sites of fat stores and not from specific areas (25).

Grapefruit Diet

Numerous myths have circulated concerning the value of eating large quantities of grapefruit to promote weight loss. One of these myths suggests that eating highly acidic grapefruit dissolves fat and results in a rapid loss of body weight. Although eating citrus fruits as part of a healthy low-calorie diet is a good idea, there is nothing magical about grapefruit that promotes fat loss. In fact, there are no magical foods that assist in weight loss.

Eating before Bedtime

Rumors exist that eating immediately prior to going to bed at night results in a greater fat gain than if the same meal were consumed during the day. These rumors are probably unfounded. Although eating a late-night meal or snack might not be a good dietary habit, this practice does not result in a greater weight gain than if the same meal had been consumed at another time during the day. Remember, it is the total daily calorie intake that determines fat gain, not the timing of the meal (4, 5).

spot reduction The false notion that exercise applied to a specific region of the body will result in fat loss in that region.

Cellulite

It is commonly believed that two kinds of body fat exist: cellulite and regular fat (18). The term **cellulite** refers to the "lumpy" hard fat that often gives skin a dimpled look. In reality, cellulite is just plain fat, not a special type of fat. The "dimpled" appearance comes from fat accumulating into small clusters and giving rise to the lumpy appearance of the skin.

Some health spas have advertised that vigorous massages provided by machines can remove cellulite and improve the appearance of your skin. Nonetheless, no scientific evidence exists that massage techniques are effective in promoting body fat loss or altering skin appearance.

Fat-Dissolving Creams

Over the years, numerous companies have marketed "weight loss creams" which are claimed to cause spot reduction of fat when applied to the skin. This is an attractive idea, as evidenced by the fact that companies have made millions of dollars from selling these products. Despite the boastful claims made by manufacturers, there is limited scientific evidence that these creams are effective in promoting fat loss.

Saunas, Steambaths, and Rubber Suits

Another hoax related to the loss of body fat is the notion that sitting in saunas or steambaths and/or running in a rubber suit melts body fat. Although saunas and steambaths do temporarily increase your metabolic rate, they do not melt away fat, nor do they significantly contribute to weight loss (7). For similar reasons, exercising in a rubber suit does not promote a greater fat loss than would be achieved by performing the same exercise in comfortable clothes.

These three methods do result in body water loss due to sweating, however. The accompanying body weight loss has been believed by some to be a loss of fat, but this is not the case. The weight temporarily lost in this way is regained as soon as body water is restored to normal levels.

Using saunas or steambaths and exercising while wearing a rubber suit may increase body temperature well above normal. This puts additional stress on the heart and circulatory system and could increase the risk of cardiac problems for older individuals or anyone with heart problems.

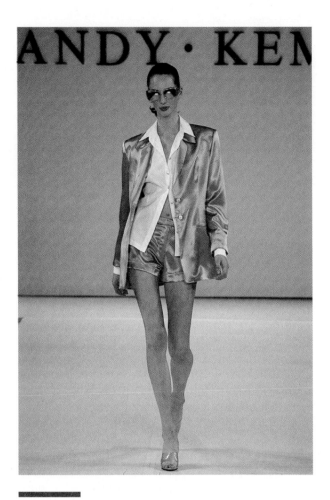

There are enormous societal pressures to be lean.

Eating Disorders

The low social acceptance of individuals with a high percentage of body fat and an emphasis on having the "perfect" body have increased the incidence of eating disorders. Two of the more common ones that affect young adults are anorexia nervosa and bulimia. Because of the relatively high occurrence of both disorders in female college students, we will discuss both the symptoms and health consequences of each.

Anorexia Nervosa

Anorexia nervosa is a common eating disorder that is unrelated to any specific physical disease. The end result of extreme anorexia nervosa is a state of starvation in which the individual becomes emaciated due to a refusal to eat. The psychological cause of anorexia nervosa is unclear, but it seems to be linked to an unfounded fear of fatness that may be related to family or societal pressures to be thin (9).

The incidence of this eating disorder has grown in recent years. Individuals with the highest probability of developing anorexia nervosa are upper middle class young women who are extremely self-critical. It is estimated that the incidence of anorexia nervosa is as high as one in every 200 adolescent girls (32, 33).

The anorexic may use a variety of techniques to remain thin, including starvation, exercise, and laxatives. The effects of anorexia include excessive weight loss, cessation of menstruation, and, in extreme cases, death. Because anorexia is a serious mental and physical disorder, medical treatment by a team of professionals (physician, psychologist, nutritionist) is necessary to correct the problem. Treatment may require years of psychological counseling and nutritional guidance. The first step in seeking professional treatment for anorexia is the recognition that a problem exists. The following are common symptoms of anorexia:

1. An intense fear of gaining weight or becoming obese

People with anorexia often have distorted body images.

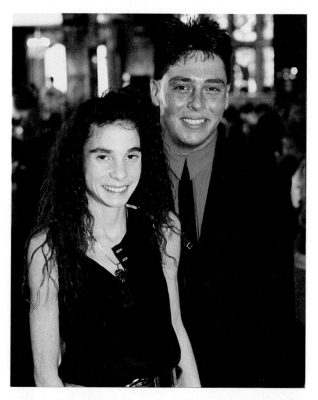

2. Feeling fat even at normal or below-normal body fatness because of a highly distorted body image

3. In women, the absence of three or more menstrual cycles

4. The possible development of odd behaviors concerning food; for example, the preparation of elaborate meals for others, but only a few low-calorie foods for their own consumption

5. About 50% of all anorexics eventually become bulimic (see next section)

Bulimia

Bulimia is overeating (called *binge eating*) followed by vomiting (called *purging*). In essence, the bulimic repeatedly ingests large quantities of food and then forces himself or herself to vomit in order to prevent weight gain. Bulimia may result in damage to the teeth and the esophagus, due to frequent vomiting of stomach acids. Like anorexia nervosa, bulimia is most common in young women, has a psychological origin, and requires professional treatment when diagnosed. Several authors have indicated that the incidence of bulimia may be as low as 1% or as high as 20% among U.S. girls and women aged 13 to 23 years (32, 33).

Most bulimics look "normal" and are of normal weight. However, even when their bodies are slender, their stomachs may protrude due to being stretched by frequent eating binges. Other common symptoms of bulimia include the following (36):

1. Recurrent binge eating.

2. A lack of control over eating behavior.

3. Regular self-induced vomiting and use of diuretics or laxatives.

cellulite The "lumpy" hard fat that often gives skin a dimpled look. Cellulite is just plain fat and not a special category of fat.

anorexia nervosa A common eating disorder that is unrelated to any specific physical disease. The end result of extreme anorexia nervosa is a state of starvation in which the individual becomes emaciated due to a refusal to eat.

bulimia An eating disorder that involves overeating (called *binge eating*) followed by vomiting (called *purging*).

4. Strict fasting or use of vigorous exercise to prevent weight gain.

5. Averaging two or more binge-eating episodes a week during a 2 to 3 month period.

6. Overconcern with body shape and weight.

Although maintaining an optimal body composition is a primary health goal, eating disorders are not appropriate means for weight loss. If you or any of your friends exhibit one or more of the symptoms cited here, please seek professional advice and treatment.

Exercise and Diet Programs to Gain Weight

The major focus of this chapter has been how to lose body fat. However, a small number of people, who consider themselves to be too thin, want to gain body weight. Both men and women can suffer from self-image problems if they feel they are too skinny. Although current social attitudes stress leanness in women, most agree that some degree of body curvature is desirable. Also, many men want a muscular body because of the improved self-image that comes with increased muscularity (9).

Body weight gain can be achieved in two ways. First, you can create a positive caloric balance and a positive fat balance and gain additional body fat. Second, you can increase your body weight by increasing your muscle mass through a weight training program. Let's discuss each of these types of body weight gain.

Gaining Body Fat

Before deciding to gain body fat, you should determine if your current body composition is within the desired range (see Chapter 2). If your percent body fat is below the recommended range (fewer than 8% of people fall into this category), it may be desirable for you to increase your body fat to reach the optimal percent body fat. Nonetheless, before looking at a dietary means for gaining fat, you should examine the cause of your being too lean (9). Several lifestyle problems could contribute to a low percentage of body fatness (9). For example, are you getting enough sleep? If not, you may be burning large amounts of energy and creating a negative caloric balance. Do you drink large amounts of coffee? Coffee can influence body weight in two ways. First, more

than three to five cups of coffee can reduce your appetite. Second, consumption of coffee or other caffeine-containing beverages increases your resting metabolism for several hours. Further, do you skip meals? Failing to eat regularly may result in a negative caloric balance and fat loss. Finally, do you have an eating disorder?

If lifestyle is not the problem, consult with your physician to rule out the possibility that the cause of your low body fat is due to hormonal imbalances or other diseases that influence body weight. After discussing with your physician your desire to gain fat and obtaining medical clearance to do so, consider the following recommendations:

1. Establish a weight gain goal that will place you at the low end of the recommended percent body fat range.

2. Create a positive energy balance. This is accomplished by increasing your total caloric intake to exceed your daily expenditure. A positive caloric balance of 3500 calories will generally result in a weight gain of 1 pound of fat. In general, a gain of about 1 pound of fat per week is a reasonable goal (positive balance of 500 calories/day).

3. To create a positive caloric balance, compute your daily caloric expenditure, and increase your caloric intake to exceed expenditure. When creating a positive caloric diet, use the basic principles of nutrition discussed in Chapter 7. That is, increase your total caloric intake by using the food pyramid, therefore adhering to the recommended guidelines for fat, carbohydrate, and protein intake.

4. Consult a physician and a nutritionist. Although anyone can gain weight while eating a positive caloric diet, the safest means of gaining body fat is with the assistance of these professionals.

Gaining Muscle Mass

If your percent of body fat is within the recommended range and you wish to increase your body mass, your goal should be to gain muscle mass, not fat. Unfortunately, there are no over-the-counter products or shortcuts for gaining muscle (see Nutritional Links to Health and Fitness 8.2). The key to gaining muscle mass is a program of rigorous weight training along with the increase in caloric intake needed to meet the increased energy expenditure and energy required to synthesize muscle. Exercise programs designed to improve muscular strength and size were discussed in Chapter 5 and will not be addressed here. The focus here is on the dietary adjustments needed to optimize gains in muscle mass. Again, in order to gain muscle mass, you need to create a small positive caloric balance to provide the energy required to synthesize new muscle protein. Nonetheless, before we provide dietary guidelines, let's discuss how much energy is expended during weight training and the energy required to promote muscle growth.

How much energy is expended during weight training? Energy expenditure during routine weight training is surprisingly small. For instance, a 70-kg man performing a 30-minute weight workout probably burns fewer than 70 calories (9). The reason for this low caloric expenditure is that during 30 minutes in the weight room, the average person spends only 8 to 10 minutes actually lifting weights; much time is spent in recovery periods between sets.

How much energy is required to synthesize 1 pound of muscle mass? Current estimates are approximately 2500 calories, of which, about 400 calories (100 grams) must be protein (9). To compute the additional calories required to produce an increase in muscle mass, you must first estimate your rate of muscular growth. This is difficult because the rate of muscular growth during weight training varies between people. While relatively large muscle mass gains are possible in some individuals, studies have shown that most men and women rarely gain more than 0.25

pounds of muscle per week during a 20-week weight training program (3 days/week, 30 minutes/day). If we assume that the average muscle gain is 0.25 pounds per week and that 2500 calories are required to synthesize one pound of muscle, a positive caloric balance of approximately 100 calories per day is needed to promote muscle growth (0.25 pounds/week × 2500 calories/pound = 625 calories/week; therefore 625 calories/week ÷ 7 days/week = 90 calories/day).

What are the dietary guidelines for gaining muscle mass? The major adjustments in diet are an increased caloric intake and assurance that you are obtaining adequate amounts of dietary protein. If you follow the dietary guidelines to produce a positive caloric balance (see Chapter 7), your diet will contain enough protein to support an increase in muscle mass. When planning your diet, consider the following points:

1. To increase your caloric intake, use the food pyramid presented in chapter 7. This will ensure that your diet meets the criteria for healthful living and provides adequate protein for building muscle.

2. Avoid intake of high-fat foods and limit your positive caloric balance to approximately 90 calories per day. Increasing your positive caloric balance above this level will not promote a faster rate of muscular growth but will result in increased body fat.

3. If you discontinue your weight training program, lower your caloric intake to match your daily energy expenditure.

8.2 Nutritional Links to Health and Fitness

Can Nutritional Supplements Promote Muscle Growth?

Numerous nutritional products are advertised as "wonder drugs" for promoting muscle growth. Many of these commodities are high-protein and often high-calorie drinks. There is no scientific evidence to support the notion that any of these products result in increased muscular strength or size. Regular weight training is the only proven and safe method of building muscle mass (see ref. 20 for a review).

Although consumption of small quantities of high-protein drinks may not be harmful, if you are eating a typical U.S. diet, increasing your protein in-

take is not necessary to promote muscle growth (9, 20). For example, let's look at the daily requirements of protein for normal growth and development. The RDA for protein is 0.8 grams per kilogram (kg) of body weight. Therefore, for a 70-kg man this would be 56 grams of protein per day (70 × 0.8 = 56). The average U.S. diet, however, contains about 100 grams of protein, which is almost twice the RDA recommendation. Therefore, protein supplements are not normally necessary to promote muscle growth.

Summary

1. Millions of people in the United States carry too much body fat for optimal health.

2. Obesity is defined as a high percentage of body fat; that is, over 25% for men and over 30% for women.

3. Obesity is linked to many diseases, including heart disease, diabetes, and hypertension.

4. The optimal percent body fat for health and fitness is believed to be 10% to 20% for men and 15% to 25% for women.

5. The energy balance theory of weight control states that to maintain your body weight, your energy intake must equal your energy expenditure.

6. Evidence suggests that creating a fat deficit is an essential factor in weight loss. This is because dietary fat is more easily stored as body fat than either carbohydrate or protein. The importance of a low-fat diet in weight control is illustrated by the fact that body fat gain is a result of a continual imbalance of fat intake and fat metabolism.

7. Total daily energy expenditure is the sum of both resting metabolic rate and exercise metabolic rate.

8. The four basic components of a comprehensive weight control program are weight loss goals; a reduced caloric diet stressing balanced nutrition; an exercise program designed to increase caloric expenditure and maintain muscle mass; and a behavior modification program designed to modify those behaviors that contribute to weight gain.

9. Weight loss goals should include both short-term and long-term goals.

10. Numerous weight loss myths exist. This chapter has discredited such weight loss methods as diet pills, spot reduction, grapefruit diets, cellulite reduction, and the use of saunas, steam baths, and rubber exercise suits.

11. Two relatively common eating disorders are anorexia nervosa and bulimia. Both are serious medical conditions and require professional treatment.

12. Weight training and a positive caloric balance are required to produce increases in muscle mass.

Study Questions

1. What is obesity? What diseases are linked to obesity?

2. Discuss several possible causes of obesity.

3. Discuss the concept of optimal body weight. How is optimal body weight computed?

4. Explain the roles of resting metabolic rate and exercise metabolic rate in determining total caloric expenditure. Which is more important in total daily caloric expenditure in a sedentary individual?

5. Outline a simple method that can be used to compute your daily caloric expenditure. Give an example.

6. List the four major components of a weight loss program.

7. Discuss the following weight loss myths: spot reduction; grapefruit diet; eating before bedtime; cellulite reduction; and saunas, steam baths, and rubber suits.

8. Define the eating disorders anorexia nervosa and bulimia.

9. Discuss the role of behavior modification in weight loss.

10. Define the following terms:

    energy balance theory of weight control
    isocaloric balance
    negative caloric balance
    positive caloric balance
    set point theory

11. Explain the fat deficit concept of weight control.

12. Compare exercise metabolic rate with resting metabolic rate.

13. What is cellulite?

14. How does creeping obesity occur?

15. Discuss the process of combining diet and exercise to increase muscle mass.

Suggested Reading

Leeds, M. *Nutrition for healthy living.* WCB-McGraw-Hill, Boston, MA, 1998.

Mole, P. Exercise and the fat balancing act. *ACSM's Health and Fitness Journal* 1(3): 18-26, 1997.

Powers, S., and E. Howley. *Exercise physiology: Theory and application to fitness and performance.* Wm. C. Brown, Dubuque, IA, 1994.

Sizer, F., and E. Whitney. *Nutrition: Concepts and controversies.* West/Wadsworth, New York, NY, 1997.

Williams, M. *Lifetime fitness and wellness.* Wm. C. Brown, Dubuque, IA, 1996.

Suggested Readings on the World Wide Web
Shape Up America
(http://www.shapup.org/sva)
Latest information about physical fitness and weight control by ex-Surgeon General, Dr. Everett Koop.
Sympatico:
(http://www.ns.sympatico.ca/healthyway)
Articles about fitness, health, book reviews, and links to nutrition, fitness, and wellness topics.

References

1. Atkinson, R. Treatment of obesity. *Nutritional Reviews* 50:338–345, 1992.

1a. National Institutes of Health technology assessment conference statement: Methods for voluntary weight loss and control. *Nutrition Reviews* 50:340–345, 1992.

2. Wadden, T., J. Sternberg, K. Letizia, A. Stunkard, and G. Foster. Treatment for obesity by very low calorie diet, behavior therapy, and their combination: A five year prospective. *International Journal of Obesity* 13(Suppl. 2):39–46, 1989.

3. American College of Sports Medicine, L. Durstine, et al., eds. *Resource manual for guidelines for exercise testing and prescription.* 2d ed. Lea and Febiger, Philadelphia, 1993.

4. Bjorntorp, P., and B. Brodoff, eds. *Obesity.* J. B. Lippincott, Philadelphia, 1992.

5. Perri, M., A. Nezu, and B. Viegener. *Improving the long-term management and treatment of obesity.* John Wiley and Sons, New York, 1992.

6. Stefanick, M. Exercise and weight control. *Exercise and Sport Science Reviews.* (J. Holloszy, ed.) Williams and Wilkie, Baltimore, pp. 363–396, 1993.

7. Stunkard, A., and T. Wadden, eds. *Obesity: Theory and therapy.* Raven Press, New York, 1993.

8. Kuczmarski, R. Prevalence of overweight and weight gain in the United States. *American Journal of Clinical Nutrition* 55:495s–502s, 1992.

9. Williams, M. *Lifetime fitness and wellness.* Wm. C. Brown, Dubuque, IA, 1996.

10. Van Itallie, T. Health implications of overweight and obesity in the United States. *Annals of Internal Medicine* 103:983–988, 1985.

11. Health implications of obesity: National Institutes of Health consensus development conference. *Annals of Internal Medicine* 103:977–1077, 1985.

12. Bouchard, C., R. Shepherd, T. Stephens, J. Sutton, and B. McPherson, eds. *Exercise, fitness, and health: A consensus of current knowledge.* Human Kinetics, Champaign, IL, 1990.

12a. Barrow, M. *Heart talk: Understanding cardiovascular diseases.* Cor-Ed Publishing, Gainesville, FL, 1992.

13. Bouchard, C., A. Tremblay, J. Despres, et al. The response to long-term overfeeding in identical twins. *New England Journal of Medicine* 322:1477–1482, 1990.

14. Stunkard, A., T. Sorensen, C. Hanis, et al. An adoption study of human obesity. *New England Journal of Medicine* 314:193–198, 1986.

15. Howley, E., and B. D. Franks. *Health fitness: Instructors handbook.* Human Kinetics, Champaign, IL, 1997.

16. Hockey, R. *Physical fitness: The pathway to healthful living.* Times Mirror/Mosby, St. Louis, 1989.

17. Getchell, B. *Physical fitness: A way of life.* Allyn and Bacon, Needham Heights, MA, 1997.

18. Corbin, C., and R. Lindsey. *Concepts of physical fitness.* Wm. C. Brown, Dubuque, IA, 1997.

19. Pollock, M., and J. Wilmore. *Exercise in health and disease.* W. B. Saunders, Philadelphia, 1990.

20. Powers, S., and E. Howley. *Exercise physiology: Theory and application to fitness and performance.* Wm. C. Brown, Dubuque, IA, 1994.

21. Bailey, J., R. Barker, and R. Beauchene. Age-related changes in rat adipose tissue cellularity are altered by dietary restriction and exercise. *Journal of Nutrition* 123:52–58, 1993.

22. Blair, S. Evidence for success of exercise in weight loss control. *Annals of Internal Medicine* 119:702–706, 1993.

23. Poehlman, E. A review: Exercise and its influence on resting energy metabolism in man. *Medicine and Science in Sports and Exercise* 21:515–525, 1989.

24. Jequier, E. Body weight regulation in humans: The importance of nutrient balance. *News in Physiological Sciences* 8:273–276, 1993.

25. King M., and F. Katch. Changes in body density, fatfolds, and girths at 2.3 kg increments of weight loss. *Human Biology* 58:709,1986.

26. Broeder, C., K. Burrhus, L. Svanevik, and J. Wilmore. The effects of either high intensity resistance or endurance training on resting metabolic rate. *American Journal of Clinical Nutrition* 55:802–810, 1992.

27. Bailey, C. *The new fit or fat*. Houghton Mifflin, Boston, 1991.

28. Romijn, J., E. Coyle, L. Sidossis, et al. Regulation of endogenous fat and carbohydrate metabolism in relation to exercise and duration. *American Journal of Physiology* 265:E380–E391, 1993.

29. Tremblay, A., S. Coveney, J. Despres, A. Nadeau, D. Prud'homme. Increased resting metabolic rate and lipid oxidation in exercise-trained individuals: Evidence for a role of beta-oxidation. *Canadian Journal of Physiology and Pharmacology* 70:1342–1347, 1992.

30. Mayer, J., N. Marshall, J. Vitale, J. Christensen, M. Mashayekhi, and F. Stare. Exercise, food intake, and body weight in normal rats and genetically obese adult mice. *American Journal of Physiology* 177:544–548, 1954.

31. Gwinup, G., R. Chelvam, and T. Steinberg. Thickness of subcutaneous fat and activity of underlying muscles. *Annals of Internal Medicine* 74:408–411, 1971.

32. Andersen, A. Anorexia nervosa and bulimia. *Journal of Adolescent Health Care* 4:15–21, 1983.

33. Borgen, J., and C. Corbin. Eating disorders among female athletes. *Physician and Sports Medicine* 15:89–95, 1987.

34. Sizer, F., and E. Whitney. *Nutrition: Concepts and controversies.* West/Wadsworth, New York, NY, 1997.

35. Mole, P. Exercise and the fat balancing act. *ACSM's Health and Fitness Journal* 1(3): 18–26, 1997.

36. Leeds, M. *Nutrition for healthy living.* WCB-McGraw-Hill, Boston, MA, 1998.

Determining Ideal Body Weight Using Percent Body Fat and the Body Mass Index

NAME _____ DATE _____

There are a number of different ways to compute an ideal body weight. In Chapter 2, we discussed percent body fat (estimated from skinfold measurements). Method A of this laboratory allows you to compute and record your ideal body weight using the percent body fat method. Method B allows you to calculate and record your ideal body weight using the body mass index procedure (see Chapter 2). Choose one of these techniques and complete the appropriate section.

Method A: Computation of Ideal Body Weight Using Percent Body Fat

Step 1: Calculate fat-free weight

100% – your percent body fat estimated from skinfold measurement = _____ % fat free weight.

Therefore,

_____ % fat-free weight expressed as a fraction × your body weight in pounds = _____ pounds fat-free weight.

Step 2: Calculate optimal weight

Remember: Optimal body fat ranges are 10% to 20% for men and 15% to 25% for women.

Optimal weight = fat-free weight/(1.00 – optimal %fat), with optimal %fat expressed as a fraction.

Therefore,

the low and high optimal weight ranges for your gender are

For low %fat: Optimal weight = _____ pounds

For high %fat: Optimal weight = _____ pounds

Method B: Computation of Ideal Body Weight Using Body Mass Index (BMI)

The BMI uses the metric system. Therefore, you need to determine your weight in kilograms (1 kilogram = 2.2 pounds) and your height in meters (1 inch = 0.0254 meters).

Step 1: Compute your BMI.

BMI = body weight (kg)/(height in meters)^2

Your BMI = _____

Step 2: Calculate Your Ideal Body Weight Based on BMI*.

The ideal BMI is 21.9 to 22.4 for men and 21.3 to 22.1 for women. The formula for computing ideal body weight using BMI is

ideal body weight (kilograms) = desired BMI × (height in meters)^2

Consider the following example as an illustration of the computation of ideal body weight. A woman who weighs 60 kilograms and is 1.5 meters tall computes her BMI to be 26.7. Her ideal BMI is between 21.9 and 22.4; therefore, her ideal body weight range is

ideal body weight = 21.9 × 2.25 = 49.3 kilograms
ideal body weight = 22.4 × 2.25 = 50.4 kilograms

Now complete this calculation using your values for BMI.

My ideal body weight range using the BMI method is _____ to _____ kilograms.

* Note: BMI may not be a good method to determine ideal body weight for a highly muscled individual.

Estimating Daily Caloric Expenditure and the Caloric Deficit Required to Lose 1 Pound of Fat Per Week

NAME _____ DATE _____

Part A. Estimation of Your Daily Caloric Expenditure

Using Table 8.1, compute your estimated daily caloric expenditure.

Estimated daily caloric expenditure = _____ calories/day.

Part B. Calculation of Caloric Intake Required to Promote 1 Pound Per Week of Weight Loss

Recall that 1 pound of fat contains approximately 3500 calories. Therefore, a negative caloric balance of 500 calories/day will result in a weight loss of 1 pound per week. Use the following formula to compute your daily caloric intake to result in a caloric deficit of 500 calories.

estimated daily caloric expenditure – 500 calories (deficit) = daily caloric intake needed to produce a 500-calorie deficit

In the space provided, compute your daily caloric intake needed to produce 1 pound/week of weight loss.

_____ (estimated caloric expenditure)

_____ – 500 _____ (caloric deficit)

= _____ target daily caloric intake

Weight Loss Goals and Progress Report

NAME _____ DATE _____

In the spaces, record your short-term and long-term weight loss goals. Then keep a record of your weight loss progress on the chart.

Ideal body weight (range): _____

Short-term weight loss goal: _____ (pounds/week)

Long-term weight loss goal: _____ pounds

Week No.	Body Weight	Date	Weight Loss
1			
2			
3			
4			
5			
6			
7			
8			
9			
10			
11			
12			
13			
14			
15			
16			
17			
18			
19			
20			
21			
22			

23_____

24_____

25_____

26_____

27_____

28_____

29_____

30_____

31_____

32_____

33_____

34_____

35_____

36_____

37_____

38_____

39_____

40_____

Exercise and the Environment

After studying this chapter, you should be able to

1 Describe how to prevent heat loss during exercise.

2 List several important guidelines for exercising in a hot environment.

3 Describe the appropriate exercise clothing for exercising in the heat.

4 Differentiate between the various types of heat injuries.

5 Discuss how heat acclimatization reduces the risk of heat injury.

6 Describe the appropriate clothing for exercise in a cold environment.

7 Explain why exercise at high altitude results in higher heart rate and elevated breathing.

8 List two major forms of air pollution.

9 Outline a strategy for coping with air pollution.

ost of us know from personal experience that environmental factors can affect exercise performance. For example, hot environments, high altitude, and air pollution can elevate exercise heart rates, promote labored breathing, and impair exercise tolerance. A general understanding of how environmental factors can influence exercise performance is important for the physically active individual. In this chapter we discuss common environmental hazards that should be considered when planning workouts and outline ways to cope with environmental stress. In particular, we focus on the following environmental concerns: heat and humidity, cold, altitude, and air pollution. Let's begin with a discussion of exercise in a hot environment.

Exercise in the Heat

Humans are **homeotherms,** which means *same temperature.* That is, body temperature is regulated around a set point; humans regulate their body temperature around the set point of 98.6°F or 37°C. Variations in body temperature can result in serious bodily injury. Indeed, heat illness can occur when body temperature rises above 105°F (41°C)(1). Cramps, dizziness, nausea, lack of sweat production, and dry, hot skin are all indications of impending heat illness. Therefore, the body must maintain precise control over temperature to avoid a life-threatening situation. Figure 9.1 illustrates both the environmental and physiological extremes of heat and cold that humans can endure.

During exercise, heat is produced as a byproduct of muscular contractions. High-intensity exercise using large muscle groups produces more body heat than low-intensity exercise involving small muscle groups. Hence, during vigorous exercise using large muscle groups, the body must eliminate excess heat in order to prevent a dangerous rise in body temperature. In the next several paragraphs we discuss heat loss during exercise and outline key factors to consider when exercising in a hot environment.

Heat Loss during Exercise

The primary means of heat loss during exercise are **convection** and **evaporation.** Convection is heat loss by the movement of air (or water)

around the body. Evaporative heat loss occurs due to the conversion of sweat (water) to a gas (water vapor). Let's discuss each of these methods individually.

Convective heat loss occurs only when the air or water molecules moving around the body are cooler than skin temperature, because the faster the flow of cool air or water around the body, the greater the heat loss. Minimal convective cooling occurs during exercise in a hot environment where there is limited air movement (riding a stationary exercise bicycle, for example). In contrast, bicycling outdoors on a cold day or swimming in cool water results in a large amount of convective cooling.

On a warm day with limited air movement around the body, evaporation is the most important means of body heat loss (1). The evaporation of sweat on the skin's surface removes heat from the body, even if the air temperature is higher than body temperature, as long as the air is dry. However, if the **humidity** is high, meaning the air is relatively saturated with water, and the air temperature is high, evaporation is retarded and body heat loss is drastically decreased. Under these conditions, heat produced by the contracting muscles is retained and body temperature increases gradually throughout the exercise session. Prolonged exercise in a hot and humid environment can result in a dangerously high increase in body temperature. Figure 9.2 on page 222, illustrates the differences in body heat gain during exercise in a high-temperature/high-humidity environment, a high-temperature/low-humidity environment, and a low-temperature/low-humidity environment.

Guidelines for Exercise in the Heat

Short-term exposure (30 to 60 min) to an extremely hot environment is sufficient heat stress to cause heat illness in some people (2). This is especially true for people at high risk for heat illness (the elderly and those with low cardiovascular fitness levels are most susceptible). Even those individuals who are physically fit and accustomed to the heat are at risk if they exercise in a hot environment.

Heat stress on the body is not simply a function of the air temperature; both the heat and humidity must be considered. As indicated in Figure 9.3 on page 223, the higher the humidity, the higher the "effective" temperature. The effective temperature can be defined as the tempera-

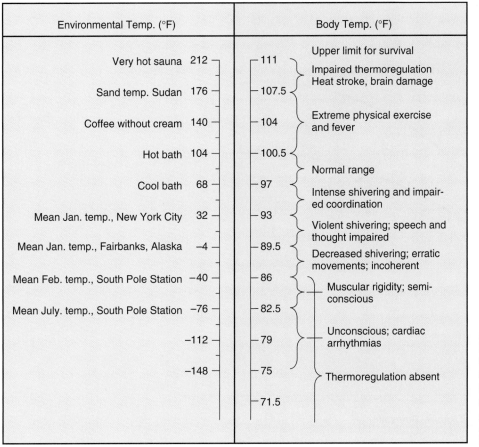

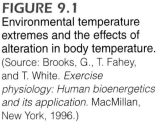

FIGURE 9.1
Environmental temperature extremes and the effects of alteration in body temperature. (Source: Brooks, G., T. Fahey, and T. White. *Exercise physiology: Human bioenergetics and its application.* MacMillan, New York, 1996.)

ture that the body senses. At high levels of humidity, evaporation is retarded and the body cannot get rid of the heat normally lost through evaporative processes. This causes the temperature in the body to increase above what it would normally be on a less humid day at the same ambient temperature.

Although it is obvious that it is extremely dangerous to exercise at high air temperatures (130°F, 55°C), it may not be obvious to most people that the body undergoes the same heat stress at only 85°F (29.5°C) when the humidity is high (~100%). In other words, the effective temperature remains at 130°F. Thus, high humidity causes a moderately high ambient temperature to be sensed by the body as extremely hot (see Figure 9.3).

The best way to determine if the environmental conditions are imposing a heat load on your body is to monitor your heart rate. An increase in body temperature during exercise in a hot environment will result in large increases in heart rate compared with exercise in a cool environment. This point is illustrated in Figure 9.4,

which shows the large differences in heart rate responses to exercise in the three different conditions. A temperature-induced increase in exercise heart rate is significant because it increases the difficulty of staying within your target heart rate zone (see Chapter 4).

homeotherms Animals that regulate their body temperature around a constant level; that is, body temperature is regulated around a set point. Humans regulate their body temperature around the set point of 98.6°F or 37°C.

convection Heat loss by the movement of air (or water) around the body.

evaporation The conversion of water (or sweat) to a gas (water vapor). The most important means of removing heat from the body during exercise.

humidity The amount of water vapor in the air. If the relative humidity is high, meaning the air is relatively saturated with water, and the air temperature is high, evaporation is retarded and body heat loss is drastically decreased.

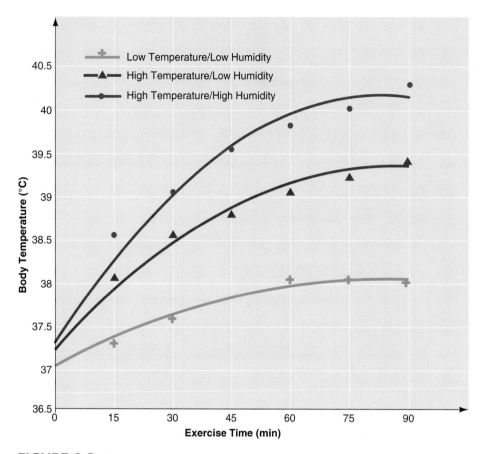

FIGURE 9.2 Body temperature responses to prolonged exercise in a high-temperature/high-humidity environment, a high-temperature/low-humidity environment, and a low-temperature/low-humidity environment.

Given the dangers of combined high heat and humidity, should you even consider exercising under these conditions? The answer is "yes," but when exercising in the heat, keep the following in mind:

1. Start exercising slowly, and keep your exercise session relatively short (15 to 20 minutes).

2. Monitor your exercise heart rate often, and keep your exercise intensity low so that you stay within your target heart rate zone.

3. Wear appropriate clothing (see the following section on exercise clothing).

4. Drink plenty of cold fluids before, during, and after the exercise session (see Nutritional Links to Health and Fitness 9.1).

5. Do not use supplemental salt tablets. Salt is lost from the body in sweat (especially in those unaccustomed to the heat). It has long been thought by those involved in athletics

that people should replace this lost salt by taking supplemental salt tablets. However, recent research suggests that this is not necessary. As discussed in Chapter 7, many people consume too much salt in the diet. In fact, supplemental salt is counterproductive to coping with heat stress. Thus, it is not necessary to take salt tablets to replace lost sodium; replacement of body water is the critical element (see A Closer Look 9.1).

6. Exercise in the coolest part of the day. Mornings are best because much of the radiant heat from the ground has been lost overnight and the air temperature is most likely the lowest of the day. After sunset would be the second best time because the radiant heat from the sun will not be a factor. If you must exercise during the heat of the day, try to find a shaded area. This might mean exercising indoors or hiking/jogging in a wooded area.

Exercise Clothing for Hot Environments

Although it may be impossible to prevent body heat gain during exercise in a hot environment, there are ways to reduce the risks of heat injury. Wearing the proper clothing is essential to minimize the possibility of overheating (3). Clothing should be minimal to maximize the body surface area exposed for evaporation. It should be lightweight and made from materials that allow air to move through them freely, such as lightweight cotton. This promotes both convective and evaporative cooling. Dry clothing retards heat exchange compared with the same clothing soaking wet. Switching to dry clothing when your clothes become saturated with sweat makes little sense from a temperature-regulation standpoint. Dry clothing simply prolongs the time between sweating and cooling. Cottons and linens are best for readily absorbing moisture. Heavy clothing and that made of rubber or plastic retard evaporative heat loss by trapping humid air next to the skin. In addition, because dark colors absorb radiant heat from the sun, light-colored clothing should be worn outdoors.

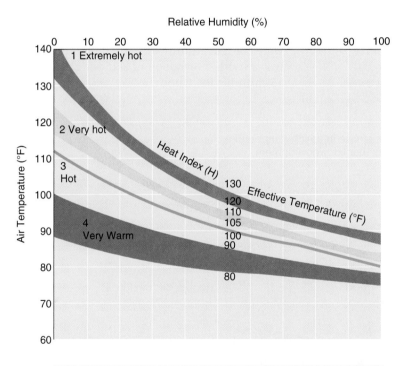

Category	Heat Index	General Effect of Heat Index on People in Higher Risk Groups
1	130° or higher	Heat/sunstroke highly likely with continued exposure
2	105°–130°	Sunstroke, heat cramps, or heat exhaustion likely and heatstroke possible with prolonged exposure and/or physical activity
3	90°–105°	Sunstroke, heat cramps, and heat exhaustion possible with prolonged exposure and/or physical activity
4	80°–90°	Fatigue possible with prolonged exposure and/or physical activity

FIGURE 9.3 The concept of "heat index" or "effective" temperature. (Source: Donatelle, R. J., and L. G. Davis. *Access to health.* Prentice-Hall, Englewood Cliffs, NJ, 1996.)

Heat Acclimatization

Exercise in a hot, or even moderately hot, environment will cause the body to adapt or **acclimatize** to this condition. *Acclimatization* refers to the physiological adaptations that occur to assist the body in dissipating heat. These changes include an earlier onset of sweating, a higher exercise sweat rate (i.e., more evaporative cooling), and an increase in blood volume (3). Interestingly, heat acclimatization occurs rapidly. Within 10 to 12 days of heat exposure, the physiological responses to exercise in the heat are drastically altered (4). The end result is that heat acclimatization promotes a decreased exercise heart rate and lower body temperature. A key point here is that heat acclimatization decreases the possibilities of experiencing heat injuries during exercise.

Heat injuries can occur when the exercise heat load exceeds the body's ability to regulate body temperature. They are serious and can result in damage to the nervous system, and in extreme cases, death. The following are the most common of the heat injuries.

Heat Cramps: Heat cramps are characterized by muscle spasms or twitching of limbs. This usually occurs in people who are unacclimatized to the heat. The person with these symptoms should be moved to a cool place, laid down, and given one to two glasses of water with one-half teaspoon of salt added to each glass.

Heat Exhaustion: Heat exhaustion results in general weakness, fatigue, a possible drop in blood pressure, blurred vision, occasionally a loss of consciousness, and profuse sweating, with pale, clammy skin. Heat exhaustion can occur in an acclimatized individual. First aid should consist of moving the victim to a cool place, removing the clothing, applying cold water or ice, administering one-half glass of water (with 1 teaspoon of salt per glass) each 15 minutes for 1 hour.

FIGURE 9.4 Heart rate responses to prolonged exercise in a high-temperature, high-humidity environment and a low-temperature, low-humidity environment.

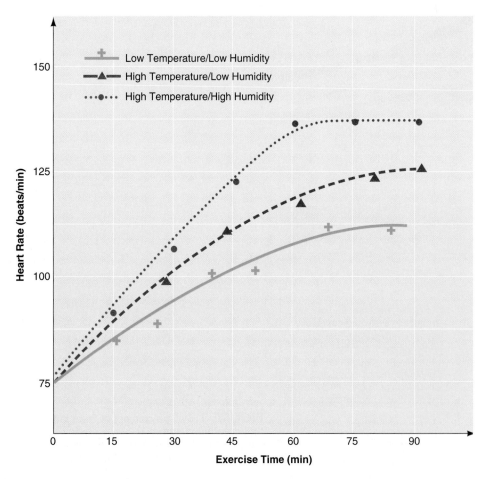

9.1 Nutritional Links to Health and Fitness

Guidelines for Fluid Intake during Exercise in a Hot Environment

Because the sweat you lose during exercise is replaced with water from the blood, the ultimate danger during prolonged exercise in the heat is the loss of blood volume. The best strategy for preventing a decrease in blood volume is maintaining a regular schedule of fluid intake during exercise. However, thirst for fluid lags behind fluid loss. This is because your body does not recognize a need for fluid until the composition of the blood is changed. Therefore, you should begin to drink within 10 to 20 minutes after beginning exercise before the fluid deficit accumulates. The following fluid replacement schedule will help in meeting your body's needs for water (15):

Contents of fluid

The drink should be:

- low in sugar (generally less than 8 grams per 100 ml of water)
- electrolytes (sodium and potassium)
- cold (approximately 45–55°F, or 8–13°C)

Fluid intake prior to workout

Drink approximately 200 ml (6 oz) of the fluid 20 to 30 minutes prior to the workout.

Fluid intake during workout

Thirst is a poor gauge of the amount of fluid needed. Drink approximately 100 to 200 ml (3–6.6 oz) every 10 to 20 minutes during exercise, regardless of whether you feel thirsty.

Fluid replacement after workout

In general, you should consume 30 ml (~1 oz) of fluid for every minute of exercise performed. Another means of estimating how much fluid you need is to weigh yourself prior to exercise and immediately after your cool-down period. The difference in body weight is a measure of how much fluid was lost via sweating, and more than that amount should be replaced. In fact, each ounce of body weight lost due to sweating is equivalent to 1 fluid ounce. For example, a pre/postexercise body weight difference of 1 pound indicates that 16 ounces of sweat were lost during exercise. Therefore, consumption of more than 16 fluid ounces (~475 ml) of fluid is required to replace body fluid stores.

Heat Stroke: Heat stroke is a life-threatening emergency. For the person experiencing heat stroke, sweating stops and the skin is hot and red. Muscles are limp. There is involuntary limb movement, seizures, diarrhea, vomiting, and a rapid, strong heart beat. The individual may hallucinate and eventually lapse into a coma. Any of these symptoms should be taken very seriously, and emergency procedures should be begun. First aid consists of moving the victim to a cool place, removing clothing, and reducing body temperature as rapidly as possible (water, ice, soft drinks, fanning). Seek emergency medical assistance immediately.

Each of these conditions has the following similarities: They are initiated by heat exposure; there is significant loss of water and electrolytes;

acclimatize Refers to the physiological adaptations that occur to assist the body in adjusting to environmental extremes. Exercise in a hot or even moderately hot environment will cause the body to adapt to these conditions.

heat injuries also called *heat illness* Bodily injury that can occur when the exercise heat load exceeds the body's ability to regulate body temperature. They are serious and can result in damage to the nervous system and, in extreme cases, death.

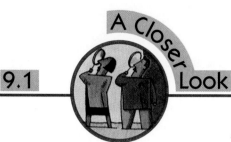

Adverse Effects of Dehydration

Exercise in the heat can be extremely danger-ous depending on the exercise intensity, ambient temperature, relative humidity, clothing, and state of hydration (water content of the body). Although some forms of heat illness can occur prior to significant weight loss due to sweating, the following table shows how weight loss during exercise can be a pre-dictor of some of the dangers associated with exer-cise in the heat. The loss of body weight during exercise in the heat is simply due to water loss through sweating. Thus, prolonged, profuse sweating is the first warning signal of impending dehydration.

% Body Weight Loss	Symptoms
0.5	Thirst
2.0	Stronger thirst, vague discomfort, loss of appetite
3.0	Concentrated blood, dry mouth, reduced urine
4.0	Increased effort for exercise, flushed skin, apathy
5.0	Difficulty in concentrating
6.0	Impaired temperature regulation, increased heart rate
8.0	Dizziness, labored breathing in exercise, confusion
10.0	Spastic muscles, loss of balance, delirium
11.0	Circulatory insufficiency, decreased blood volume, kidney failure

and there is an increase in heat storage by the body, as indicated by a high core temperature. The most important of these is the loss of water, a factor that can be prevented by drinking plenty of fluids. Inattention to any of the signs of heat ill-ness can lead to heat stroke and finally to death. Do not take these symptoms lightly!

Exercise in the Cold

Exercising below an effective temperature of ~80°F (see Figure 9.3) increases your ability to lose heat and therefore greatly reduces the oppor-tunity for heat injury. However, exercising at am-bient temperatures below ~60°F dictates that some combination of warm clothing and produc-tion of muscle heat is required to prevent too much body heat loss. If these two factors are not

combined properly in extremely cold tempera-tures, the chances for developing a large decrease in body temperature (hypothermia) could be life threatening (1). Indeed, exercise in the cold for long periods (e.g., 1–4 hours) or swimming in cold water may overpower the body's ability to prevent heat loss, resulting in hypothermia. Se-vere hypothermia can result in a loss of judg-ment, which increases the risk of further cold injury. It can be avoided by limiting the duration of exercise in a cold environment, dressing ap-propriately, and avoiding cold water (water can be considered too cold if it makes you start to shiver).

A question that is often asked is, "Can you damage your lungs by breathing cold air during exercise?" Research suggests that exercise in cold weather 15 to 32°F (-10–0°C) does not present a major risk to lung tissues (5). Indeed, inhaled cold air is rapidly warmed by the nasal passages and airways so that by the time the gas reaches the lungs, it is close to body temperature.

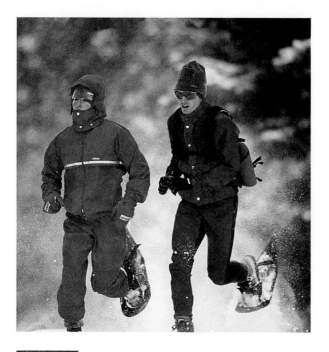

Exercise in the cold can be enjoyable if the proper clothing is worn.

Exercise Clothing for Cold Environments

The key to exercising in the cold is wearing the proper clothing (6). The ideal clothing permits sweat to be transferred from the skin to the outer surface of the clothing so that some of the heat produced during exercise will be lost and normal body temperature maintained. Your strategy should be to insulate the body just enough to trap only the amount of heat necessary for maintenance of body temperature, but not enough to overheat.

Trapping heat is best accomplished by wearing multiple layers of clothing. *Layering,* or dressing in multiple layers of clothing, reduces heat loss by trapping air between the layers. This is because air is an excellent insulator, and layers of clothing are very effective at trapping air. The thicker the zone of trapped air next to the body, the more effective the insulation. Therefore, several layers of light clothing provide much greater insulation than a single bulky coat. To provide layering, as well as the ability to transport moisture from the skin, the best materials are wool or synthetics such as polypropylene. Also, remem-

A Closer Look

9.2

Exercise in the Cold — But Don't Get Wet!

Exercise in a cool or cold environment can be safe as well as pleasurable if the proper clothing is worn. If the intensity of the exercise causes a person to sweat or if a person gets wet in the rain, a dangerous condition would occur. A recent study (14) examined the effects of cold, rain, and wind on exercise tolerance and hypothermia. Subjects were asked to attempt a 5-hour walk at 5° C (41° F) at a brisk pace. At the end of 1 hour the subjects were exposed to constant rain and wind in addition to the cold. These conditions were severe enough that only 5 of 16 subjects could complete the 5-hour walk.

During the first hour of walking, body temperature actually rose 1 degree! However, with the onset of wind and rain, body temperature started to decrease even when some subjects began shivering. The shivering produced weakness and loss of manual dexterity. Over the last 2 hours, body temperature

was variable in those completing the walk. Of the 5 subjects that completed the walk, 2 experienced a severe decrease in body temperature because they were not able to maintain the walking pace due to fatigue from shivering.

This study illustrates several important concepts. It illustrates the interaction between air temperature, wind, and water. If clothing gets wet, it conducts heat from the body so fast that heat production during exercise may not be sufficient to maintain body temperature. It is important to note that the subjects in this study were not wearing protective rainwear. Any type of waterproof clothing would have given them significant additional time to exercise in the wind and rain. In contrast, a very fit individual who was capable of increasing exercise intensity in the conditions of this study may have been able to complete the 5 hours without rainwear.

	Ambient Temperature, °F*														
	40	35	30	25	20	15	10	5	0	-5	-10	-15	-20	-25	-30
	Effective Temperature, °F														
Calm	40	35	30	25	20	15	10	5	0	-5	-10	-15	-20	-25	-30
5	37	33	27	21	16	12	6	1	-5	-11	-15	-20	-26	-31	-35
10	28	21	16	9	4	-2	-9	-15	-21	-27	-33	-38	-46	-52	-58
15	22	16	11	1	-5	-11	-18	-25	-36	-40	-45	-51	-58	-65	-70
20	18	12	3	-4	-10	-17	-25	-32	-39	-46	-53	-60	-67	-76	-81
25	16	7	0	-7	-15	-22	-29	-37	-44	-52	-59	-67	-74	-83	-89
30	13	5	-2	-11	-18	-26	-33	-41	-48	-56	-63	-70	-79	-87	-94
35	11	3	-4	-13	-20	-27	-35	-43	-49	-60	-67	-72	-82	-90	-98
40	10	1	-6	-15	-21	-29	-37	-45	-53	-62	-69	-76	-85	-94	-101

(Wind Speed, mph — left axis)

Little Danger   Danger   Great Danger

*°C = 0.556 (°F −32)

Convective heat loss at wind speeds above 40 mph have little additional effect on body cooling.

FIGURE 9.5 The "wind-chill" index. (Source: McArdle, W. D., F. I. Katch, and V. L. Katch, *Exercise physiology: Energy, nutrition, and human performance.* 4th ed. Lea and Febiger, Malvern, 1996.)

ber to cover your head because 30% to 40% of body heat is lost through the head.

However, too much clothing may limit your freedom of movement as well as result in body heat gain. An increase in body heat can lead to sweating, which causes the clothing to lose its insulating properties. In addition, wet clothing can actually facilitate the loss of body heat and, during extreme cold, could lead to a decrease in body temperature, which would be fatal (4). The proper amount of clothing to provide comfort during exercise varies with the temperature and the speed of the wind as well as with the intensity and duration of exercise. Indeed, wind is a major complicating factor in the cold. The greater the speed of the wind in a cold environment, the colder it feels. This effect of wind to cause a colder "feel" than the air temperature is referred to as the *wind chill factor*. In other words, the wind makes the effective temperature colder than the measured air temperature.

Exercise and Altitude

Each year, more and more people go to high altitudes to participate in recreational activities such as skiing, hiking, and camping. How does the body respond to exercise at high altitudes, and how can you adjust your exercise prescription?

The primary concern with exercise at high altitude (e.g., altitudes >5000 feet) is that the lower barometric pressure limits the amount of oxygen transported in arterial blood (7). This results in a reduction in oxygen transport to the exercising muscles, and therefore both exercise tolerance and VO_2 max are reduced. The magnitude of the reduction increases as a function of the altitude. That is, the higher the altitude, the greater the reduction in VO_2 max and exercise tolerance. This point is illustrated in Figure 9.6. Note that there is little change in VO_2 max until the altitude of approximately 5000 feet above sea level is reached (e.g., the elevation of Denver, Colorado). Above 5000 feet, there is a progressive decrease in VO_2 max.

To cope with this lowered oxygen delivery to the exercising muscles, the body makes several physiological adjustments (Figure 9.7). Breathing becomes deeper and faster in an attempt to maximize oxygen transfer from the lungs to the blood. Exercise heart rate rises to increase blood flow and oxygen delivery to the exercising muscles. To stay within your target heart rate zone during exercise at a high altitude, it is necessary to lower your exercise intensity to a level below your normal (sea level) intensity. In general, there is little need to alter your duration or frequency of training during a brief stay at a high altitude. However, the air is very dry at high altitudes, which

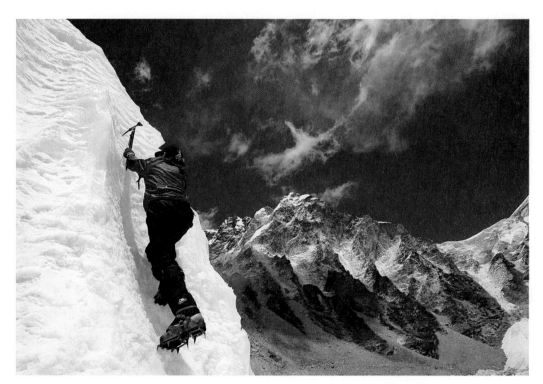

Altitude presents a significant, long-lasting challenge to the body.

results in increased loss of water with breathing (7). In addition, the body decreases its water content as a way to cope with the stress of altitude exposure. Be sure to drink plenty of fluids during and after exercise.

FIGURE 9.6 The effects of altitude on maximal exercise capacity.

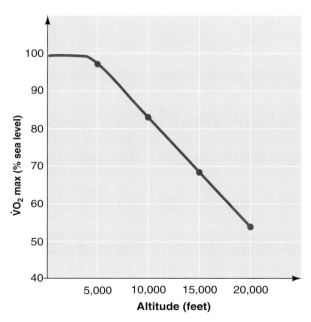

Exercise and Air Pollution

Air pollution is a growing problem in many parts of the world. In this section we examine the effects of air pollution on exercise performance and establish guidelines for minimizing its effects.

Major Forms of Air Pollution

Two major pollutants that affect exercise performance are ozone and carbon monoxide (8, 9, 10). **Ozone** is primarily produced by a chemical reaction between sunlight and the hydrocarbons emitted from car exhausts. This form of pollution is extremely irritating to the lungs and airways. It causes tightness in the chest,

ozone A gas produced by a chemical reaction between sunlight and the hydrocarbons emitted from car exhausts. This form of pollution is extremely irritating to the lung and airways. It causes tightness in the chest, coughing, headaches, nausea, throat and eye irritation, and, worst of all, bronchoconstriction.

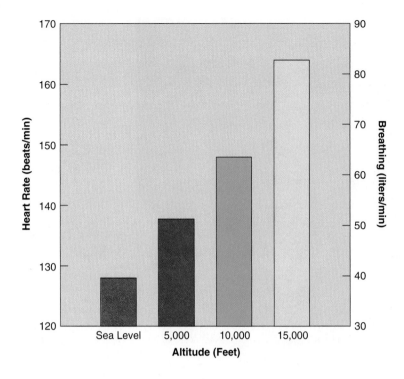

FIGURE 9.7 Heart rate and ventilation responses to moderate exercise at sea level, 5,000, 10,000, and 15,000 feet in altitude. Exercise workload is constant at each altitude.

coughing, headaches, nausea, throat and eye irritation, and, worst of all, bronchoconstriction (11). In fact, exposure to ozone can trigger an asthma attack.

In an effort to protect citizens from air pollution, many cities monitor air quality and issue health alerts when it is poor. Stage 1 health alerts are issued when ozone reaches 0.2 ppm (parts per million) and stage 2 alerts at 0.35 ppm. These alerts suggest that anyone with lung problems, such as asthma, should not exercise outdoors.

Many large metropolitan areas now have stage 1 alerts on more than 100 days out of the year. Although the long-term effects of ozone exposure are not clear, recent research suggests that chronic exposure to ozone results in diminished lung function (11).

Carbon monoxide is a gas produced during the burning of fossil fuels, such as gasoline and coal, and it is also contained in cigarette smoke. This pollutant binds to hemoglobin in the blood and reduces the blood's oxygen-carrying capacity.

carbon monoxide A gas produced during the burning of fossil fuels such as gasoline and coal; also contained in cigarette smoke. This pollutant binds to hemoglobin in the blood and reduces the blood's oxygen carrying capacity.

High levels of carbon monoxide can impair exercise performance by reducing oxygen delivery to the exercising muscles (12). In cities where traffic is heavy and congested, carbon monoxide can be a serious deterrent to exercise. For example, research suggests that runners in large metropolitan areas attain carbon monoxide levels in the blood that are twice the level necessary to negatively affect exercise performance (13).

Coping with Air Pollution

The only way to deal with air pollution is to avoid exercising when ozone or carbon monoxide levels are high (Figure 9.8). On hot summer days, ozone levels are highest during midday (11 A.M. to 3 P.M.) when the sun's ultraviolet rays are strongest. Avoid exercising during this time and again when automobile traffic is heavy. Carbon monoxide levels reach approximately 35 ppm in moving traffic and can rise to greater than 100 ppm in slow and congested conditions (2). These levels can extend 20 to 30 yards away from traffic. Exercisers should avoid heavily traveled roads and/or stay at least 30 yards away from the road if possible. Exposure to carbon monoxide (from sitting in traffic with the window down or being in a smoke-filled room) can be detrimental before exercise, too, because carbon monoxide leaves the blood so slowly. In fact, it may take over 6 hours to remove significant amounts of carbon monoxide from the blood (2).

Remember: Air pollution is not always visible. Therefore, you must be aware of the times of day at which various pollutants are in highest concentrations and avoid exercise. Pollutants not only affect exercise performance but also are hazardous to your health with chronic exposure. So, don't simply try to avoid pollution; do what you can to reduce pollution in order to have a cleaner environment in which to exercise. Walk or take the bus when possible, recycle waste, don't burn leaves or garbage; these are just a few things that we can do to make a better environment in which to live and exercise.

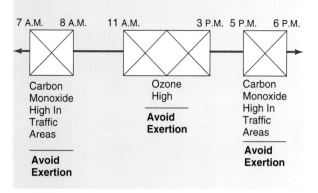

FIGURE 9.8 Hours at which to avoid exercise due to high levels of ozone and carbon monoxide.

Summary

1. Evaporation is the primary means of heat loss during exercise in a hot environment.

2. Although it is generally safe to exercise in a hot environment, the following guidelines need consideration:

- Start slowly and reduce your total exercise time.

- Adjust your exercise intensity to avoid exceeding your target heart rate.

- Wear loose, light-colored clothing.

- Drink plenty of fluids before, during, and after the exercise session.

3. Heat acclimatization occurs after several days of exposure to a hot environment. It results in a greater ability to lose body heat and reduces the chance of heat injury.

4. Although long-term exercise in a cold environment could result in hypothermia, in general, short-term exercise in a cold environment does not pose a serious threat to heat balance.

5. Exercise at high altitude results in a reduced amount of oxygen in the arterial blood, which reduces oxygen transport to the working muscles and lowers both VO_2 max and exercise tolerance.

6. At high altitude, it is necessary to reduce the intensity of exercise below normal in order to stay within your target heart rate range. However, there is little need to reduce your duration or frequency of exercise training during brief stays at moderate altitudes.

7. Ozone is produced by a chemical reaction between sunlight and automobile exhaust. Carbon monoxide is produced by the burning of fossil fuels. Both forms of air pollution can impair exercise tolerance.

8. The best way to deal with air pollution is to avoid exercising when ozone or carbon monoxide levels are high. Ozone levels are highest during hot summer days. Carbon monoxide levels are highest when automobile traffic is heavy.

Study Questions

1. Define the term *homeotherm.*

2. How is body heat lost during swimming?

3. What is the primary means of heat loss during exercise in a hot environment?

4. List key guidelines for exercising in the heat.

5. List guidelines for fluid intake during and after exercise in hot environments.

6. Describe the appropriate exercise clothing for exercise in hot and cold environments.

7. Outline the major types of heat injury, and list the symptoms of each.

8. Why does exercise at high altitude result in higher heart rates and breathing than the same exercise performed at sea level?

9. Discuss the effects of air pollution on exercise tolerance.

10. What guidelines should you follow to minimize your exposure to air pollution?

11. Define the term *acclimatize.*

12. Distinguish between the terms *ozone* and *carbon monoxide.*

13. Describe the difference between *convection* and *evaporation.*

Suggested Reading

Fox, E., R. Bowers, and M. Foss. *The physiological basis for exercise and sport.* Brown and Benchmark, Dubuque, IA, 1993.

Maughan, R. J., and S. M. Shirreffs. Recovery from prolonged exercise: Restoration of water and electrolyte balance. *Journal of Sports Science* 15(3):297–303. 1997.

Neiman, David C. *Fitness and sports medicine: An introduction.* 3rd ed. Bull Publishing, Palo Alto, CA, 1995

Powers, S. K., and E. T. Howley. *Exercise physiology: Theory and application to fitness and performance.* Brown and Benchmark, Dubuque, IA, 1997.

Terrados, N., and R. J. Maughan. Exercise in the heat: Strategies to minimize the adverse effects on performance. *Journal of Sports Science* 13: S55–S62, 1995.

West, J. B., and S. Lahiri, eds. *High altitude and man.* Williams and Wilkins, Baltimore, 1984.

Suggested Readings on the World Wide Web

Gatorade Sports Science Institute (http://www.gssiweb.com/library/) Many articles relating to fluid replacement during exercise. Sign up to be on a mailing list for new articles.

Marathoning: Start to Finish (http://www.teamoregon.com.publications/ marathon/) Guides to exercise in heat and cold, training for racing, ergogenic aids, and sports nutrition.

Winter Exercise (http://webmentor.com/mwrop/ winter.html) Guidelines for exercise, injuries and dressing in the cold.

Northern Outfitters (http://www.galapagostravel.com/northern/high-html) Cold weather clothing outfitters.

References

1. Brooks, G. A., T. D. Fahey, and T. White. *Exercise physiology: Human biogenetics and its applications.* 3rd ed. MacMillan, New York, 1996.

2. Neiman, David C. *Fitness and sports medicine: An introduction.* Bull Publishing, Palo Alto, CA, 1995.

3. Fox, E., R. Bowers, and M. Foss. *The physiological basis for exercise and sport.* Brown and Benchmark, Dubuque, IA, 1993.

4. McArdle, W. D., F. I. Katch, and V. L. Katch. *Exercise physiology: Energy, nutrition, and human performance.* 4th ed. Lea and Febiger, Malvern, 1996.

5. McFadden, E. R. Respiratory heat and water exchange: Physiological and clinical implications. *Journal of Applied Physiology* 54:331, 1984.

6. Claremont, A. D. Taking winter in stride requires proper attire. *Physician and Sports Medicine* 4:65, 1976.

7. Pandolf, K. B., M. N. Sawka, and R. R. Gonzalez. *Human performance physiology and environmental medicine at terrestrial extremes.* Benchmark Press, Indianapolis, IN, 1988.

8. Adams, W. C. Effects of ozone exposure at ambient air pollution episode levels on exercise performance. *Sports Medicine* 4:395–424, 1987.

9. Foxcraft, W. J., and W. C. Adams. Effects of ozone exposure on four consecutive days on work performance and VO_2 max. *Journal of Applied Physiology* 61:960–966, 1986.

10. Pierson, W. E., et al. Implications of air pollution effects on athletic performance. *Medicine and Science in Sports and Exercise* 18:322–327, 1986.

11. Lippmann, M. Effects of ozone on respiratory function and structure. *Annual Review of Public Health* 10:49–67, 1989.

12. Klausen, K., C. Anderson, and A. Nandrup. Acute effects of cigarette smoking and inhalation of carbon monoxide during maximal exercise. *European Journal of Applied Physiology* 51:371–379, 1983.

13. Nicholson, J. P., and D. B. Case. Carboxyhemoglobin levels in New York City runners. *Physician and Sports Medicine* 11:135–138, 1983.

14. Thompson, R. L. and J. S. Hayward. Wet-cold exposure and hypothermia: Thermal and metabolic responses to prolonged exercise in the rain. *Journal of Applied Physiology* 81(3): 1128–37, 1996.

15. Maughan, R. J. and S. M. Shirreffs. Recovery from prolonged exercise: Restoration of water and electrolyte balance. *Journal of Sports Science* 15(3): 297–303, 1997.

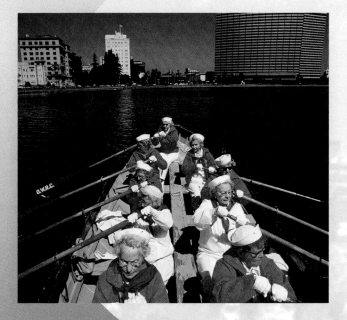

10

Exercise for Special Populations

Learning Objectives

After studying this chapter, you should be able to

1 Describe factors to consider when developing an exercise program for an individual with orthopedic problems.

2 Outline the exercise guidelines for an obese individual.

3 Discuss exercise training programs for type I and type II diabetics.

4 Discuss the benefits of exercise for asthmatics.

5 Outline the considerations for beginning or continuing an exercise program during pregnancy.

6 Discuss the physiological changes that come with aging and list the general guidelines for maintaining an exercise program throughout life.

Many people with special medical concerns want and need to participate in an exercise program. For most of these individuals, it is both safe and healthy to exercise. Although the exercise program may or may not have a direct benefit on the condition in question, in almost all cases, exercise training will result in increased energy levels, increased stamina, enhanced quality of life, and other health benefits, which will indirectly benefit the condition.

People with special medical concerns may need to use certain precautions when beginning an exercise program. There are even a few conditions that necessitate medical supervision during exercise and some in which exercise may be ill advised. In most instances, the decision should be made in consultation with a physician.

For example, people with serious heart problems are likely to need medical supervision while exercising. Usually, exercise is performed under the direct supervision of nurses and exercise specialists in a hospital or other institutional setting. In contrast, an individual with an orthopedic problem (e.g., joint problems) or diabetes, after consulting with the physician, often needs only to modify the "standard" exercise prescription (discussed in Chapter 4).

In this chapter, we will provide exercise guidelines for individuals with some of the more common health concerns that do not require medical supervision. There are certainly many other special concerns, too numerous to mention, that may dictate a modification in an exercise program. If you have special health concerns that are not discussed here, consult your physician before beginning an exercise program.

Orthopedic Problems

Individuals with orthopedic problems, such as bone or joint disorders, often need to take special care when designing an exercise program. The objective of the exercise prescription is to find an exercise mode that uses large muscle groups that are not associated with the problem area. For example, if the orthopedic problem is in the lower leg, this would mean undertaking exercise other than running, walking, or any other weight-bearing activity. Riding a stationary exercise bicycle, swimming, and using a rowing machine are non–weight-bearing exercises that use large muscle groups and are considered excellent for developing aerobic fitness. In addition, the muscles of the upper body and the uninjured leg could undergo resistance training exercises.

By using alternate modes of exercise, fitness levels can be maintained, even during times when injury makes exercise difficult.

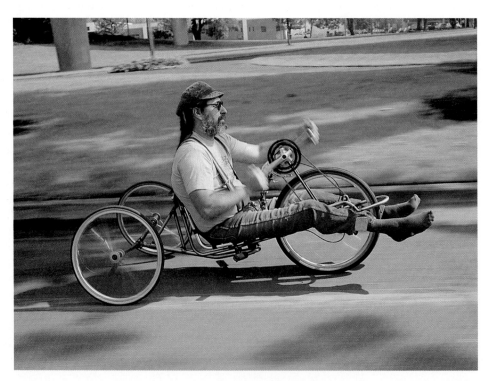

The exercise prescription is made somewhat easier if the problem is in the arm. In this instance, the individual could exercise using the legs as well as the uninjured arm. Because arm movement provides balance in many whole-body exercises, it would be wise to select exercises in which maintenance of balance is not a problem. Examples of these exercises are stationary cycling, walking, and stair-climbing.

Obesity

Although it is well established that exercise is an important factor in promoting weight loss (see Chapter 8), the exercise prescription for obese individuals requires special attention. For example, obese individuals have the following exercise limitations: heat intolerance, shortness of breath during heavy exercise, lack of flexibility, frequent musculoskeletal injuries, and a lack of balance during weight-bearing activities such as walking or running (1, 2).

When designing an exercise program for the obese individual, activities that can be sustained for long periods of time (30+ minutes), such as walking, swimming, or bicycling, should be emphasized. Further, obese people should avoid exercise in a hot or humid environment. The initial goal of the exercise program should not be to improve cardiovascular fitness but rather to increase voluntary energy expenditure and to establish a regular exercise routine. Therefore, the beginning exercise intensity should be below the typical target heart rate range for improving cardiorespiratory fitness, and the initial duration of exercise should be low (about 5–10 min/day) to reduce the risk of soreness and injury (3). The duration can be gradually increased in 1-minute increments to achieve an energy expenditure of approximately 300 kcals per workout. As the musculoskeletal system adapts to the exercise regimen, the intensity, too, can gradually be increased.

Diabetes

Diabetes is a metabolic disorder characterized by high blood glucose levels. Chronic elevation of blood glucose is associated with increased inci-

dence of heart disease, kidney disease, nerve dysfunction, and eye damage (4). In fact, diabetes is one of the leading causes of death in the United States and its incidence is increasing (4).

There are two types of diabetes. Type I diabetes usually occurs in the young and is due to abnormally low levels of the hormone insulin; it is often called *insulin-dependent diabetes.* This type of diabetes is now thought to be caused by the body's immune system attacking the pancreas and destroying those cells that produce insulin. Type II diabetes often occurs in overweight, middle-aged adults due to a reduction in the ability of insulin to transport glucose from the blood into cells. This form of diabetes generally is due to the lack of sensitivity of the cells to the action of insulin. Although the specific cause of the problem is not known, it is clear that obesity causes the disease to increase in severity (5). Because type II diabetics generally do not have a problem producing insulin, they generally do not require insulin treatment and are referred to as *non–insulin-dependent diabetics.*

There are three important tools for managing diabetes: diet, exercise, and insulin (5, 6). Although about three-fourths of known diabetics are taking insulin, it is estimated that 90% of non–insulin-dependent diabetes can be prevented with proper diet and exercise regimens (7, 8). There is great motivation to use diet and exercise to control blood glucose because there is considerable trouble, expense, and even danger associated with taking insulin. The danger is associated with the possibility of taking too much, which could result in a coma or, for those taking oral medication to control blood glucose, an increased risk of cardiovascular disease (9).

How can exercise benefit the diabetic individual? There are four reasons why exercise training can be beneficial. First, exercise training may help control blood glucose in the non–insulin-dependent diabetic. Exercise training improves the transport of glucose into cells and therefore reduces insulin requirements. Although this effect has been thought to last only a short time after an exercise bout (10), there is mounting evidence that the effect may be long lasting for the non–insulin-dependent diabetic (11, 12). It may be that simply learning to control blood glucose for the duration of the exercise bout alone is motivation enough to make exercise beneficial (see Nutritional Links to Health and Fitness 10.1).

Second, it may be that the most beneficial use of exercise is to help in controlling body weight (5, 7). One of the single most important objectives

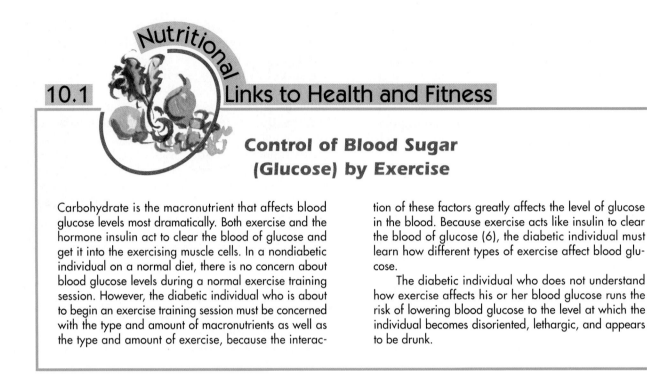

10.1 Nutritional Links to Health and Fitness

Control of Blood Sugar (Glucose) by Exercise

Carbohydrate is the macronutrient that affects blood glucose levels most dramatically. Both exercise and the hormone insulin act to clear the blood of glucose and get it into the exercising muscle cells. In a nondiabetic individual on a normal diet, there is no concern about blood glucose levels during a normal exercise training session. However, the diabetic individual who is about to begin an exercise training session must be concerned with the type and amount of macronutrients as well as the type and amount of exercise, because the interac-

tion of these factors greatly affects the level of glucose in the blood. Because exercise acts like insulin to clear the blood of glucose (6), the diabetic individual must learn how different types of exercise affect blood glucose.

The diabetic individual who does not understand how exercise affects his or her blood glucose runs the risk of lowering blood glucose to the level at which the individual becomes disoriented, lethargic, and appears to be drunk.

---

of the individual with diabetes is not to become overweight. This leads to higher blood glucose levels as well as increased blood lipids and elevated blood pressure. If an overweight person with diabetes loses weight, glucose levels may return to normal without taking insulin or oral hypoglycemic drugs (13). Obviously, exercise can play an important role in weight management for the diabetic.

Third, the individual with diabetes is at high risk for heart disease. As we have seen, a lack of exercise is now considered to be a primary risk factor for heart disease. Exercise leads to reduced blood pressure, total cholesterol, LDLs, and triglycerides, and to increased HDLs in overweight diabetic individuals (14). Thus, the importance of exercise in lowering their risk of heart disease cannot be overlooked.

Last, but certainly not least, are the psychosocial benefits associated with exercise training. Regular exercise results in many psychological and social benefits that act to enhance the daily lives of individuals with diabetes (15). Improvements in self-confidence, self-control, self-esteem, vigor, and general well-being are especially important.

Because the guidelines for developing the exercise prescription differ for the two categories of diabetes, we will examine each separately.

Exercise for Type I Diabetics

Before beginning an exercise program, the insulin-dependent diabetic must work with a personal physician to learn to manage resting blood glucose levels. This is important because exercise, like insulin, acts to lower blood glucose (10). Indeed, the combination of exercise and insulin can produce low blood glucose levels, which can lead to seizures or loss of consciousness.

Generally, the type I diabetic can participate in the same activities as nondiabetics. The recommended training intensity for type I diabetics is identical to the recommended values for healthy individuals (see chapters 4–6). However, exercise should be performed daily so that a regular pattern can be established for glucose control. Thus, the daily exercise duration should be only 20 to 30 minutes. Insulin-dependent diabetics should adopt the following guidelines when beginning an exercise training program.

- Do not exercise alone.
- Get a thorough medical examination, and tell your physician about your plans to begin an exercise program.
- Use footwear designed for the planned activity, and maintain good foot hygiene.

- Consume a meal 1 to 3 hours prior to exercise.
- Consume a snack of complex carbohydrates after exercise.
- If advised by your physician, reduce your insulin dose before the exercise session (the amount will depend on the type of insulin you take and the amount of exercise you do).
- Avoid exercising the muscle in which a short-acting insulin injection is given.
- Avoid late-evening exercise, because the exercise may alter blood sugar which cannot be monitored while you are asleep.
- Monitor blood glucose before, during, and after exercise.
- Carefully monitor your blood glucose alterations to different forms of exercise.

Exercise for Type II Diabetics

The most important change for type II diabetics is in exercise duration. Because one of the major objectives of exercise for the type II diabetic is to assist in the reduction of body fat, the recommended exercise duration is longer than that for the type I diabetic. It is generally short at the start (5–10 min/day) and is gradually increased over a period of weeks, reaching a total workout time of 40 to 60 minutes/session. The frequency of exercise should be increased gradually from 3 to 5 days per week in an effort to maximize energy expenditure and promote weight loss. Because of the long duration and relatively high frequency of exercise, the type II diabetic should maintain an exercise intensity near the lower end of the target range (40% to 60% of aerobic capacity) to reduce the risk of injury (16).

Asthma

Asthma is a disease that reduces the size of airways leading to the lungs and can result in a sudden difficulty in breathing. It is promoted by a number of factors, such as air pollution, pollen, and exercise. Unfortunately, the incidence of asthma is on the rise (especially in children) and, although solid evidence is lacking, it is thought to be due to an increase in pollution of indoor air (e.g., mold, mildew). Fortunately, asthma can be controlled by proper medication.

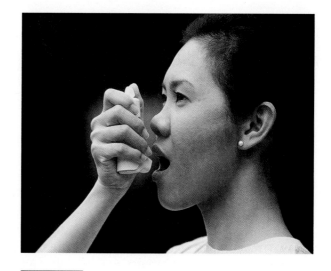

Exercise can be both safe and healthy for the asthmatic who takes the proper precautions.

It is generally agreed that asthmatics can safely participate in all types of exercise training. However, a prerequisite for planning exercise programs for asthmatics is that they have the proper medication program to control the asthma (17). Once the asthma is under control, the exercise prescription is identical to that for individuals without asthma. However, a wise precaution is to exercise with others and keep an inhaler of asthma medication handy during training in case of a sudden asthma attack.

The following guidelines should be followed by asthmatics who are beginning an exercise training program.

- Work with your personal physician to develop the proper medical protocol to control your asthma.
- Never exercise alone.
- Avoid cold weather exercise.
- Carry your inhaler while you exercise.
- Avoid exercise in polluted environments (properly filtered indoor air may be preferable to outdoor air).

asthma A disease that reduces the size of airways leading to the lungs and can result in a sudden difficulty in breathing. It is promoted by a number of factors, such as air pollution, pollen, and exercise.

Pregnancy

Can women continue an exercise program safely during a normal pregnancy? The answer is generally "yes," but the decision to exercise during pregnancy must be made by the individual after consultation with her physician. To date, most of the evidence suggests that short-duration, low- to moderate-intensity exercise does not pose a serious risk to the health of the fetus or the mother (18, 18a). However, prolonged or high-intensity exercise may impair fetal development. The best evidence suggests that intense exercise during pregnancy results in reduced birth weights (19). The reason is unknown but may be related to decreased blood flow to the fetus or the increase in body temperature during exercise (18a). It is recommended that pregnant women choosing to exercise perform low-intensity, short-duration exercise (10–20 minutes).

The following guidelines should be followed while performing exercise during pregnancy.

- Consult your physician about your exercise plan.
- Do not increase the amount of exercise normally performed prior to your pregnancy.
- Do not participate in sports that have a high risk of injury (e.g., contact sports).
- Do not use exercises that require lying on the back for more than 5 minutes. The weight of the fetus may reduce blood flow through vessels supplying blood to the lower extremities.
- Avoid exercises that place major importance on balance, such as dancing or treadmill walking.
- In the last 3 months of the pregnancy, avoid exercises that use quick, jerking movements because they may cause joint strains.
- Wear good supportive footwear and adequate breast support.
- Avoid exercise in the heat. Remember: The primary dangers of exercise during pregnancy are increased body temperature and lack of blood flow to the baby. Because water removes heat from the body better than does air, aquatic exercise is an excellent means of preventing large amounts of body heat gain.
- Monitor your pulse and stay at the low end of your target heart rate zone. Don't exceed 140 beats/minute.
- Concentrate on non–weight-bearing exercises, such as cycling or swimming.
- Drink plenty of fluids.
- If you experience any of the following, stop exercising immediately and call your doctor: shortness of breath, dizziness, numbness, tingling, abdominal pain, or vaginal bleeding.

Exercise during pregnancy can be beneficial for the mother and pose little risk for the fetus.

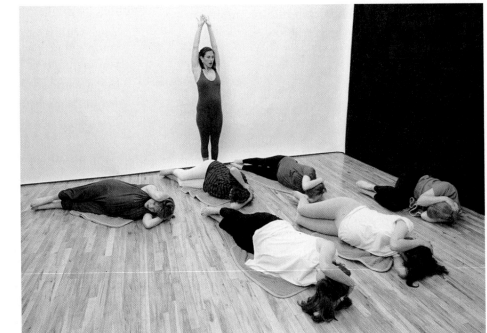

Aging

Throughout this text, we have focused on the young individual (about 18–25 years of age). In this section, we shift our focus to consider exercise for older individuals. Who are the elderly? Usually, the defining age for elderly is considered to be 65 because this is the age when retirement and Social Security benefits begin. However, when considering exercise capacity, we cannot equate ability with age. There are many individuals above 65 years of age who have the exercise capacity of people one-third their age; and their number is growing.

Sedentary individuals experience a significant decline in VO_2 max with age (Figure 10.1). However, recent research has shown that older individuals engaging in a regular program of vigorous physical activity can maintain the aerobic capacity of someone one-third their age (20). Note in Figure 10.1 that a 75-year-old individual may have the aerobic capacity of a 25-year-old! Although this may seem like a new idea, the adaptability of the human body has been known for centuries. About 400 B.C. Hippocrates said,

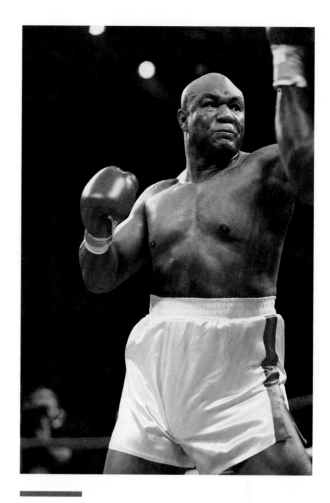

Chronological age and physiological age are not necessarily equivalent. George Foreman continues to box at a world-class level in his mid-forties.

FIGURE 10.1 The decline in VO_2 max with age. There is a decline of approximately 10% per decade after age 25. (Source: Neiman, David C. *Fitness and sports medicine: A health-related approach.* Bull Publishing Co., Palo Alto, CA, 1995. Reprinted with permission.)

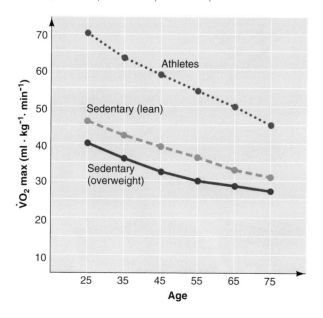

All parts of the body which have a function, if used in moderation and exercised in labors in which each is accustomed, become thereby healthy, well-developed and age more slowly, but if unused and left idle they become liable to disease, defective in growth, and age quickly.

Obviously the normal biological changes that take place during aging are inevitable. However, recent scientific evidence suggests that an active lifestyle can delay the aging process and result in a longer, healthier, and happier life (21).

Physiological Changes with Aging

Aging results in a gradual decline in biological function. Many of the age-related changes in the body begin to appear between the ages of 30 and 40 (20, 22). As illustrated in Figure 10.2, the physiological changes that accompany aging are similar to those seen with inactivity or prolonged weightlessness, such as experienced by astronauts.

The most common functional changes with aging are decreased cardiorespiratory function, increased body fat, and musculoskeletal fragility (23). What causes these age-related changes? Interestingly, approximately one-half of the decline in functional capacity is due to a decrease in physical activity (24). Therefore, regular exercise may improve cardiorespiratory function, assist in maintaining a satisfactory percent body fat, and maintain the mineral content of bone during the aging process.

Guidelines for Exercise

It is important for everyone to remain physically active. However, older individuals should seek exercise advice from their physicians and avoid physical activities that present a high risk of introducing orthopedic problems. Activities such as walking, cycling, swimming, and light weight training are generally recommended. When designing the exercise prescription for older individuals, the basic principles for the development of fitness apply (see Chapter 3). The following guidelines outline some specific con-

siderations for exercise after age 40 for men and age 50 for women.

- Due to the risks of heart disease associated with age, it is wise for men over 40 and women over 50 to perform a physician-supervised, graded exercise stress test before engaging in a vigorous physical fitness program.

- Non–weight-bearing exercises are recommended to reduce the risk of musculoskeletal problems.

- Exercise intensity should be at the lower end of the target heart rate range.

- Exercise frequency should be limited to 3 to 4 days per week to reduce the risk of injury.

- Exercise duration should be modified to meet the needs (and abilities) of the aging individual. For example, in the beginning stages of the exercise program, it is likely that many unconditioned elderly individuals cannot exercise for more than 5 to 10 minutes per exercise session. In this case, the individual may exercise several times per day for short durations (three 10-minute sessions/day). As the program progresses, the individual can slowly increase the duration of each session and begin to have fewer sessions (two 15-minute sessions/day).

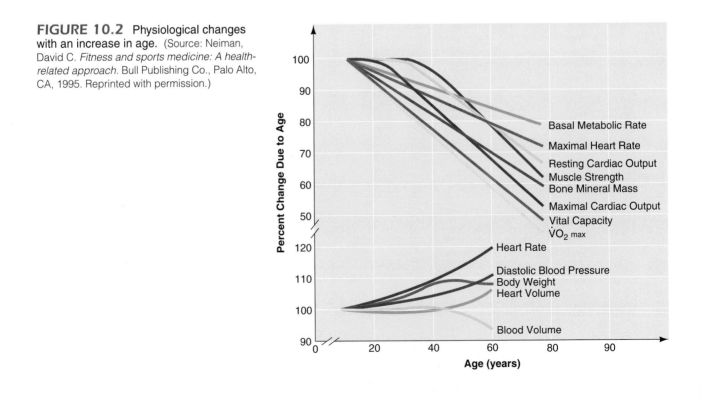

FIGURE 10.2 Physiological changes with an increase in age. (Source: Neiman, David C. *Fitness and sports medicine: A health-related approach.* Bull Publishing Co., Palo Alto, CA, 1995. Reprinted with permission.)

Summary

1. Individuals with orthopedic problems often require special considerations when designing an exercise program. The objective of the exercise prescription is to find an exercise mode that increases physical fitness but does not aggravate the existing orthopedic condition.

2. The obese individual should emphasize the use of non–weight-bearing activities (e.g., swimming, cycling). In addition, the exercise should be of lower than normal intensity.

3. Diabetes results from a deficiency in the amount or effectiveness of the hormone insulin, which acts to transfer glucose from the blood into the cells.

4. The key to developing a sound exercise program for a type I diabetic is to learn to manage blood glucose levels during exercise. If blood glucose can be managed, the diabetic individual can participate in the same activities as the nondiabetic individual.

5. Only minor differences exist between the exercise guidelines for the type I and the type II diabetic. The most important difference is the recommended duration of exercise (type II diabetics generally perform a longer duration).

6. Asthma is a disease that results in a sudden reduction in the size of the airways. Asthmatics who can control their asthma medically can safely participate in an exercise training program.

7. Aging is not a sudden process but is a slow, gradual decline in biological function. The common functional changes seen with both aging and inactivity are decreased cardiorespiratory function, obesity, and musculoskeletal fragility. Approximately one-half of the decline in functional capacity observed with aging is due to a decrease in physical activity.

8. Pregnancy does not prevent women from exercising. Short-duration, low-to-moderate intensity exercise does not pose a serious risk to the health of the fetus or the mother.

Study Questions

1. What exercises may be prescribed for an individual with an orthopedic problem in the lower extremity? The upper extremities? The back?

2. List the problems likely to be encountered by an obese individual who is beginning an exercise program.

3. Distinguish between type I and type II diabetes.

4. Contrast the special guidelines to be followed by type I and type II diabetics who wish to start an exercise program.

5. What physiological changes occur during exercise that may have detrimental effects on the fetus?

6. List the guidelines to be followed for starting or maintaining an exercise program during pregnancy.

7. List the primary physiological changes seen with aging.

8. List the guidelines for establishing a fitness program for an older individual.

9. What special considerations should be taken by an individual with asthma who is starting an exercise program?

10. What is the purpose of the hormone insulin?

Suggested Reading

Artal, R., and R. A. Wiswell. *Exercise in pregnancy.* Williams and Wilkins, Los Angeles, 1986.

Botti, J. J., and R. L. Jones. Aerobic conditioning, nutrition, and pregnancy. *Clinical Nutrition* 4:14–17, 1985.

Bouchard, C., L. Perusse, and C. Leblanc. Inheritance of the amount and distribution of human body fat. *International Journal of Obesity* 12:205–215, 1988.

Graham, C. et al. *The diabetes sports and exercise book.* Lowell House, Los Angeles, 1996.

Kulpa, P. J., B. M. White, and R. Visscher. Aerobic exercise in pregnancy. *American Journal of Obstetrics and Gynecology* 156:1395–1403, 1987.

Larson, E. B., and R. A. Bruce. Health benefits of exercise in an aging society. *Archives of Internal Medicine* 147:353–356, 1987.

Morton, M. J., M. S. Paul, and J. Metcalfe. Exercise during pregnancy. *Medical Clinics of North America* 69:97–107, 1985.

Neiman, David C. *Fitness and sports medicine: An introduction.* 3rd ed. Bull Publishing, Palo Alto, CA, 1995.

Pollock, M. *Exercise in health and disease.* W. B. Saunders, Philadelphia, PA, 1998.

Powers, S. K., and E. T. Howley. *Exercise physiology: Theory and application to fitness and performance.* Brown and Benchmark, Dubuque, IA, 1994.

Roberts, J. A. Exercise-induced asthma in athletes. *Sports Medicine* 6:193–196, 1988.

Stamford, B. A. Exercise and the elderly. *Exercise and Sports Sciences Reviews* 16:341–379, 1988.

Suggested Readings on the World Wide Web

Diabetes Monitor: Information about Diabetes (http://www.mdcc.com/dr-00005.html). Suggestions for exercise and nutrition for those with diabetes.

Sympatico: Healthyway (http://www.ns.sympatico.ca/healthyway/) Numerous articles, book reviews, and links to nutrition, fitness, and wellness topics.

World Health Network: Exercise and Aging (http://www.worldhealth.net/) Site for the American Academy of Anti-Aging Medicine. Numerous articles about exercise and aging.

Babyzone: Pregnancy and Your Health (http://siteguider.com/health.htm) Guidelines and articles for safe exercise during pregnancy.

Canadian Lung Association: Exercise & Asthma (http://www.lung.ca/asthma/exercise/index.html) Guidelines for exercising for people with asthma.

Health Net (http://www.health-net.com/) Weight training, low back disorders, exercise programming, heart health, nutrition, mind and body, sports medicine, managing stress, wellness, men's health, women's health, diabetes, and arthritis.

Healthfinder (http://www.healthfinder.gov/) Search engine of the National Institutes of Health. Find the latest information on any health-related topic from the most respected health organization in the world.

References

1. Zelasko, C. Exercise for weight loss: What are the facts? *Journal of the American Dietetic Association* 95(12):1414–17, 1995.

2. Jakicic, J., et al. Prescription of exercise intensity for the obese patient: The relationship between heart rate, VO_2 and perceived exertion. *International Journal of Obesity and Related Metabolic Disorders* 19(6): 382–387, 1995.

3. American College of Sports Medicine: The recommended quantity and quality of exercise for developing and maintaining fitness in healthy adults. *Sports Medicine Bulletin* 13:1, 1992.

4. Kovar, M. F., M. I. Harris, and W. C. Hadden. The scope of diabetes in the United States population. *American Journal of Public Health* 77:1549–1550, 1987.

5. Horton, E. S. Role and management of exercise in diabetes mellitus. *Diabetes Care* 11(2):201–211, 1988.

6. Spelsberg, A., and J. E. Manson. Physical activity in the treatment and prevention of diabetes. *Comprehensive Therapy* 21(10): 559–562, 1995.

7. Franz, M. J. Exercise and the management of diabetes mellitus. *Journal of the American Dietetic Association* 87:872–882, 1987.

8. Cantu, R. C. *Diabetes and exercise.* Mouvement Publications, Ithaca, NY, 1982.

9. American Diabetes Association. *The fitness book for people with diabetes.* G. Hornsby, ed. American Diabetes Association, 1995.

10. Ivy, J. L. The insulin-like effect of muscle contraction. *Exercise and Sport Sciences Reviews* 15:29–54, 1987.

11. Oshida, Y., K. Yamanouchi, S. Hayamizu, Y. Sato. Long-term mild jogging increases insulin action despite no influence on body mass index or VO_2 max. *Journal of Applied Physiology* 66:2206–2210, 1989.

12. Rogers, M. A., C. Yamamoto, D. S. King, J. M. Hagberg, A. A. Ehsani, and J. O. Holloszy. Improvement in glucose tolerance after 1 week of exercise in patients with mild NIDDM. *Diabetes Care* 11:613–618, 1988.

13. National Institutes of Health. Consensus development conference on diet and exercise in non-insulin-dependent diabetes mellitus. *Diabetes Care* 10:639–644, 1987.

14. U.S. Department of Health and Human Services. The Surgeon General's report on nutrition and health. DHHS (PHS) Publication No. 88–50211. U.S. Government Printing Office; Washington D.C., 1994.

15. Leon, A. S. Diabetes. In: J. S. Skinner, ed. *Exercise testing and exercise prescription for special cases.* Williams and Wilkins, Baltimore, 1992.

16. Richter, E. A., and H. Galbo. Diabetes, insulin and exercise. *Sports Medicine* 3:275–288, 1986.

17. Katz, R. M. Prevention with and without the use of medications for exercise-induced asthma. *Medicine and Science in Sports and Exercise* 18:331–333, 1986.

18. Wong, S. C., and D. C. McKenzie. Cardiorespiratory fitness during pregnancy and its effect on outcome. *International Journal of Sports Medicine* 8:79–83, 1987.

18a. Bell, R., and M. O'Neill. Exercise and pregnancy: A review. *Birth* 21(2):85–95, 1994.

19. Clapp, J. F., and S. Dickstein. Endurance exercise and pregnancy outcome. *Medicine and Science in Sports and Exercise* 16:556–562, 1984.

20. Allison M., and C. Keller. Physical activity in the elderly: Benefits and intervention strategies. *Nurse Practitioner* 22(8):53–58, 1997.

21. Paffenbarger, P. S., R. T. Hyde, and A. L. Wing. Physical activity, all-cause mortality, and longevity of college alumni. *New England Journal of Medicine* 314:605–613, 1986.

22. Hagberg, J. M. A hemodynamic comparison of young and old endurance athletes during exercise. *Journal of Applied Physiology* 58:2041–2046, 1985.

23. Shephard, R. J. Nutrition and the physiology of aging. In: E. A. Young, ed. *Nutrition, aging, and health.* Alan R. Liss, New York, 1986.

24. Meredith, C. N., M. J. Zackin, W. R. Frontera, and W. J. Evans. Body composition and aerobic capacity in young and middle-aged endurance-trained men. *Medicine and Science in Sports and Exercise* 19:557–563, 1987.

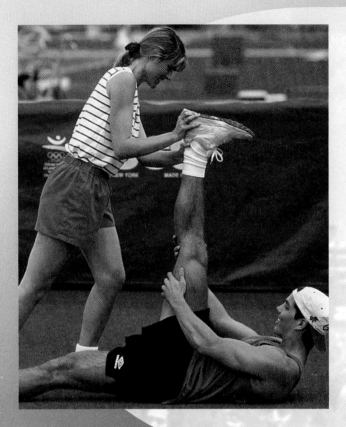

11

Prevention and Rehabilitation of Exercise-Related Injuries

After reading this chapter, you should be able to

1 Discuss the role of overtraining in causing an increase in the risk of exercise-related injury.

2 List the symptoms of overtraining.

3 Define acute and delayed-onset muscle soreness.

4 Discuss possible causes of muscle strains and ways in which they can be avoided.

5 Define tendonitis and discuss how it should be treated.

6 Discuss ligament sprains and how to avoid them.

7 Describe the most common injuries to the lower extremities.

8 Outline a general plan to reduce the incidence of exercise-related injuries.

9 Discuss the general guidelines for the treatment of injuries.

10 Define *cryokinetics* and discuss its use in the rehabilitation process.

People in the United States are now participating in fitness programs in record numbers. Unfortunately, in the quest for fitness many people abide by the old adage, "No pain, no gain." The problem with this approach to fitness is that excessive or improper exercise increases the risk of injury to joints, muscles, tendons, and ligaments. Bone injuries and soft-tissue injuries are painful and result in lost training time. Further, research has shown that exercise-related injuries contribute to the high number of drop-outs from personal fitness programs (1).

Although many training-related injuries can be prevented, almost everyone who engages in regular physical activity is going to experience one or more exercise-related injuries during his or her lifetime. In this chapter we will discuss the cause, prevention, and treatment of exercise-related injuries.

The Risk and Causes of Injury from Increased Physical Activity

Because running is involved in most physical activities, let's first examine the risk of injury involved with this mode of exercise. More than one-third of runners develop orthopedic injuries serious enough to reduce weekly running mileage (1). Approximately 60% of those injuries involve the foot and knee. One of the major factors responsible for this type and number of injuries is the severity of stress on the legs and feet. In fact, the impact of the foot on the running surface is approximately 2.5 times the body weight of the runner (2). In addition, the incidence of injury increases with running mileage (1). The following "rule of thumb" may help you gauge your risk of injury due to running: If you run 15 miles a week, you can expect one injury every 2 years. Although there have been many factors blamed for the injuries encountered by runners, there is convincing evidence that only a few play a significant role in causing injuries.

The factors most closely correlated with running injuries are improper training techniques (e.g., excessive distance, changed training routine), inadequate shoes, and alignment abnormalities in the legs and feet (1). Although all of these

factors should be considered, the most important factor seems to be improper training techniques; they account for two-thirds of all injuries (3). Figure 11.1 illustrates the results of one study which determined the factors associated with running injuries. The graph shows that increases in miles run per workout and number of days run per week were the major causes of injury.

Improper training techniques not only are responsible for increased injuries (72% in one study) (4), but also are responsible for the overtraining syndrome. The overtraining syndrome is a major cause of exercise-related injuries. Overtraining results from too much exercise and not enough recovery time between workouts. The symptoms may include increased resting heart rate, reduced appetite, weight loss, irritability, disturbed sleep, elevated blood pressure, frequent injuries, increased incidence of infections, and chronic fatigue.

To prevent overtraining, a good rule of thumb is to increase your exercise intensity or duration no more than 10% over a 2-week period. In addition, listen to your body. If you notice any of the overtraining symptoms, reduce your training intensity and/or duration and increase your rest intervals. Avoidance of overtraining can greatly reduce your chance of injury and help maintain a positive attitude about fitness.

FIGURE 11.1 Factors associated with injuries during running. (Source: Neiman, David C. 1995. *Fitness and sports medicine: An introduction.* 2d ed. Bull Publishing Co., Palo Alto, CA. Reprinted with permission.)

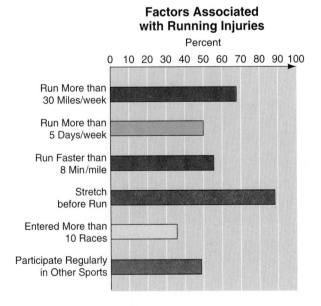

Factors Associated with Running Injuries

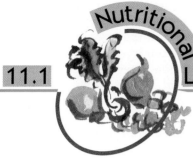

Nutritional

11.1 Links to Health and Fitness

Does Nutrition Have a Role in Repair of Exercise-Induced Injuries?

There are two aspects of nutrition that may be important to exercise-related injuries. First, when muscle is damaged, the repair systems of the body remove the damaged fibers so that new fibers can grow as replacements. The growth of muscle fibers requires dietary protein to provide amino acids as building blocks for the new fibers. This does not mean that supplemental protein in the diet is necessary for adequate repair to damaged muscle. By following the guidelines in Chapter 7 you are assured of adequate protein for repair of damaged muscle.

The second important aspect is the notion that antioxidants may play a role in minimizing the extent of damage caused by injury. Injury to tissue causes the repair system of the body to release chemicals in the injured area, which may cause inflammation and further destruction to tissue before the rebuilding phase begins. Antioxidants may play a role in preventing this further injury by acting as a scavenger of the free radicals produced during the injury. Although much more research is needed in this area to define nutrition's role in repair of injuries, it is obviously wise to ensure that the RDA of all vitamins and minerals is consumed daily.

Although little can be done about some of the alignment abnormalities in the legs and feet, a change in shoes can have an impact on injury prevention in many cases. Approximately one-third of runners show a decrease in injuries with a change to the proper shoe (1) (see Chapter 16 for discussion of proper shoes). This is due to the increased cushioning provided by the shoe as well as increased support for the arch of the foot. This is also true of specialized shoes used in other activities such as tennis and aerobic dance.

Another activity associated with high rates of injury is aerobic dance. Aerobic dance became popular in the early 1970s with routines consisting of dance and calisthenic-type exercises. Today, it has evolved into specialized aerobic programs such as water aerobics, low-impact aerobics, step aerobics, and specific dance aerobics. Approximately one-half of all participants in traditional aerobic dance classes report injuries (5). Injuries to participants occur at a rate of approximately one injury per 100 hours of dancing. One study found that more than three sessions per week, improper shoes, and nonresilient surfaces were the primary causes of injury (6).

In summary, improper training techniques (e.g., excessive distance, drastic changes in the training routine) are the major causes of injuries. Excessive distance may cause wear to tissues, such as connective tissue in joints, while drastic changes in training routines may put greater stress on tissues and result in injury by tearing tissues (see Nutritional Links to Health and Fitness 11.1).

overtraining syndrome A phenomenon resulting from improper training techniques which results in exercise-related injuries. Overtraining results from too much exercise and not enough recovery time between workouts. The symptoms may include increased resting heart rate, reduced appetite, weight loss, irritability, disturbed sleep, elevated blood pressure, frequent injuries, increased incidence of infections, and chronic fatigue.

Common Injuries: Cause and Prevention

Although many injuries can occur as a result of exercise, some are more common than others. This section discusses the cause and prevention of many general types of injuries associated with exercise training.

Back Pain

Cause One of the most important health concerns in the United States is back pain. Over 50% of the population complains of recurring back pain, and over two million people are unable to work because of it (7). There are many causes of back pain, including improper lifting techniques, weak muscles, poor posture, and bone disorders (see Table 11.1). Treatments include pain-killers, muscle relaxants, antiinflammatory drugs, bracing, traction, bed rest, surgery, and therapeutic exercises. Even without any form of treatment, approximately 80% of back patients recover spontaneously (7). Thus, it is not clear whether the treatments for back pain only serve to lessen the pain or are beneficial in speeding recovery.

Back problems are of critical concern when beginning an exercise program. Depending on the exact nature of the problem, exercise may be extremely helpful or extremely harmful. You should attempt to find the cause before starting an exercise program. It is possible that certain types of exercise may compound the problem and, thus, should be avoided.

In contrast, exercise has been effectively used in pain clinics for treating back pain (8). In addition, exercise can be used to prevent or correct some back problems by strengthening weak muscles and stretching the stronger ones. If you have a problem with your back, consult your physician before beginning an exercise program in order to determine what complications or benefits may be realized by your exercise program.

Prevention Exercise can play a key role in prevention of back pain. Exercises to increase flexibility and strength, reduce body fat, improve muscle balance between the trunk flexors and extensors, and prevent osteoporosis can decrease your risk of developing back problems (9). In addition, in consultation with your physician, you may decide that these exercises can help alleviate back pain that you may already be experiencing.

If muscles on one side of a joint are stronger than those on the other side, the resulting imbalance of forces can pull the associated body parts out of alignment. Exercises should be performed which strengthen the longer, weakened muscles and stretch the short, stronger ones. For example, individuals with an exaggerated curvature in the lower back will need to strengthen the abdominal muscles and stretch the muscles of the lower back and hips (Figure 11.2).

Use the following guidelines to help prevent irritation of back problems or to prevent the onset of back pains.

- Maintain a healthy body weight and body composition. Obesity puts great strain on the lower back.
- Warm up before engaging in any physical activity.
- Do exercises to strengthen the abdominal muscles.
- Do exercises to stretch the lower back and hamstring muscles.
- When lying down, lie on your side with your knees and hips bent. Try to avoid lying on your back, but if you do, place a pillow under your knees.
- During prolonged standing, try to take the strain off of the lower back by bending one

---

Table 11.1

Risk Factors for Back Pain
In most cases, back pain is preventable. A knowledge of the following factors, which lead to a higher than normal risk of recurring back pain, may help in alleviating back pain or preventing future back problems.

Poor posture
Improper lifting of heavy loads
Frequent bending from the waist
Weak lower back muscles
Being overweight
Lack of flexibility in lower back
Lack of flexibility in hamstring muscles
Quick, jerking movements of the spine
Osteoporosis
Increasing age

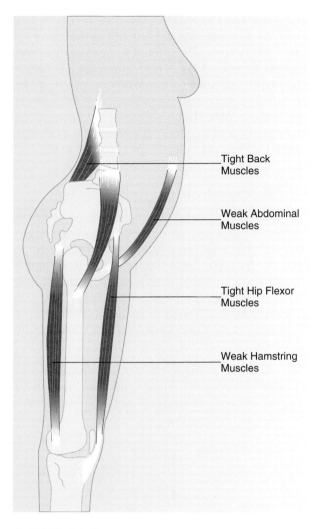

Tight Back Muscles

Weak Abdominal Muscles

Tight Hip Flexor Muscles

Weak Hamstring Muscles

FIGURE 11.2 Bad posture will lead to muscle imbalance, which may result in back pain.

leg at the hip and knee to prop one foot on an object such as a rail or box.
- Avoid quick, jerking movements of the spine.
- Do not overextend the neck or lower back or overflex the neck.
- Avoid stretching the long/weak muscles (abdominal muscles).
- Be especially careful when using passive stretches by another person. Avoid passive back or neck stretches or any ballistic passive stretches (see Chapter 6).
- Avoid movements that place forces on spinal disks, such as extending and rotating the spine simultaneously, trunk and neck circling, and double leg lifts.
- Avoid forceful hyperextension and flexion of the spine.

- Avoid improper lifting. Squat to lift any object, and never bend at the waist.

Acute Muscle Soreness

Cause **Acute muscle soreness** may develop during or immediately following an exercise bout that has been too long or too intense. Popular belief has linked the build-up of lactic acid to acute muscle soreness. However, lactic acid is not the cause of this type of soreness (10). Instead, it is more likely caused by other alterations in the chemical balance within muscle, increased fluid accumulation in muscle, or injury to muscle tissue.

Prevention Exercise that is more strenuous or prolonged than normal is likely to cause the aforementioned changes in muscle which result in acute muscle soreness. Novice exercisers should be particularly cautious in this regard when beginning an exercise training program. These changes can be further prevented by gradually beginning and ending the exercise session. All exercise sessions should begin slowly with a warm-up period of 5 to 15 minutes (see Chapter 3). This is necessary to allow muscles to increase the internal temperature slowly to avoid damage during the more stressful exercise training session. Finally, a postexercise cool-down regimen is important in allowing the muscles to return to their normal, pre-exercise physiological condition.

Delayed-Onset Muscle Soreness

Cause Delayed-onset muscle soreness (DOMS) develops within 24 to 48 hours of a bout of exercise that is excessive in duration or intensity (11). It is also common following new or unique physical activities that use muscle groups

acute muscle soreness This condition may develop during or immediately following an exercise bout that has been too long or too intense. Acute muscle soreness is likely caused by alterations in the chemical balance within muscle, increased fluid accumulation in muscle, or injury to muscle tissue.

delayed-onset muscle soreness (DOMS) This condition develops within 24 to 48 hours after a bout of exercise that is excessive in duration or intensity. It is common following new or unique physical activities that use muscle groups unaccustomed to exercise.

unaccustomed to exercise. For example, it is not unusual for a runner to experience soreness in the upper body following the initiation of a weight training program.

DOMS is likely caused by microscopic tears in the muscle (11). This form of exercise-induced soreness results in swelling and pain within the damaged muscles. Many investigators believe that this type of injury occurs primarily during the lengthening phase of muscular contraction (eccentric portion of the contraction; see Chapter 5). The damage apparently is due to the greater force placed on the muscle during this phase of the contraction. For example, downhill running (which emphasizes such contractions) by an individual unaccustomed to this type of exercise will generally produce soreness in the leg muscles within 24 to 48 hours after the exercise session. Similarly, in people unaccustomed to walking up and down steps, DOMS also occurs 24 to 48 hours after such exercise.

Prevention As with acute muscle soreness, DOMS can be prevented by refraining from exercise that is more strenuous or prolonged than normal. Start with a warm-up and limit both the intensity and duration of the first several workouts. Remember that eccentric contractions are more likely to result in muscle damage than concentric (shortening) contractions. Therefore, in the beginning stages of an exercise program, try to avoid exercises that involve large amounts of eccentric contractions (e.g., walking down steps, running downhill, eccentric contraction during weight lifting, etc.).

Muscle Strains

Cause If a muscle is overstretched or forced to shorten against an extremely heavy weight, such as when lifting a heavy box, muscle fibers may be damaged. This damage is referred to as a **strain** and can range from a minor separation of fibers to a complete tearing of fibers (12). The following classification system has been developed for categorizing the degree of muscle damage due to strain.

1st Degree: Only a few muscle fibers are stretched or torn. Movement is painful, but a full range of motion is still possible (Figure 11.3A).

FIGURE 11.3 A strain can result in tears in a muscle of varying degrees of severity. **(A)** First degree strain with minimal disruption of muscle fibers. **(B)** Second degree strain with significant tearing and hemorrhage. **(C)** Third degree strain with complete tear and loss of function.

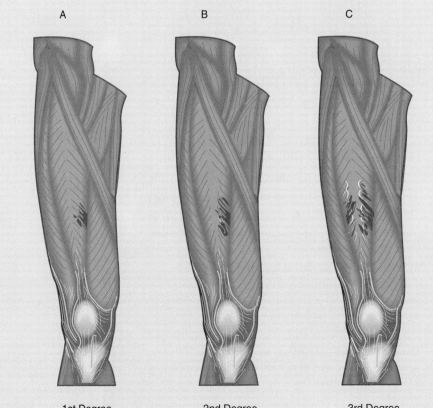

A   B   C

1st Degree   2nd Degree   3rd Degree

2nd Degree: Many muscle fibers are torn, and movement is extremely painful and limited. The torn area may cause a soft, sunken area in the muscle. Swelling may occur around the tear due to hemorrhage (bleeding) (Figure 11.3B).

3rd Degree: The muscle is torn completely. The tear can be in the belly of the muscle, in the tendon, or at the point where the tendon attaches to the bone. Movement is generally impossible. Initial pain is intense but quickly subsides because nerve fibers are also damaged. Surgery is usually necessary for repair (Figure 11.3C).

Prevention Because strains occur when muscles must generate excessive force, it is logical that strains can be prevented by limiting the amount of stress placed on muscles, for example, by avoiding lifting extremely heavy objects and avoiding quick, jerking movements. A warm-up is also critical in avoiding muscle strains. A warmed muscle is more pliable; that is, it is more easily stretched and less likely to tear. Therefore, predicting how much force will cause muscle damage is impossible because it depends on how much the muscle has been warmed up. Before lifting a heavy object or engaging in activities that require quick, jerking kinds of movements, go through a thorough warm-up for 5 to 15 minutes. Although a good warm-up should prevent muscle strains, remember, however, that muscle contractions more strenuous than normal may result in DOMS.

Tendonitis

Cause Tendons are the tissue that connect muscles to bone. Tendonitis is one of the most common of the exercise-related injuries (12). The term *tendonitis* means inflammation or swelling of a tendon. As muscles shorten and pull on tendons, the tendons move across other tendons, muscles, and soft tissue. This movement, if unaccustomed, can cause irritation and swelling in the tendon. Once tendonitis develops, pain associated with movement is the first symptom. Swelling, redness, and warmth generally follow. Tendonitis can occur in a number of areas, such as the elbow and shoulder, and is a common injury of runners, tennis players, and weight lifters.

Prevention Tendonitis is generally caused by strenuous, prolonged muscle contractions to which an individual is unaccustomed. Therefore,

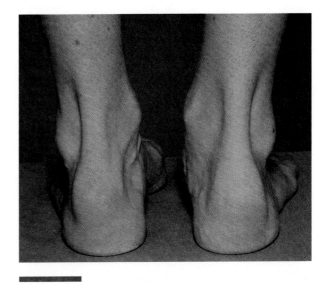

Tendonitis is an inflammation of the connective tissue between muscle and bone. Here the Achilles tendon of the left leg is inflamed and swollen.

the best prevention of tendonitis is to avoid overuse. If you feel tendon pain or discomfort during a workout, stop exercising. This will prevent further irritation and reduce the severity of tendon damage. If you cannot stop using the muscle and tendon causing the pain, follow the "Management of Injuries" measures listed at the end of this chapter.

Ligament Sprains

Cause A **sprain** is caused by damage to a ligament (12). Ligaments are tough, inelastic bands of connective tissue that connect the bones, provide joint support, and determine the direction and range of motion of joints. Ligament damage can occur if excessive force is applied to a joint. One of the most common sites of ligament damage is the ankle. When walking or running on an uneven surface it is easy to "turn" the ankle. This means that the ankle joint is rotated such that much of the body weight is placed on the

strain Damage to a muscle that can range from a minor separation of fibers to a complete tearing of fibers.

tendonitis Inflammation or swelling of a tendon. One of the most common exercise-related injuries.

sprain Damage to a ligament that occurs if excessive force is applied to a joint.

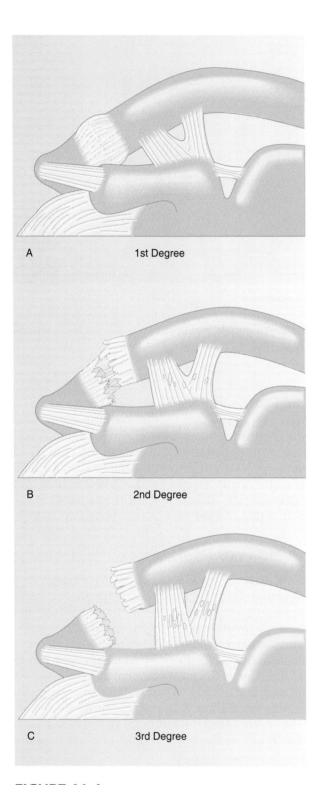

A   1st Degree

B   2nd Degree

C   3rd Degree

FIGURE 11.4 A sprain involves damage to the ligaments that support joints. **(A)** First degree sprain with minimal disruption of tendons in the shoulder. **(B)** Second degree sprain with significant tearing. **(C)** Third degree sprain with complete tear and loss of stability of joint.

side of the foot. Because the ankle joint is not designed to rotate to that degree, the stress on the joint causes the ligaments to be damaged. Like muscle strains, the degrees of ligament damage are classified as follows:

1st Degree: Stretching and separation of a limited number of ligament fibers, resulting in minor instability of the joint (Figure 11.4A). Minor pain and swelling will likely result.

2nd Degree: Tearing and separation of a significant number of ligament fibers (Figure 11.4B). Moderate instability of the joint with definite pain, swelling, and stiffness will occur.

3rd Degree: Total tearing or separation of the ligament, causing major instability of the joint (Figure 11.4C). Nerves may be damaged and pain may subside quickly. A high level of swelling generally occurs.

Prevention The development of high-tech, lightweight metal alloys have made it possible to construct braces that provide added support to joints and therefore offer some protection from ligament damage. These braces are commonly used in football, a sport recognized for inducing knee damage. Without these expensive, high-tech devices, the best protection against torn ligaments is to refrain from activities that may subject a joint to high stress, such as tennis, soccer, racquetball, basketball, and so on. In addition, if you have a particular joint that has been injured previously or is weak, maintain maximum strength in the muscles surrounding the joint, because strong muscles provide additional support.

Torn Cartilage

Cause Cartilage is tough, connective tissue that forms a pad on the end of bones in certain joints, such as the elbow, knee, and ankle. Cartilage acts as a shock absorber to cushion the weight of one bone on another and to provide protection from the friction due to joint movement. Although this pad is the toughest of connective tissue, it can be damaged and torn (12). Unusually high forces or unusual movements can cause tearing of cartilage. This results in joint pain which is normally corrected with surgery (see A Closer Look 11.1).

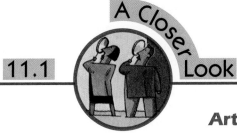

11.1

Arthroscopic Surgery: A High-Tech Approach to Joint Repair

Severe ligament and cartilage damage around a joint usually requires surgery. Knee injuries are common in many sports, such as football, soccer, and basketball, and traditional surgical techniques are expensive, cause trauma to the joint, and result in prolonged recuperation and rehabilitation. However, a commonly used surgical procedure called **arthroscopic surgery** can repair joint injuries without causing undue trauma to the joint. It is performed in the following way. Small micro-optic devices are inserted to allow surgeons to look inside the joint, along with a microsurgery tube that is capable of cutting and removing small pieces of damaged tissue as well as sewing the remaining tissue together. Arthroscopic surgery can take place with only two or three minor incisions, resulting in less damage and demanding less recovery and rehabilitation time than conventional surgery whereby the joint is cut open and repaired.

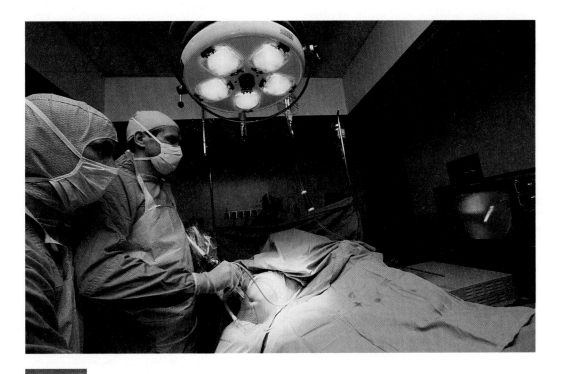

Arthroscopic surgery is relatively painless and requires much less recovery time than conventional surgery, which requires opening the joint capsule.

arthroscopic surgery A common type of surgery that can repair joint injuries without causing undue trauma to the joint.

Prevention There are no preventive measures for torn cartilage other than eliminating those activities that are likely to cause the problem. Again, activities that may result in torn cartilage include any that produce excess stress on the joint or forceful movements that take the joint outside the normal range of motion.

Common Injuries to the Lower Extremities

We have discussed the cause and prevention of several general exercise-related injuries. Because many fitness programs involve weight-bearing activities such as running, walking, and aerobic dance, let's take a closer look at some specific injuries involving the legs. In general, walking does not result in a large number of injuries. However, more than one-third of all runners develop one or more leg injuries as a result of overtraining. Further, recent studies have reported that approximately 50% of all participants in aerobic dance classes develop leg injuries. Most of these running and dance injuries are to the foot and the knee, due to the stress placed on the legs and feet. The force of the foot on the running surface (or dance floor) is approximately 2.5 times greater than the body weight of the person. In the case of a 150-pound runner, the amount of force generated when the foot strikes the pavement is 375 pounds! It is easy to see how injuries might occur with this level of stress. In the following paragraphs we will discuss the cause and prevention of the most common lower extremity injuries.

Patella-Femoral Pain Syndrome

Cause Patella-femoral pain syndrome **(PFPS),** sometimes called "runner's knee" (also known as **chondromalacia**), is a common exercise-induced injury which is manifest as pain behind the knee cap (patella)(12). In sports injury clinics, PFPS may account for almost 10% of all visits, or 20% to 40% of all knee problems (13). The basic cause of PFPS is still unknown, but there are several predisposing factors. These include overuse,

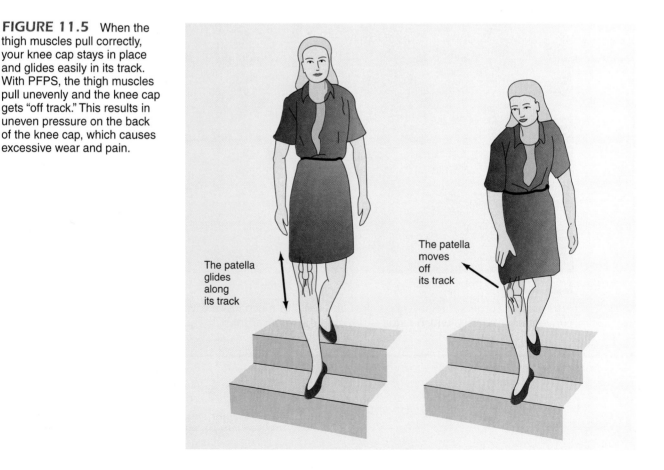

FIGURE 11.5 When the thigh muscles pull correctly, your knee cap stays in place and glides easily in its track. With PFPS, the thigh muscles pull unevenly and the knee cap gets "off track." This results in uneven pressure on the back of the knee cap, which causes excessive wear and pain.

The patella glides along its track

The patella moves off its track

immobilization, acute trauma, overweight, genetic predisposition, and malalignments of knee extensor muscles (Figure 11.5).

When these factors are present, the increased forces and repetitive movements of exercise result in pain and may result in cracking and popping sounds during movement. Over time and with increased use, the articular (joint) cartilage may begin to degenerate and may lead finally to osteoarthritis.

Prevention PFPS can be prevented by avoiding stress on the knee due to excessive amounts of running, jumping, aerobic dancing, and stair climbing. In some cases, antiinflammatory drugs may alleviate the pain. Further, the chances of developing PFPS can be reduced by strengthening the front thigh muscles (quadriceps); this improves the tracking of the patella and reduces wear on the patellar surface. An aggressive rehabilitation program that includes quadriceps exercises, rest, and antiinflammatory drugs has proved beneficial for over 70% of patients with PFPS.

The two best exercises seem to be knee extension exercises over the last 20° of extension and/or isometric contractions of the quadriceps muscles with the leg fully extended (try to press the back of the knee to the floor while lying on your back)(12). Although ice will not help prevent PFPS or rehabilitate the joint, it may provide some relief from pain and inflammation. Remember, avoid unnecessary stresses on the knee, such as squatting, and excessive amounts of activities such as running, jumping, step aerobics, and stair climbing.

Finally, proper athletic footwear may reduce the chances of developing PFPS. If you develop any of the symptoms of PFPS, see your physician or a podiatrist to discuss the possibility that footwear may be contributing to the problem.

Shin Splints

Cause *Shin splints* is a generic term referring to pain associated with injuries to the front of the lower leg (12). Three of the most common injuries that cause shin splints are strain to one or several muscles located in the lower leg (see Figure 11.6); inflammation of tissue connecting the two bones of the lower leg, the tibia and the fibula; and microscopic breaks (called *stress fractures* and discussed later) in either the tibia or the fibula.

Prevention Shin splints can be avoided by running on soft surfaces; by wearing well-

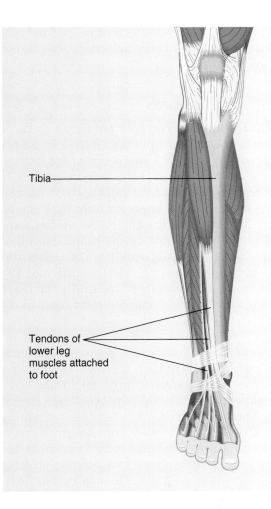

FIGURE 11.6 Shin splints are often caused by irritation of muscles and tendons in the front of the lower leg.

Tibia

Tendons of lower leg muscles attached to foot

padded, shock-absorbing shoes; and by slowly advancing exercise intensity from walking to running. If shin pain develops, it could be due to a fracture or break of bones and therefore should not be regarded lightly. High-impact activities such as running should be stopped; substitute low-impact activities such as cycling or swim-

---

patella-femoral pain syndrome (PFPS) A common exercise-induced injury that is manifest as pain behind the knee cap (patella).

chondromalacia Sometimes called "runner's knee"; it is a common exercise-induced injury which is manifest as pain behind the knee cap. In sports injury clinics, chondromalacia may account for almost 10% of all visits, or 20% to 40% of all knee problems.

ming. Stretching muscles located in the front and back of the lower leg may help in prevention of the problem.

Stress Fractures

Cause **Stress fractures** are tiny cracks or breaks in bone. Although stress fractures can occur in any leg bone, the long bones of the foot extending from the ankle to the toes are especially susceptible (Figure 11.7). Indeed, these are the most common sites of stress fractures in the body. Stress fractures result from excessive force applied to the leg and foot during running or other types of weight-bearing activities (14). Individuals with high arches or low flexibility of the lower body and people who rapidly increase training intensity or duration are the most likely candidates for this injury.

Prevention People with high arches should seek exercise advice from their physicians or a podiatrist (foot specialist), who might prescribe arch supports, which aid in preventing a stress-related problem. Again, a key factor in preventing stress fractures is to avoid overtraining by increasing your training load gradually. Remember, increase your exercise intensity or duration no more than 5% to 10% per week. Often, a lack of flexibility in the hips and back of the legs will cause the body's weight to be shifted such that some bones become chronically overloaded and frac-

FIGURE 11.7 A stress fracture in the metatarsal area results in pain with any weight-bearing movement.

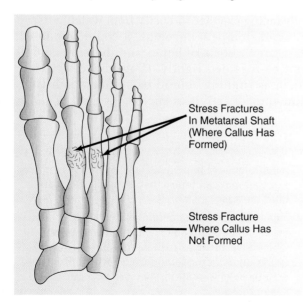

Stress Fractures In Metatarsal Shaft (Where Callus Has Formed)

Stress Fracture Where Callus Has Not Formed

ture. Thus, maintaining flexibility in the back of the legs and hips will reduce your chances of developing a stress fracture. If pain in the foot or leg makes you suspect a stress fracture, stop activities that involve the injured area. See your physician to get an X-ray of the area. If it is a stress fracture, only rest can assist the healing process.

Reducing Your Risk of Injury

To this point, we have discussed the cause and prevention of both general and specific exercise-related injuries. Here we summarize five key steps for reducing your risk of injury due to exercise training.

1. Engage in a program of muscle-strengthening exercises using all major muscle groups. Maintaining a balance of muscular strength around joints will prevent muscular imbalance and reduce the incidence of injury.

2. Warm up before and cool down after all workouts. Remember: Stretching during the warm-up may help prevent injuries, and stretching during the cool-down will help maintain flexibility.

3. Use the proper equipment. Good shoes are obviously important for activities such as running and aerobic dance. Proper footwear can reduce your chance of injury.

4. Do not overtrain! The most important factor in promoting exercise-related injuries is improper training techniques. Gradual progression of exercise intensity and duration is essential in preventing injuries.

5. Incorporate the proper amount of recovery time into your training routine. Rest is an important part of any successful training program.

Management of Injuries

As mentioned earlier, almost everyone who engages in regular physical activity will experience some type of injury. In the following sections, we will discuss injury treatment and provide an overview of the rehabilitation process.

Any injury that results in extreme pain or in which there could be a broken bone should be examined by a physician and X-rays taken to determine if there are any broken bones. The following treatment regimen should be followed for less severe injuries (strains, sprains, tendonitis, etc.).

Initial Treatment

The objectives of the initial treatment of exercise-related injuries are to decrease pain, limit swelling, and prevent further injury (15). These objectives can be met by a combination of rest, ice, compression, and elevation. The acronym **R.I.C.E.** is an easy way to remember this treatment protocol (R-rest, I-ice, C-compression, E-elevation). The R.I.C.E. principle should be applied as soon as possible after the injury. The logic behind using it is as follows.

Rest is required to prevent further injury. Movement of injured tissues will aggravate the injury and result in further damage. Any movement that causes pain should be avoided.

Application of ice to an injury reduces swelling by reducing blood flow to the cooled area. Minimizing swelling around an injury will reduce the pain and lead to more rapid healing. Ice should be placed in a cloth wrap to guard against skin damage due to frostbite and be applied for 30-minute periods, three to four times a day for 2 days after the injury.

Compression of the injured area also reduces swelling. The amount of compression applied is important. It should be enough to reduce fluid collection around the damaged area but should not be severe enough to inhibit blood flow. A snug wrap with an elastic bandage around the injured area is sufficient to control swelling.

Finally, while resting, it is beneficial to elevate the injured area, above the level of the heart if possible. Elevation reduces blood pressure and may therefore reduce swelling. Approximately 3 days following the injury, start an exercise rehabilitation program, as outlined in the next section. If there is any question about the injury's being ready for rehabilitation, delay another 24 to 48 hours.

Rehabilitation

The rehabilitation of minor injuries occurs naturally. That is, after an injury has healed and swelling has subsided, most people will begin to move the injured area at a rate that depends on the pain involved. As the pain subsides, more movement can occur until a normal range of motion is returned. However, there are several negative aspects to this rehabilitation regimen. First, it is very slow. The natural rehabilitation process, depending on the injury, may take five to ten times as long as an aggressive rehabilitation program. Second, the damaged area may be reinjured because many people attempt to return to full use of the injured area too quickly. This secondary injury results in much greater damage than the first injury and can even weaken the tissue and lead to recurring injuries throughout life. Third, without an aggressive rehabilitation program, full function of the injured tissue may never return. For example, in many types of injury, scar tissue can develop which limits the normal range of motion. Fortunately, these problems may be overcome by an active rehabilitation process.

Cryokinetics is a relatively new rehabilitation technique which is implemented after the R.I.C.E. procedures have been followed (16). It uses approximately 12 minutes of ice application followed by 3 minutes of light exercise followed by another 3 minutes of cold. This regimen should be repeated for five cycles. Exercising of the injured limb during this treatment must be guided by the pain associated with its use. Start with an exercise intensity that provides little or no pain. Intensity can be increased gradually as long as there is no increase in pain. If pain increases during the cryokinetic therapy, stop the treatment and resume the R.I.C.E. procedures until the pain subsides (see Figure 11.8).

The initial management of an injury is critical and determines the time required for completion of the rehabilitation process. For example, a regimen of cryokinetics initiated after a third degree ankle sprain (2–3 days postinjury) results in complete recovery within 2 weeks. In contrast, if the cryokinetic treatment starts late (5–7 days postinjury), the recovery may take 4 to 5 weeks.

stress fractures Tiny cracks or breaks in the bone.

R.I.C.E. An acronym representing a treatment protocol for exercise-related injuries. It stands for a combination of rest-*R*, ice-*I*, compression-*C*, and elevation-*E*.

cryokinetics A relatively new rehabilitation technique which is implemented after the acute injury and healing period have been completed. It incorporates varying periods of treatment using ice, rest, and exercise.

FIGURE 11.8 The stages of the cryokinetics procedure for injury rehabilitation.

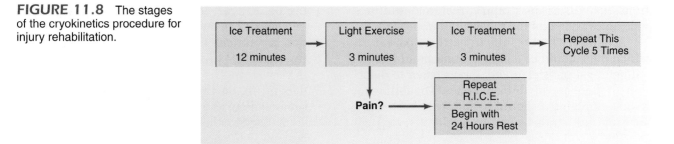

As pain subsides and the range of motion returns, full recovery may be accelerated if a program of weight training and flexibility is added to the treatment process. This is especially true of muscle injuries because the healing process may cause the muscle to shorten and thereby limit flexibility. A key point to remember is that an in-jury that does not heal properly may cause recurring pain during activity and persist for years. Therefore, for stubborn injuries, seeking the treatment advice of a trained professional (athletic trainer, physical therapist, or physician) is often recommended.

Summary

1. Injuries involved with running occur primarily in the foot and knee. This is due to the excessive stress placed on the legs and feet. The factors most closely associated with running injuries are improper training techniques, inadequate shoes, and alignment problems in the legs and feet.

2. Factors associated with injuries in aerobic dance are the number of sessions per week, improper shoes, and nonresilient surfaces.

3. Overtraining is the greatest risk to developing an exercise-related injury.

4. Back pain is a multifactoral problem that usually subsides without any medical intervention. Exercise, however, can play an important role in preventing back pain and rehabilitation of some back problems. Exercises to increase flexibility and strength, reduce body fat, improve muscle balance between the trunk flexors and extensors, and prevent osteoporosis can decrease your risk of developing back problems.

5. Acute muscle soreness may occur during or immediately after an exercise bout. This type of injury may be due to muscle damage, accumulation of fluid within the muscle, and/or chemical imbalances within the muscle itself.

6. Delayed-onset muscle soreness (DOMS) sometimes occurs 24 to 48 hours after a bout of exercise. Eccentric exercise increases the chance of DOMS.

7. When muscle is forced to contract against excessive resistance, fibers are damaged. This damage is referred to as a *strain* and can range from a minor separation of fibers to a complete tear.

8. Tendonitis is one of the most common of all overuse problems associated with physical activity. The term literally means inflammation of a tendon.

9. A sprain is caused by damage to a ligament, connective tissue that provides support for joints. In contrast, torn cartilage refers to damage to the tough, connective tissue that serves as a pad between the ends of bones.

10. Common injuries to the lower extremities are PFPS, in which the articular cartilage on the back of the knee cap (patella) may be damaged by chronic use during exercise; shin splints, which encompasses several different injuries to the front of the lower leg; and stress fractures, microscopic breaks in the bone.

11. The following steps reduce your risk of developing an exercise-related injury:

1. Engage in a program of muscle-strengthening exercises to keep a balance in strength around joints.
2. Warm up before and cool down after each workout.
3. Use the proper equipment (including proper footwear).
4. Increase your exercise intensity and duration slowly throughout your exercise training program.
5. Maintain the proper rest-to-exercise ratio. Do not overtrain!
6. For treating injuries, remember the R.I.C.E. principle: rest, ice, compression and elevation.
7. Recently, an effective new technique for injury rehabilitation called *cryokinetics* has come into use. This treatment calls for alternating cold applications and exercise.

Study Questions

1. Discuss the risk of injury involved in running.
2. What are thought to be the primary causes of running injuries?
3. Discuss the risk of injury associated with aerobic dance and the factors thought to cause the injuries.
4. Differentiate between acute and delayed-onset muscle soreness.
5. Compare and contrast a strain and a sprain.
6. Define *tendonitis* and the best method of prevention/treatment.
7. What is the cause of PFPS and how should it be treated?
8. What causes shin splints and how can they be prevented?
9. List the steps that should be followed to minimize the risk of injury from increased physical activity.
10. Define the R.I.C.E. principle and discuss its use.
11. Discuss the use of cryokinetics as a rehabilitation technique.
12. Define the following terms:
    arthroscopic surgery
    cartilage
    edema
    ligament
    stress fracture
    overtraining syndrome

Suggested Reading

Arnheim, D. D., and W. E. Prentice. *Principles of athletic training.* 8th ed. Mosby Year-Book, St. Louis, 1993.

Clarkson, P. M. and D. J. Newham. Association between muscle soreness, damage, and fatigue. *Advances in Experimental Medicine and Biology* 384:457–469, 1995.

Jones, B. H., J. M. Harris, T. N. Vinh, and C. Rubin. Exercise-induced stress fractures and stress reactions of bone: Epidemiology, etiology, and classification. *Exercise and Sports Sciences Review* 17:379–422, 1989.

Kibler, W. B., J. Chandler, and E. S. Stracener. Musculoskeletal adaptations and injuries due to overtraining. *Exercise and Sports Sciences Review* 20:99–126, 1992.

Neiman, David C. *Fitness and sports medicine: An introduction.* 3rd ed. Bull Publishing, Palo Alto, CA, 1995.

Twellaar, M., F. T. Verstappen, A. Huson, and W. van-Mechelen. Physical characteristics as risk factors for sports injuries: A four year prospective study. *International Journal of Sports Medicine* 18(1): 6–71, 1997.

Suggested Readings on the World Wide Web

Fitness Files
(http://www2.webpoint.com/augusta_fitness/)
Fitness fundamentals, flexibility and contraindicated exercises, exercise nutrition, and
treating exercise injuries.

Penn Health
(http://www.med.upenn.edu/health/hi_files/pha/
sports.html)
Provides 1–800 numbers for describing and
treating exercise-related injuries.

The Running Page
(http://sunsite.unc.edu/drears/running/
running.html)
Contains information about racing, running clubs,
places to run, running-related products, magazines,
treating running injuries, etc.

Fitness and Sports Medicine
(http://www.meriter.com/living/library/sports/
index.html)
Injury prevention and treatment, weight training,
flexibility, exercise prescriptions, and more.

References

1. Nieman, David C. *Fitness and sports medicine: An introduction.* 3rd ed. Bull Publishing, Palo Alto, CA, 1995.
2. Robbins, S. E., and A. M. Hanna. Running-related injury prevention through barefoot adaptations. *Medicine and Science in Sports and Exercise* 19:148–156, 1987.
3. Messier, S. P., and K. A. Pittala. Etiologic factors associated with selected running injuries. *Medicine and Science in Sports and Exercise* 20:501–505, 1988.
4. Lysholm, J., and J. Willnader. Injuries in runners. *American Journal of Sports Medicine* 15:168–178, 1987.
5. Garrick, J. G., and R. K. Requa. Aerobic dance: A review. *Sports Medicine* 6:169–179, 1988.
6. Richie, D. H., S. F. Kelso, and P. A. Bellucci. Aerobic dance injuries: A retrospective study of instructors and participants. *Physician Sports Medicine* 13:130–140, 1985.
7. Reuler, J. B. Low back pain. *Western Journal of Medicine* 143:259–265, 1985.
8. Mayer, T. G., R. J. Gatchel, and H. Mayer. A prospective two-year trial of functional restoration in treating industrial low back injuries. *Journal of the American Medical Association* 258:1763–1767, 1987.
9. Leino, P., S. Aro, and J. Hasan. Trunk muscle function and low back disorders: A ten-year follow-up study. *Journal of Chronic Diseases* 40:289–296, 1987.
10. Powers, S., and E. Howley. *Exercise physiology: Theory and application to fitness and performance.* 2d ed. Wm. C. Brown, Dubuque, IA, 1994.
11. Clarkson, P. M. Causes and consequences of delayed onset muscle soreness. A*CSM's Health and Fitness Journal* 1(3):12–17, 1997.
12. Arnheim, D. D., and W. E. Prentice. *Principles of athletic training.* 8th ed. Mosby Year-Book, St. Louis, 1993.
13. Kibler, W. B., J. Chandler, and E. S. Stracener. Musculoskeletal adaptations and injuries due to overtraining. *Exercise and Sports Sciences Review* 20:99–126, 1992.
14. Jones, B. H., J. M. Harris, T. N. Vinh, and C. Rubin. Exercise-induced stress fractures and stress reactions of bone: Epidemiology, etiology, and classification. *Exercise and Sports Sciences Review* 17:379–422, 1989.
15. Kellett, J. Acute soft tissue injuries—A review of the literature. *Medicine and Science in Sports and Exercise* 18:489–500, 1986.
16. Meeusen, R., and P. Lievens. The use of cryotherapy in sports injuries. *Sports Medicine* 3:398–414, 1986.

Prevention of Injuries during Exercise

NAME _____ DATE _____

Purpose:

The following lab experience is designed to find and eliminate ways in which your exercise program may cause injuries.

Procedure:

Check each of the following factors associated with prevention of injury that you have included in your exercise program. For those not checked, list the ways in which you can eliminate these risks by substituting alternative exercises or performing the same exercises in a different manner.

Preventive Measure	Check here if included	Alternate
Use of proper shoes for the activity	_____	_____
Use of warm-up	_____	_____
Stretch all muscle groups involved in the activity	_____	_____
Avoid over-stretching of the neck and back	_____	_____
Avoid extension and rotation of the spine	_____	_____
Avoid lifting extremely heavy objects	_____	_____
Avoid quick, jerking movements	_____	_____
Strengthen and balance all muscle groups involved in the activity	_____	_____
Use of properly designed training program	_____	_____
Frequency	_____	_____
Intensity	_____	_____
Duration	_____	_____
Use of proper exercise techniques	_____	_____
For running—use of level, firm surface	_____	_____
Use of proper cool-down	_____	_____
Use support device for muscle or joint if you can't stop training	_____	_____

Prevention of Cardiovascular Disease

Learning Objectives

After reading this chapter, you should be able to

1 Name the number one cause of death in the United States.

2 Identify four common cardiovascular diseases.

3 Discuss the major and contributory risk factors associated with the development of coronary heart disease.

4 Identify which coronary heart disease risk factors can be modified by lifestyle alterations.

5 List the steps involved in reducing your risk of coronary heart disease.

6 Describe the link between dietary sodium and hypertension.

7 Identify total blood cholesterol levels associated with low, moderate, and high risk of developing coronary heart disease.

8 Discuss the relationship between diet and elevated blood cholesterol levels.

diovascular diseases are a major health problem around the world and account for millions of deaths each year. The incidence of cardiovascular disease is greatest in industrialized countries, with the United States having one of the world's highest death rates (1). Although it is impossible to place a dollar value on human life, the economic cost of cardiovascular disease in the United States is great (see Figure 12.1). Estimates of lost wages and medical expenses exceed 95 billion dollars every year (1); therefore, developing a national strategy to reduce the risk of cardiovascular disease is a major health priority. This chapter focuses on lifestyle changes (e.g., exercise and diet) that can reduce your risk of cardiovascular diseases. Let's begin our discussion with an overview of cardiovascular disease in the United States.

Cardiovascular Disease in the United States

Although public awareness is currently more focused on diseases such as cancer and AIDS, cardiovascular disease remains the number one cause of death in the United States, accounting for nearly one of every two deaths. Current data

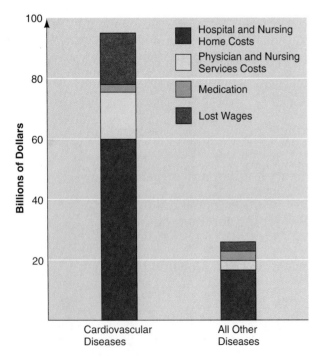

FIGURE 12.1 Annual economic costs of cardiovascular diseases and other diseases in the United States.

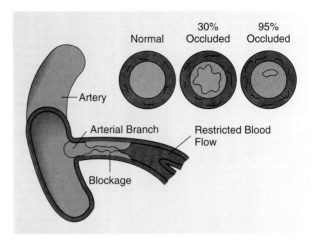

FIGURE 12.2 Stages of atherosclerosis. The "normal" artery on the left has no blockage due to plaque. However, the two arteries on the right have 30% and 95% blockage, respectively, due to the progressive collection of atherosclerotic plaque.

indicate that over 60 million adults have one or more forms of cardiovascular disease and that approximately one million die annually from cardiovascular disorders (1). Equally alarming is the fact that cardiovascular disease is not restricted to the elderly. It is the leading cause of death in men between the ages of 35 and 44 (1). Although the death rate from cardiovascular disease has always been higher for men than women, the incidence of cardiovascular disease in women has increased dramatically in recent years (1). Fortunately, it is possible to reduce your risk of developing cardiovascular disease, but before discussing how to do this, we will define the major types of cardiovascular disease.

Cardiovascular Diseases

Cardiovascular disease refers to any disease that affects the heart or blood vessels. Although there are literally hundreds of diseases that impair normal cardiovascular function, only four common cardiovascular diseases warrant discussion here.

Arteriosclerosis

Arteriosclerosis is not a single disease but rather a group of diseases characterized by a narrowing or "hardening" of the arteries. The end re-

Heart and Coronary Arteries

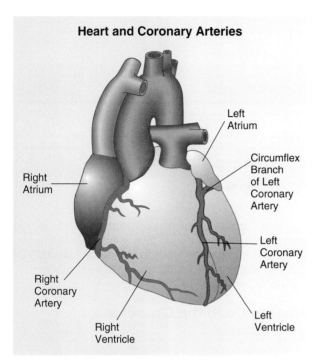

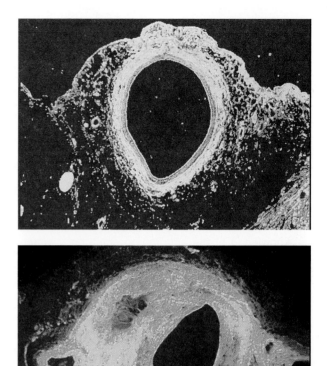

FIGURE 12.3 The coronary arteries carry blood to the working heart muscle. The photographs illustrate a normal **(top)** and an atherosclerotic coronary artery **(bottom)**. As plaque builds up in the walls of coronary arteries, the risk of heart attack increases. (Source: From Melvin H. Williams, *Lifetime Fitness and Wellness,* 3rd edition. Copyright © 1993 Wm. C. Brown Communications, Inc. Reprinted by permission of Times Mirror Higher Education Group, Inc. Dubuque, Iowa. All rights reserved.)

sult of any form of arteriosclerosis is that blood flow to vital organs may be impaired due to a progressive blockage of the artery. **Atherosclerosis** is a special type of arteriosclerosis that results in arterial blockage due to collection of a fatty deposit (called *atherosclerotic plaque*) inside the blood vessel. This plaque deposit is typically composed of cholesterol, cellular debris, fibrin (a clotting material in the blood), and calcium. Atherosclerosis is a progressive disease that begins in childhood, with symptoms appearing later in life. Figure 12.2 illustrates blocked arteries caused by atherosclerosis. Note that atherosclerosis is not an "all or none" disease but occurs in varying degrees, with some arteries exhibiting little blockage and others exhibiting major obstruction. Development of severe atherosclerosis within arteries supplying blood to the heart is the cause of almost all heart attacks.

Coronary Heart Disease

Coronary heart disease is the major disease of the cardiovascular system. **Coronary heart dis-**

ease **(CHD)**, also called *coronary artery disease*, is the result of atherosclerotic plaque forming a blockage of one or more coronary arteries (the blood vessels supplying the heart; see Figure 12.3 and corresponding photo). When the degree of blockage of a major coronary artery reaches 75%,

cardiovascular disease Any disease that affects the heart or blood vessels.

arteriosclerosis A group of diseases characterized by a narrowing or "hardening" of the arteries. The end result of any form of arteriosclerosis is that blood flow to vital organs may be impaired due to a progressive blockage of the artery.

atherosclerosis A special type of arteriosclerosis that results in arterial blockage due to collection of a fatty deposit (called *atherosclerotic plaque*) inside the blood vessel.

coronary heart disease (CHD); also called *coronary artery disease* CHD is the result of atherosclerotic plaque forming a blockage of one or more coronary arteries (the blood vessels supplying the heart).

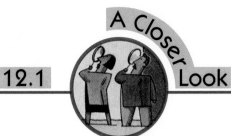

12.1

Heart Attack:
Recognition of Symptoms
and Emergency Action

Recognition of heart attack symptoms and knowledge of the appropriate emergency action could save your life or that of someone else. The following is a discussion of the symptoms of a heart attack and the correct emergency procedure to follow.

Warning Signals of a Heart Attack

Some of the most common symptoms of a heart attack (2) are

1. Mild to moderate pain in your chest that may spread to your shoulders, neck, or arms
2. Uncomfortable pressure or sensation of fullness in your chest
3. Severe pain in the chest, dizziness, fainting, sweating, nausea, or shortness of breath

Note that not all of these symptoms occur in every heart attack. Therefore, if you or someone you're with experiences any one of these symptoms for 2 minutes or more, follow the emergency procedures described next.

What to Do in the Case of a Heart Attack

If you or someone near you experiences any of the aforementioned symptoms for 2 minutes or longer, call the emergency medical service or get to the nearest hospital that offers emergency cardiac care. If you are trained in cardiopulmonary resuscitation (CPR) and the patient is not breathing or does not have a pulse, call for help and then start CPR immediately. In any cardiac emergency, rapid action may mean the difference between life and death.

Because 40% of heart attack victims die within the first hour, immediate medical attention is vital to a patient's survival.

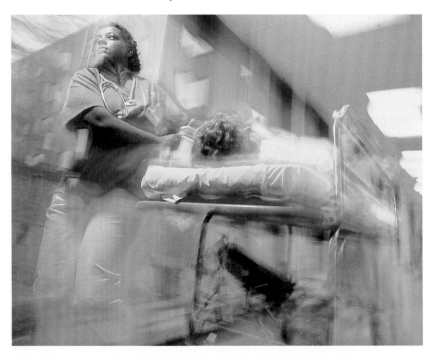

the resulting lack of blood flow to the working heart muscle causes chest pain. This type of chest pain, called *angina pectoris*, occurs most frequently during exercise or emotional stress (2).

Severe blockage of coronary arteries may result in a blood clot forming around the layer of plaque. When this happens, there is a complete blockage of heart blood flow, resulting in a **heart attack** (also called a **myocardial infarction**). Figure 12.4 illustrates what happens during a heart attack caused by complete blockage of the left coronary artery. The end result is the death of heart cells in the left ventricle; the severity of the heart attack is judged by how many heart cells are damaged. A "mild" heart attack may only damage a small portion of the heart, whereas a "major" heart attack may destroy a large number of heart cells. In general, it is the number of heart cells that are destroyed during a heart attack that determines the patient's chances of recovery (see A Closer Look 12.1).

Stroke

It is estimated that each year two million Americans suffer from a stroke (1). A **stroke** occurs when the blood supply to the brain is re-

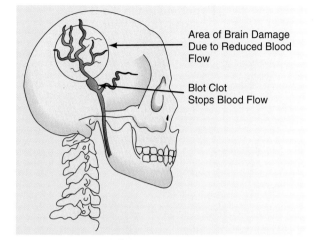

FIGURE 12.5 Illustration of brain damage due to a stroke. During a stroke, blood flow is halted to the brain, resulting in death to brain cells in the area. The circled area in the upper portion of this figure illustrates the area of the brain damaged as a result of the stroke.

duced for a prolonged period of time. A common cause of stroke is blockage of arteries (by atherosclerosis) leading to the brain (see Figure 12.5). However, strokes can also occur when a cerebral (brain) blood vessel ruptures and disturbs normal blood flow to that region of the brain.

Similar to a heart attack, which results in death of heart cells, a stroke results in death of brain cells. The severity of the stroke may vary from slight to severe, depending on location and the number of brain cells damaged. Minor strokes may involve a loss of memory, speech problems, disturbed vision, and/or mild paralysis in the extremities. In contrast, severe strokes may result in major paralysis or death.

Hypertension

Hypertension is an abnormally high blood pressure. Clinically, hypertension is generally defined as a resting blood pressure over 140 mm Hg systolic or 90 mm Hg diastolic (2). Approximately 10% of hypertension cases are caused by

FIGURE 12.4 Example of a myocardial infarction (heart attack). Note that the shaded area of the heart is damaged due to a reduction in blood flow during the heart attack.

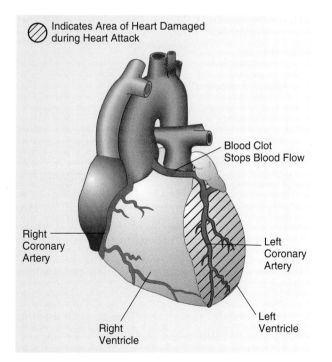

heart attack; also called *myocardial infarction* Stoppage of blood flow to the heart, resulting in the death of heart cells.

stroke Brain damage that occurs when the blood supply to the brain is reduced for a prolonged period of time.

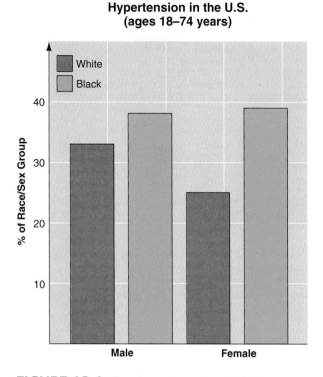

Hypertension in the U.S.
(ages 18–74 years)

FIGURE 12.6 The percentage of people in the United States with hypertension.

a specific disease (such as kidney disease). This type of hypertension is called *secondary hypertension*, because the hypertension is secondary to a primary disease. Nonetheless, in 90% of cases, the exact cause of the high blood pressure is unknown; this type of hypertension is called *essential hypertension.*

The incidence of hypertension in the United States is remarkably high (see Figure 12.6). The factors that increase your risk of hypertension include lack of exercise, a high-salt diet, obesity, chronic stress, family history of hypertension, gender (men have a greater risk than women), and race (Blacks have a greater risk than Whites).

Hypertension is a health problem for several reasons. First, high blood pressure increases the work load on the heart; this may eventually damage the heart muscle's ability to pump blood effectively throughout the body (2). Second, high blood pressure may damage the interior of arteries, resulting in the development of atherosclerosis and therefore increasing the risk of CHD and stroke (2).

Although exercise causes acute increases in blood pressure, this type of blood pressure elevation is transient and is not hypertension (i.e., hypertension is chronically elevated blood pres-

sure). Further, the increase in blood pressure during exercise does not damage the heart or blood vessels.

The American Heart Association estimates that in the United States, approximately one of every four people suffers from hypertension; that is, more than 62 million people (1). Unfortunately, because they lack symptoms, many people are not aware that they are hypertensive. Although severe hypertension may result in headaches and dizziness, these symptoms are often absent. Therefore, without annual medical checkups or blood pressure screenings, hypertension may go undiagnosed for many years. For this reason, hypertension is often called *the silent killer.*

Risk Factors Associated with Coronary Heart Disease

In an effort to identify the cause and reduce the occurrence of CHD, researchers have identified a number of major and contributory risk factors that increase the chance of developing both CHD and stroke. **Major risk factors** (also called *primary risk factors*) are factors considered to be directly related to the development of CHD and stroke. In contrast, **contributory risk factors** (also called *secondary risk factors*) are those that increase the risk of CHD, but their direct contribution to the disease process has not been precisely determined.

Major Risk Factors

Each year the American Heart Association publishes new information concerning the major risk factors associated with the development of CHD and stroke. The most recent list includes cigarette smoking, hypertension, high blood cholesterol levels, physical inactivity, heredity, gender, and increasing age (1) (Figure 12.7). The greater the number of CHD risk factors that an individual has, the higher the chances he or she has of developing CHD (see Figure 12.8 for examples). Let's discuss each of the major risk factors for CHD and stroke.

Smoking It is estimated that over 50 million people in the United States smoke (3). Many U.S. health care workers believe that cigarette smoking is the single largest cause of disease and premature death. Cigarette smoking has been linked to over 30 health problems including cancer, lung disease, and cardiovascular disease (1–4). In regard to smoking and cardiovascular disease, a smoker's risk of developing CHD is twice that of a nonsmoker (1) (see Figure 12.8). Smoking is also considered the biggest risk factor for sudden cardiac death (i.e., sudden death due to cardiac arrest, a heart attack, or irregular heart beats). In addition, smoking promotes the development of atherosclerosis in peripheral blood vessels (arterial blockage in the arms or legs). Finally, smokers who have a heart attack are more likely to die suddenly (within an hour after the attack) than are nonsmokers.

Can nonsmokers increase their risk of cardiovascular disease by breathing "second hand" cigarette smoke? Unfortunately, the answer is "yes." Numerous studies have concluded that passive inhalation of cigarette smoke can increase your risk for both cardiovascular and lung disease (3). This has prompted the banning of smoking in many public places, including airplanes, restaurants, and shopping malls.

There are at least four major ways that cigarette smoking can influence your risk of cardiovascular disease. First, cigarette smoke contains the drug nicotine, which increases both heart rate and blood pressure (3). Second, smoking increases your blood's ability to clot; an elevated

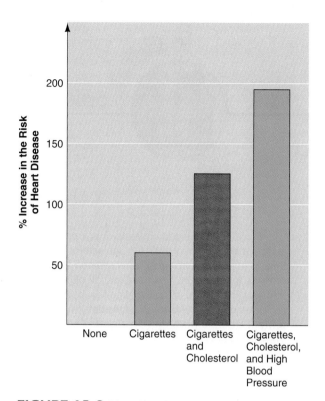

FIGURE 12.8 Your risk of developing coronary heart disease increases as the number of risk factors increase.

possibility of a blood clot raises your risk of heart attack (3). Third, nicotine also influences the way your heart functions, leading to irregular heart beats (called *arrhythmias*) (3). These arrhythmias can lead to sudden cardiac death. Finally, cigarette smoking increases your chance of developing atherosclerosis by elevating the amount of cholesterol in the blood and encouraging fat deposits around arterial walls (3).

When someone stops smoking, his or her risk of heart disease rapidly declines. It is believed that within 10 years after quitting smoking, a person's risk of death from CHD is reduced to a level equal to that of someone who has never smoked (1). Strategies to stop smoking are discussed in Chapter 14.

FIGURE 12.7 Coronary heart diesease risk factors.

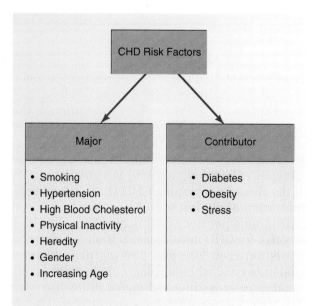

major risk factors; also called *primary risk factors* Factors considered to be directly related to the development of CHD and stroke.

contributory risk factors; also called *secondary risk* factors. Factors that increase the risk of CHD, but their direct contribution to the disease process has not been precisely determined.

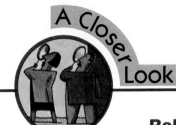

Relationship between Blood Cholesterol and Coronary Heart Disease

Elevated total blood cholesterol is a primary risk factor for development of CHD. Cholesterol is not soluble in the blood and must be combined with blood proteins for transport. This combination of cholesterol and proteins occurs in the liver and results in two major forms of blood cholesterol: **low-density lipoproteins** (LDL) and **high-density lipoproteins** (HDL). The association between elevated total blood cholesterol and the increased risk of CHD is due primarily to LDL cholesterol. Research has shown that individuals with high blood LDL cholesterol levels have an increased risk of CHD, whereas individuals with high blood HDL cholesterol levels have a decreased risk of CHD (1, 2). Because of this relationship, LDL cholesterol has been labeled "bad cholesterol" and HDL cholesterol "good cholesterol." Another method of calculating the risk of developing CHD is to use the total cholesterol to HDL cholesterol ratio; the risks for men and women are contained in Table 12.1.

Debate continues as to whether regular endurance exercise lowers blood LDL cholesterol, with some studies reporting exercise-induced reductions and others reporting no influence (5, 6). In contrast, it is clear that regular endurance exercise (running, cycling, swimming) results in an elevation of blood HDL cholesterol and reduces the risk of CHD (5, 6). The mechanism that links endurance exercise to increased HDL cholesterol is unknown and remains an active area of research.

Table 12.1

Risk of Cardiovascular Disease in Men and Women Based on the Total Cholesterol to HDL Cholesterol Ratio

Risk	Total Cholesterol to HDL Cholesterol Ratio	
	Men	Women
Low	3 to 1	3 to 1
Moderate	5 to 1	4.5 to 1
High	>9 to 1	>7 to 1

Data from Barrow (2).

Hypertension Hypertension is a unique risk factor because it is both a disease and a risk factor for stroke and CHD. As mentioned earlier, hypertension is considered a disease because it forces the heart to work harder than normal, which can eventually damage the heart muscle. As a CHD risk factor, it contributes to the development of CHD by accelerating the rate of atherosclerosis development (2, 4a).

High Blood Cholesterol Levels Cholesterol is a type of fat that can be synthesized in the body or consumed in our diet. The risk of CHD increases as blood cholesterol levels rise. Like other fats, cholesterol is not soluble in blood and must be combined with blood proteins for transport, which results in several types of blood cholesterol (see A Closer Look 12.2). Although the risk of developing CHD is related to the types of cholesterol present in the blood, research suggests that total blood cholesterol (i.e., the sum of all types of blood cholesterol) is a good predictor of the risk of developing CHD (1, 2). Blood concentration of cholesterol of less than 200 mg/dl (milligrams per deciliter) is considered to be a low risk for CHD development. Blood cholesterol levels between 200 and 239 mg/dl indicate a moderate risk, whereas blood cholesterol levels equal to or exceeding 240 mg/dl indicate a high risk of developing CHD (see Figure 12.9). Unfor-

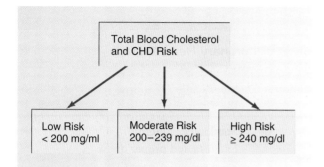

FIGURE 12.9 Total blood cholesterol levels and your risk of CHD.

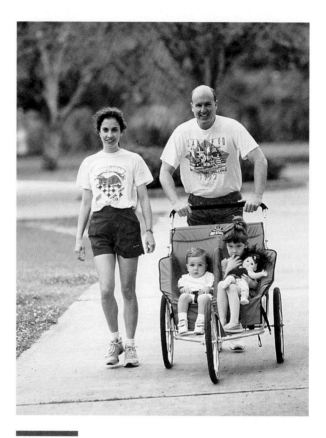

Even modest physical activity (walking for 20–30 minutes per day, three to five times per week) can reduce your risk of developing cardiovascular disease.

tunately, due to high-fat diets and a lack of exercise, over 21% of people in the United States have blood cholesterol levels over 240 mg/dl (2).

Physical Inactivity In 1992, the American Heart Association added physical inactivity (defined as a lack of regular exercise) to the list of major risk factors for the development of CHD. The addition of physical inactivity to the list of major risk factors for CHD is based on a large volume of research which suggests that the incidence of CHD is much greater in people who do not engage in regular physical activity (7–9). Thus, exercise has gained new importance in the prevention of CHD.

Heredity It is firmly established that inherited traits can increase your risk of CHD and stroke (1, 2). This means that children of parents with CHD are more likely to develop CHD than are children of parents who do not have CHD. Current evidence suggests that the familial risk for CHD may be linked to factors such as high blood cholesterol, hypertension, diabetes, and obesity (2).

Race is also a consideration because African Americans develop hypertension two to three times more often than Whites. Therefore, because hypertension increases the chances of developing CHD, African Americans have a greater risk for CHD than Whites. The reason for the high rate of hypertension among African Americans is unknown.

Gender Men have a greater risk of developing CHD and stroke than women. Much of the female protection against CHD is linked to the female sex hormone estrogen, which may elevate HDL cholesterol. Although the risk of CHD increases in women after menopause, it never becomes as great as for men (2).

low-density lipoproteins (LDL) A combination of protein, triglycerides, and cholesterol in the blood, composed of relatively large amounts of cholesterol. Promotes the fatty plaque accumulation in the coronary arteries of the heart that leads to heart disease. The association between elevated total blood cholesterol and the increased risk of CHD is due primarily to LDL cholesterol. Research has shown that individuals with high blood LDL cholesterol levels have an increased risk of CHD. Because of this relationship, LDL cholesterol has been labeled "bad cholesterol."

high-density lipoproteins (HDL) A combination of protein, triglycerides, and cholesterol in the blood, composed of relatively large amounts of protein. Protects against the fatty plaque accumulation in the coronary arteries of the heart that leads to heart disease. Research has shown that individuals with high blood HDL-cholesterol levels have a decreased risk of CHD. Therefore, HDL-cholesterol is often called "good cholesterol."

Table 12.2

Major and Contributory Risk Factors for the Development of Coronary Heart Disease

Risk Factor	Risk Factor Classification	Is Modification Possible?	Modification Required to Reduce Risk
Smoking	Major	Yes	Smoking cessation
Hypertension	Major	Yes	Exercise and proper diet
High blood cholesterol	Major	Yes	Exercise and proper diet
Physical inactivity	Major	Yes	Exercise
Heredity	Major	No	
Gender	Major	No	
Increasing age	Major	No	
Diabetes	Contributory	Yes	Proper nutrition, exercise
Obesity	Contributory	Yes	Weight loss, proper nutrition, exercise
Stress	Contributory	Yes	Stress management, exercise

Data from *Heart Facts,* American Heart Association, 1993.

Increasing Age Advancing age increases the risk of developing CHD. The explanation for this observation is that the collection of arterial plaque is an ongoing process; the longer one lives, the greater the collection. This is illustrated by the statistic that over 50% of all heart attack victims are 65 or older (1).

Contributory Risk Factors

Contributory risk factors are those that increase your risk of CHD, but their direct contribution to the disease process is unclear. You can think of contributory risk factors as those that increase your risk of developing a *major* risk factor. At present, the American Heart Association recognizes diabetes, obesity, and stress as contributory risk factors (see Table 12.2).

Diabetes As we saw in Chapter 1, diabetes is a disease that results in elevated blood sugar levels due to the body's inability to use blood sugar properly. Diabetes occurs most often in middle age and is common in people who are overweight. In addition to increasing your risk of kidney disease, blindness, and nerve damage, diabetes increases your risk of CHD and stroke. The link between diabetes and CHD is well established; more than 80% of all diabetics die from some form of cardiovascular disease. The role of diabetes in increasing your risk of CHD may be tied to the fact that diabetics

often have elevated blood cholesterol levels, hypertension, and are inactive (8).

Obesity Compared with individuals who maintain their ideal body weight, obese individuals are more likely to develop CHD, even if they have no other major risk factors (8). Further, obesity is often associated with elevated blood cholesterol levels and may contribute to hypertension (8).

Of particular interest is the fact that a person's fat distribution pattern affects the risk of CHD. As discussed in Chapter 2, a waist-to-hip circumference ratio greater than 1.0 for men and 0.8 for women indicates a significant risk for development of CHD. The physiological reason for the link between CHD and regional fat distribution is not well established but may be due to the fact that people with high waist/hip circumferences often eat high-fat diets which elevate blood cholesterol levels.

The fact that obesity is associated with a high incidence of hypertension is well established; however, the exact physiological link between obesity and hypertension is less clear. Possible causes of hypertension in obesity include a high-salt diet which elevates blood pressure and increased vascular resistance, resulting in the need for higher pressure to pump blood to the tissues (2). The role of sodium in promoting hypertension is discussed later in Nutritional Links to Health and Fitness 12.1.

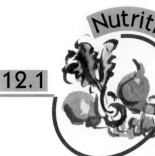

12.1 Links to Health and Fitness

High Sodium Intake Increases the Risk of Hypertension

A key factor in regulating blood pressure is dietary sodium. High sodium intake results in an elevated blood volume, which promotes higher blood pressure. Therefore, monitoring sodium intake is an important factor in preventing or controlling hypertension.

As mentioned in Chapter 7, sodium (contained in table salt) is a required micronutrient, but the daily requirement for most people is small (less than one-fourth teaspoon or 400 mg). Even athletes or laborers who lose large amounts of water and electrolytes via sweat rarely require more than 1.5 teaspoons (3000 mg) of salt per day. Currently, many U.S. citizens consume more than 6 teaspoons (12,000 mg)

of salt per day; clearly, this level of sodium intake is unhealthy and can lead to hypertension.

What is the maximum amount of dietary sodium that the body can tolerate without developing hypertension? A definitive answer to this question is not available; however, hypertension is rare in countries where sodium intake is less than 1 teaspoon per day.

The key to lowering your sodium intake is avoiding foods that are high in salt. Table 12.3 illustrates some common foods that are high in sodium. Take the time to learn which foods contain high sodium and limit your intake of sodium to less than 1 teaspoon per day.

Table 12.3

Common Foods That Contain High Sodium Content

Food	Serving Size	Sodium Content (mg)
Bologna	2 oz	700
Cheese		
American	1 oz	305
Cheddar	1 oz	165
Parmesan	1 oz	525
Deviled crab	1	2085
Frankfurter	1	495
Hamburger patty	1 small	550
Pickles (dill)	1 medium	900
Pizza (cheese)	1 (14" diameter)	600
Potato chips	20	300
Pretzels	1 oz	890
Salami	3 oz	1047
Soup		
Chicken noodle	1 cup	1010
Vegetable beef	1 cup	1046
Soy sauce	1 tablespoon	1320

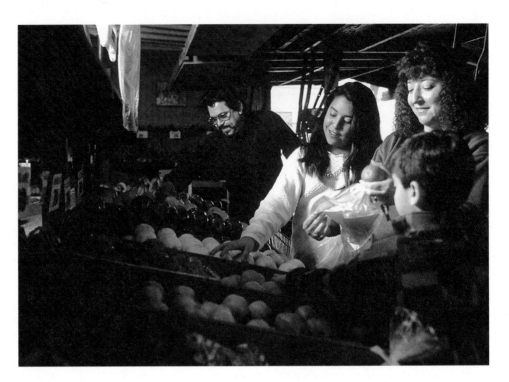

Parents should impress on their children the importance of good dietary habits in preventing cardiovascular disease.

Stress Stress increases your risk of CHD; however, the exact link between stress and CHD is unclear and continues to be studied. Nonetheless, it seems likely that stress contributes to the development of several major CHD risk factors. For example, stress may be linked to smoking habits. People under stress may start smoking in an effort to relax, or stress could influence smokers to smoke more than they normally would. Further, stress increases the risk of developing both hypertension and elevated blood cholesterol. The physiological connection between stress and hypertension appears to be the stress-induced release of "stress" hormones which elevate blood pressure. Currently, it is unclear how stress is linked to high blood cholesterol.

Reducing Your Risk of Heart Disease

Although it remains the number one killer in the United States, the incidence of cardiovascular disease has declined over the past 30 years (1). This drop is due primarily to people reducing their risk factors for CHD. Table 12.2 on page 274 contains a list of the major and contributory CHD risk factors discussed earlier in the chapter. Note that four of the seven major risk factors and two of the contributory factors can be modified. Therefore, of the ten CHD risk factors presented in Table 12.2, 70% of these factors can be modified to reduce your risk of developing cardiovascular disease.

How does one implement a CHD risk reduction program? The first step is the identification of your risk status. This can be done by completion of Laboratory 12.1 and by careful examination of Table 12.2. The next step is to implement a positive healthy lifestyle to modify those CHD risk factors that can be altered.

Modification of Major Risk Factors

The four major CHD risk factors that can be modified are smoking, hypertension, high blood cholesterol, and physical inactivity. The risk of CHD decreases as soon as smokers "kick" the habit. Clearly, smoking cessation is an important means for reducing CHD risk. The well-known fitness and wellness expert, Dr. Melvin Williams,

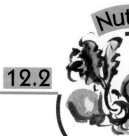

12.2 Nutritional Links to Health and Fitness

Diet and Blood Cholesterol Levels

One of the easiest dietary means of reducing your blood cholesterol is to reduce your intake of saturated fat and cholesterol. Saturated fats stimulate cholesterol synthesis in the liver and therefore contribute to elevated blood cholesterol. Saturated fats are found mostly in meats and dairy products; avoiding high intake of these foods can reduce your blood cholesterol levels. (See Table 12.4 for a partial listing and the Appendix for a complete listing of the cholesterol content of various foods.)

offers the following advice on smoking (10): "If you don't smoke, don't start! If you smoke, quit!" Unfortunately, for most people, smoking is a difficult habit to break. Chapter 14 provides guidelines to assist in smoking cessation.

Hypertension can be reduced in several ways. In some instances, medication may be required to control high blood pressure. However, in many hypertension cases, exercise and a proper diet that features low sodium intake may assist in the reduction of blood pressure (see Nutritional Links to Health and Fitness 12.1 on page 275).

High blood cholesterol may be lowered by diet, exercise, and drug treatment (including increasing your niacin intake) (2). One of the simplest means of reducing cholesterol is through diet. Decreasing your intake of saturated fats and cholesterol may significantly reduce your blood cholesterol levels (see Nutritional Links to Health and Fitness 12.2).

Table 12.4

Common Foods That Are High in Cholesterol and Saturated Fat

Food	Serving Size	Cholesterol (mg)	Saturated Fat (g)
Bacon	2 slices	30	0.7
Beef (lean)	8 oz	150	12
Butter	1 tablespoon	32	0.4
Cheese			
American	1 oz	27	5.4
Cheddar	1 oz	30	5.9
Egg	1 boiled	113	2.8
Frankfurter	1	30	5.2
Hamburger patty	1 small	68	5.9
Milk (whole)	1 cup	33	5
Milkshake	10 oz	54	8.2
Pizza (meat)	2 slices	31	8
Sausage	3 oz	42	8.6

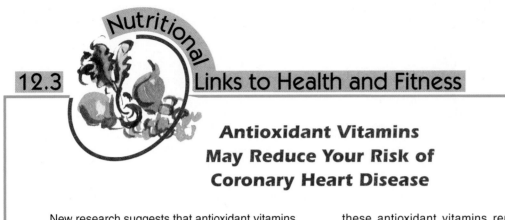

Nutritional 12.3 Links to Health and Fitness

Antioxidant Vitamins May Reduce Your Risk of Coronary Heart Disease

New research suggests that antioxidant vitamins (i.e., vitamins E, C, and beta carotene) may reduce your risk of CHD. Specifically, several comprehensive studies have shown that diets high in antioxidant vitamins reduce the risk of arteriosclerosis. The mechanism to explain this observation is reduction by these antioxidants of the buildup of LDL (bad) cholesterol on arterial walls (11).

While it appears that a diet high in antioxidants may reduce your risk of CHD, the optimal intake of

these antioxidant vitamins remains controversial. Most studies showing protective effects of antioxidants have used vitamin supplements at doses above the recommended daily allowances (RDA). This has raised concern by many nutritionists who argue that high doses of these vitamins may result in toxic side effects. Until additional research is performed, the best advice is to eat plenty of fresh fruits and vegetables to obtain as many antioxidants as possible from your diet (11).

Further, new evidence suggests that a diet high in antioxidant vitamins E and C may also reduce your risk of developing CHD (see Nutritional Links to Health and Fitness 12.3).

The addition of exercise to your daily routine is another simple way to reduce your CHD risk. Even modest levels of exercise (i.e., 20–30 minutes of walking performed three to five times per week) have been shown to reduce the risk of CHD development due to physical inactivity (1, 7–9). In addition, regular aerobic exercise has been shown to modify other CHD risk factors by positively influencing blood pressure, body composition, and blood cholesterol levels.

Modification of Contributory CHD Risk Factors

The two contributory CHD risk factors that can be modified are obesity and stress. Body weight loss can be achieved by a combination of diet modification and exercise (see Chapter 8). For example, a diet low in calories and fat coupled with an increase in physical activity will help reduce

excess body fat. Relaxation techniques (discussed in Chapter 14) can help in counteracting the effects of a stressful lifestyle and therefore reduce the risk for development of CHD.

Lowering Your Risk of Coronary Heart Disease: A Final Word

Regardless of your family history of cardiovascular disease, by positively modifying CHD risk factors, you can reduce your risk of disease. The more changes you make to lower your CHD risk, the better your chances are of preventing cardiovascular disease. Be prepared for occasional backsliding (e.g., eating a high-fat meal); however, when this occurs, quickly regain your focus and return to a healthy lifestyle. Proper CHD risk factor management can add both quality and years to your life. Take action today and lower your CHD risk.

Summary

1. Heart disease is the number one cause of death in the United States. Almost one out of every two deaths in the United States is due to heart disease.

2. Cardiovascular disease refers to any disease that influences the heart and blood vessels. Common cardiovascular diseases include arteriosclerosis, coronary artery disease, stroke, and hypertension.

3. Coronary risk factors are those that increase your risk for the development of coronary heart disease.

4. Coronary risk factors are classified as either major or contributory. Major risk factors are defined as those that directly increase your risk of coronary heart disease. Contributory risk factors may increase your chance of developing coronary heart disease by promoting the development of a major risk factor.

5. Major risk factors for the development of coronary heart disease include smoking, hypertension, high blood cholesterol, physical inactivity, heredity, gender, and increasing age.

6. Contributory risk factors for the development of coronary heart disease include diabetes, obesity, and stress.

7. Your risk of developing coronary heart disease can be reduced by modification of the following risk factors: smoking, hypertension, high blood pressure, physical inactivity, obesity, and stress.

Study Questions

1. Identify the number one cause of death in the United States.

2. Define the following terms:
   cardiovascular disease
   coronary heart disease
   coronary artery disease
   hypertension

3. List the major and contributory risk factors for the development of coronary heart disease.

4. Discuss the difference between *major* and *contributory* risk factors for the development of coronary heart disease.

5. High-density and low-density lipoproteins have been labeled as being "good" and "bad" cholesterol, respectively. Explain.

6. Which major coronary heart disease risk factors can be modified?

7. Which contributory coronary heart disease risk factors can be modified?

8. How does a high-salt diet contribute to hypertension?

9. What is the link between diet and blood cholesterol?

10. How does smoking increase your risk of developing cardiovascular disease?

11. How are arteriosclerosis and atherosclerosis related?

Suggested Reading

American Heart Association. *Heart and stroke facts.* Dallas, 1997.

Donatelle, R., and L. Davis. *Access to health.* Allyn and Bacon, Needham Heights, MA, 1996.

Leeds, M., *Nutrition for healthy living.* WCB-McGraw-Hill, Boston, MA, 1998.

Pollock, M., and D. Schmidt. *Heart disease and rehabilitation.* Human Kinetics. Champaign, IL, 1995.

Suggested Readings on the World Wide Web

Health Net

(http://www.health-net.com/)

Information on exercise training, heart health, nutrition, managing stress, and wellness.

Healthy Way: Heart Disease

(http://www.ns.sympatico.cahealthyway/LISTS/ B2-C06-01_all1.html)

Links to sites about prevention, diagnosis, and determining your risk of heart disease.

American Heart Association

(http://www.nahrt.org/indexto.html)

Facts and statistics about heart and cardiovascular diseases.

References

1. American Heart Association. *Heart and stroke facts,* 1996 Statistical Supplement, Dallas.

2. Barrow, M. *Heart talk: Understanding cardiovascular diseases.* Cor-Ed Publishing, Gainesville, FL, 1992.

3. American Cancer Society. *Fifty most often asked questions about smoking and health and the answers.* The American Cancer Society. New York, 1990.

4. American Cancer Society. *1996 cancer facts and figures.* Atlanta, The American Cancer Society, 1993.

4a. Pollock, M., and D. Schmidt. *Heart disease and rehabilitation.* Human Kinetics. Champaign, IL, 1995.

5. Wood, P. Physical activity, diet, and health: independent and interactive effects. *Medicine and Science in Sports and Exercise* 26:838–843, 1994.

6. Durstine, J., and W. Haskell. Effects of training on plasma lipids and lipoproteins. *Exercise and Sport Science Reviews* 22:477–521, 1994.

7. Blair, S. N., H. W. Kohl, R. S. Paffenbarger, D. G. Clark, K. H. Cooper, and L. W. Gibbons. Physical fitness and all-cause mortality: A prospective study of healthy men and women. *Journal of the American Medical Association* 262:2395–2401, 1989.

8. Bouchard, C., R. Shephard, T. Stephens, J. Sutton, and B. McPherson, eds. *Exercise, fitness, and health: A consensus of current knowledge.* Human Kinetics, Champaign, IL, 1990.

9. Paffenbarger, R. S., R. T. Hyde, A. L. Wing, and C. C. Hsieh. Physical activity, all-cause mortality of college alumni. *New England Journal of Medicine* 314:605–613, 1986.

10. Williams, M. *Lifetime fitness and wellness.* Wm. C. Brown, Dubuque, IA, 1996.

11. Leeds, M. *Nutrition for healthy living.* WCB-McGraw-Hill, Boston, MA, 1998.

Assessment of Your Risk of Heart Disease

NAME _____ DATE _____

The following RISKO questionnaires were developed by the American Heart Association as a tool to evaluate your risk of developing coronary heart disease. Risko scores are based on four of the most important modifiable factors that contribute to the development of heart disease. These factors include weight (obesity), hypertension, blood cholesterol levels, and smoking.

The RISKO score you compute for yourself estimates your risk of developing coronary heart disease over the next several years. Note that the RISKO heart appraisal is not a substitute for a thorough medical examination. Rather, it is designed to increase your awareness of heart disease risk and to assist you in reducing your risk.

RISKO

The purpose of this lab is to give you an estimate of your chances of suffering a heart attack.

Rules

Choose the table appropriate for your sex and study each of the four risk factors. Enter your score for each factor. Total the four scores and enter the figure at the bottom of the table. This total—your score—is an estimate of your risk.

To Calculate Cholesterol

A cholesterol blood level is best. If you can't get one from your doctor, then estimate your total cholesterol as 200 (mg/100ml) and your HDL as 40 (mg/100ml).

To Calculate Blood Pressure

If you have no recent reading but have passed an insurance or industrial examination, chances are you are 140 or less.

What Your Score Means

Note: If you're diabetic, you have a greater risk of heart disease. Add 7 points to your total score.

0–2	You have a low risk of heart disease for a person of your age and sex.
3–4	You have a low-to-moderate risk of heart disease for a person of your age and sex. That's good, but there's room for improvement.
5–7	You have a moderate-to-high risk of heart disease for a person of your age and sex. There's considerable room for improvement in some areas.
8–15	You have a high risk of developing heart disease for a person of your age and sex. There's lots of room for improvement in all areas.
16 & Over	You have a very high risk of developing heart disease for a person of your age and sex. You should act now to reduce all your risk factors.

(Source: Reproduced with permission from *RISKO, A Heart Health Appraisal,* 1994. Copyright American Heart Association.)

RISKO FOR Women

NAME _____ DATE _____

1. Systolic Blood Pressure

SCORE ☐

If you **are not** taking anti-hypertensive medications and your blood pressure is...

125 or less	0 points
between 126 and 136	2 points
between 137 and 148	4 points
between 149 and 160	6 points
between 161 and 171	8 points
between 172 and 183	10 points
between 184 and 194	12 points
between 195 and 206	14 points
between 207 and 218	16 points

If you **are** taking anti-hypertensive medications and your blood pressure is...

117 or less	0 points
between 118 and 123	2 points
between 124 and 129	4 points
between 130 and 136	6 points
between 137 and 144	8 points
between 145 and 154	10 points
between 155 and 168	12 points
between 169 and 206	14 points
between 207 and 218	16 points

2. Blood Cholesterol

SCORE ☐

Locate the number of points for your total and HDL cholesterol in the table below.

HDL

Total	25	30	35	40	50	60	70	80
140	2	1	0	0	0	0	0	0
160	3	2	1	0	0	0	0	0
180	4	3	2	1	0	0	0	0
200	4	3	2	2	0	0	0	0
220	5	4	3	2	1	0	0	0
240	5	4	3	3	1	0	0	0
260	5	4	4	3	2	1	0	0
280	5	5	4	4	2	1	0	0
300	6	5	4	4	3	2	1	0
340	6	5	5	4	3	2	1	0
400	6	6	5	5	4	3	2	2

3. Cigarette Smoking

SCORE ☐

If you...

do not smoke	0 points
smoke less than a pack a day	2 points
smoke a pack a day	5 points
smoke two or more packs a day	9 points

4. Weight

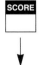

Locate your weight category in the table below. If you are in...

weight category A	0 points
weight category B	1 point
weight category C	2 points
weight category D	9 points

FT	IN	A	B	C	D
4	8	up to 139	140–161	162–184	185+
4	9	up to 140	141–162	163–185	186+
4	10	up to 141	142–163	164–187	188+
4	11	up to 143	144–166	167–190	191+
5	0	up to 145	146–168	169–193	194+
5	1	up to 147	148–171	172–196	197+
5	2	up to 149	150–173	174–198	199+
5	3	up to 152	153–176	177–201	202+
5	4	up to 154	155–178	179–204	205+
5	5	up to 157	158–182	183–209	210+
5	6	up to 160	161–186	187–213	214+
5	7	up to 165	166–191	192–219	220+
5	8	up to 169	170–196	197–225	226+
5	9	up to 173	174–201	202–231	232+
5	10	up to 178	179–206	207–238	239+
5	11	up to 182	183–212	213–242	243+
6	0	up to 187	188–217	218–248	249+
6	1	up to 191	192–222	223–254	255+

TOTAL SCORE ☐

RISKO FOR Men

NAME _____ DATE _____

1. Systolic Blood Pressure

SCORE ☐

If you **are not** taking anti-hypertensive medications and your blood pressure is...

124 or less	0 points
between 125 and 134	2 points
between 135 and 144	4 points
between 145 and 154	6 points
between 155 and 164	8 points
between 165 and 174	10 points
between 175 and 184	12 points
between 185 and 194	14 points
between 195 and 204	16 points
between 205 and 214	18 points
between 215 and 224	20 points

If you **are** taking anti-hypertensive medications and your blood pressure is...

120 or less	0 points
between 121 and 127	2 points
between 128 and 135	4 points
between 136 and 143	6 points
between 144 and 153	8 points
between 154 and 163	10 points
between 164 and 175	12 points
between 176 and 190	14 points
between 191 and 204	16 points
between 205 and 214	18 points
between 215 and 224	20 points

2. Blood Cholesterol

SCORE ☐

Locate the number of points for your total and HDL cholesterol in the table below.

	HDL							
	25	30	35	40	50	60	70	80
140	4	2	0	0	0	0	0	0
160	5	3	2	0	0	0	0	0
180	6	4	3	1	0	0	0	0
200	7	5	4	3	0	0	0	0
220	7	6	5	4	1	0	0	0
240	8	7	5	4	2	0	0	0
260	8	7	6	5	3	1	0	0
280	9	8	7	6	4	2	0	0
300	9	8	7	6	4	3	1	0
340	9	9	8	7	6	4	2	1
400	10	9	9	8	7	5	4	3

(Total column label at left of cholesterol rows)

3. Cigarette Smoking

SCORE ☐

If you...

do not smoke	0 points
smoke less than a pack a day	2 points
smoke a pack a day	5 points
smoke two or more packs a day	9 points

4. Weight

SCORE ☐

Locate your weight category in the table below. If you are in...

weight category A	0 points
weight category B	1 point
weight category C	2 points

FT	IN	A	B	C
5	1	up to 162	163–250	251+
5	2	up to 167	168–257	258+
5	3	up to 172	173–264	265+
5	4	up to 176	177–272	273+
5	5	up to 181	182–279	280+
5	6	up to 185	186–286	287+
5	7	up to 190	191–293	294+
5	8	up to 195	196–300	301+
5	9	up to 199	200–307	308+
5	10	up to 204	205–315	316+
5	11	up to 209	210–322	323+
6	0	up to 213	214–329	330+
6	1	up to 218	219–336	337+
6	2	up to 223	224–343	344+
6	3	up to 227	228–350	351+
6	4	up to 232	233–368	369+
6	5	up to 238	239–365	366+
6	6	up to 241	242–372	373+

TOTAL SCORE ☐

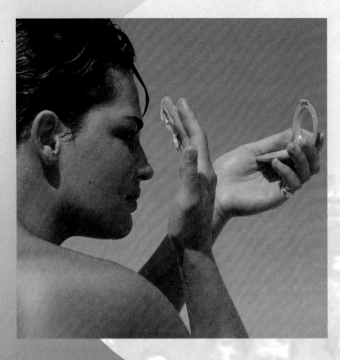

13

Prevention of Cancer

Learning Objectives

After reading this chapter, you should be able to

1 Discuss the incidence of cancer in the United States.

2 Define *cancer*.

3 Identify factors that influence your risk of developing cancer.

4 Discuss several types of occupational carcinogens.

5 List the most common types of cancer.

6 Outline ways to reduce your risk of skin cancer due to exposure to ultraviolet light.

7 Discuss the role of diet and exercise in reducing your cancer risk.

8 Explain how free radicals increase your risk of cancer.

Cancer is the second leading cause of death in the United States, and the number of deaths from cancer is increasing steadily. Current predictions are that cancer will strike approximately three of four families, and it is estimated that during 1999 over 1.4 million new cases of cancer will be diagnosed in the United States (1). Cancer can strike at any age, although it occurs more frequently in older people. Current statistics forecast that about 30% of all U.S. citizens will eventually develop cancer (1). Although the number of cancer cases is on the rise, due to modern medical advances cancer is no longer a death sentence. New detection and treatment regimens have essentially become a cure for many cancers. According to the American Cancer Society, more than eight million Americans alive today have successfully survived cancer. The key to survival is early detection. If more cancers were diagnosed earlier, over one-half of cancer patients could be saved! See A Closer Look 13.1 for identification of the seven warning signals of cancer.

Many experts believe that the rise in cancer may be linked to cancer-causing chemicals in water and food supplies as well as to dangerous lifestyle habits such as smoking, eating high-fat diets, drinking excessively, and sunbathing (1–3). This chapter provides information about the various types of cancers and how to reduce your risk of developing cancer. Let's begin with an overview of cancer.

What Is Cancer?

Cancer is not a single disease, but a class of over 100 different diseases that can influence almost every body tissue (4). Cancer is caused by the uncontrolled growth and spread of abnormal cells. A group of cancer cells, called a **tumor,** can be either benign or malignant. Generally, a benign tumor is not a serious health threat; it does not grow rapidly or spread to other parts of the body. In contrast, when a malignant tumor invades an organ of the body, cancerous cells attach to the organ and begin to divide rapidly. As the malignant tumor grows in size, the cancer cells interfere with normal organ function, which may eventually result in organ failure and possibly death.

An important difference that separates malignant tumors from benign tumors is that malignant tumors can spread throughout the body. This process, known as *metastasis,* makes malignant cancers extremely dangerous. For example, a ma-

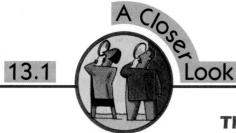

A Closer Look

13.1

The Seven Warning Signs of Cancer

Everyone should know the seven warning signals of cancer, which can be remembered as the word *caution.* If you develop any of the following signs, see a physician immediately for a cancer screening test.

Change in the size or color of a wart or mole

A sore that does not heal or heals slowly

Unusual or unexplained bleeding from the bowel, nipples, or vagina, or the presence of blood in the urine

Thickening or lump in the breast or on the lip or tongue

Indigestion that persists or loss of appetite

Obvious change in bowel or bladder habits

Nagging or persistent cough or hoarseness and difficulty in swallowing

lignant cancer that begins in the breast might spread to the pancreas and other organs involved in digestion and absorption of food (Figure 13.1). This type of rapidly spreading cancer reduces the chances of survival because of the difficulty in treating multiple cancer sites.

When an abnormal growth is discovered in the body, the only way to determine if the growth is a benign or malignant tumor is through biopsy. A biopsy is the surgical removal of a small sample of the tumor for subsequent laboratory analysis.

Types of Cancer

Cancer can develop in almost any tissue (4). Skin cancer is the most common of all cancers (1). Other common sites for cancer include the mouth, lung, stomach, colon, kidney, liver, bone, prostate

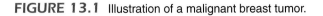

FIGURE 13.1 Illustration of a malignant breast tumor.

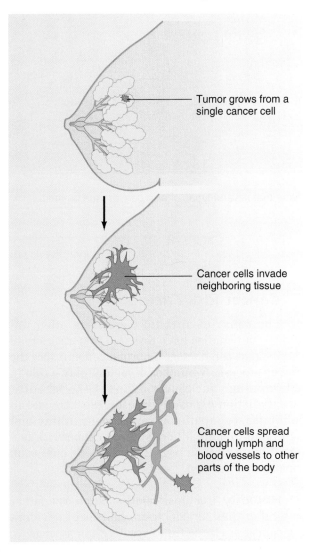

Tumor grows from a single cancer cell

Cancer cells invade neighboring tissue

Cancer cells spread through lymph and blood vessels to other parts of the body

gland, and breast (Figure 13.2 on page 288). Excluding skin cancer, the most common types of cancer are prostate cancer in men and breast cancer in women (1). Over 95% of all breast cancers are discovered by women themselves; a routine breast self-examination should be a monthly practice by all women (see A Closer Look 13.2 and Figure 13.3 on page 289).

Although most cancers occur in people over the age of 40, testicular cancer is one of the most common cancers in young men (1), with those between the ages of 15 and 34 at greatest risk. In general, testicular tumors are first noticed as a painless enlargement of the testis. Early detection of testicular cancer is the key to survival, so it is important that all young men perform a routine self-examination (see A Closer Look 13.3 on page 290). If a suspicious lump is found, medical advice should be sought at once.

Recently, the largest increase in cancer has been in a deadly form of skin cancer known as malignant melanoma (1). The increase in this type of cancer is likely due to the diminishing layer of ozone around the earth which protects us from the sun's ultraviolet rays. These rays are the primary cause of skin cancers.

In addition, there has been a tremendous increase in lung cancer in both men (90%) and women (500%) since 1960 (1). The reason for the increased incidence of lung cancer in men is unknown but may be linked to poor air quality (i.e., airborne carcinogens) in many cities. The rise in lung cancer in women is likely due to the rise in the number of female smokers over this time period. The increase is significant because lung cancer is very dangerous, resulting in more deaths among both men and women than any other form of cancer.

How Do Normal Cells Become Cancerous?

Cell growth and division is controlled by DNA located within the cell. Normal DNA carefully regulates cell growth and division in a slow and steady fashion. Cancer occurs when DNA is damaged and cell division increases out of control.

cancer A class of over 100 different diseases that can influence almost every body tissue. Cancer is caused by the uncontrolled growth and spread of abnormal cells.

tumor A group of cancer cells.

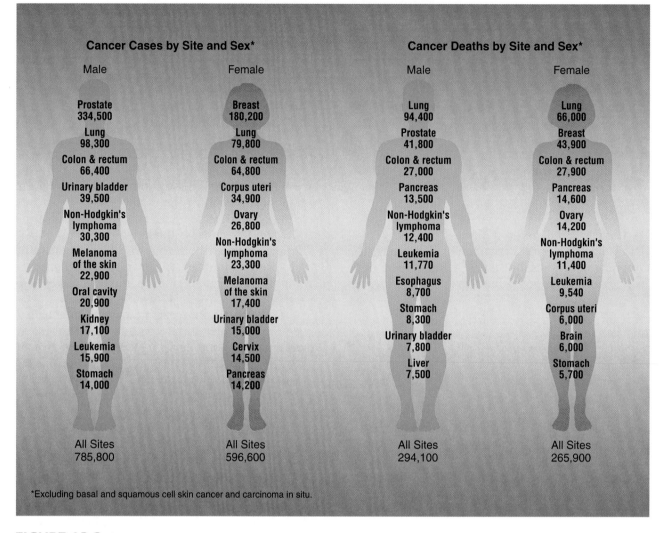

FIGURE 13.2 Cancer incidence and death rate by site and sex. Note that several types of skin cancers are omitted. (Data from the American Cancer Society, 1997.)

DNA damage, resulting in cancer, can occur in response to a number of environmental agents. These cancer-causing agents, called **carcinogens,** include radiation, chemicals, drugs, and other toxic substances (4). When a carcinogen enters the cell, it damages the DNA, which results in a normal cell becoming an abnormal cancer cell (Figure 13.5 on page 291).

carcinogens Cancer-causing agents which include radiation, chemicals, drugs, and other toxic substances.

Cancer Risk Factors

The cause of specific cancers is often unknown, but studies have revealed that a variety of carcinogens can damage a normal cell and start the cancer process. A number of factors play a role in determining your cancer risk (1, 5–7); heredity, race, radiation exposure, viruses, tobacco use, alcohol use, occupational carcinogens, ultraviolet light, and diet are all considered cancer risk factors (Figure 13.6 on page 292). Let's discuss each separately.

Heredity If a close relative (such as a father or mother) has cancer, your chances of developing cancer are three times greater than average (5,

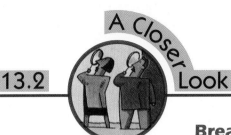

A Closer Look

13.2

Breast Self-Examination

Do you know that 95% of all breast cancers are discovered first by women themselves? And that the earlier breast cancer is detected, the better the chance of complete cure?

Of course, most lumps or changes are not cancer. But you can help safeguard your health by making a habit of examining your breasts once a month—a day or two after your period or, if you're no longer menstruating, on any given day. And if you notice anything changed or unusual—a lump, thickening, or discharge—contact your doctor right away. See Figure 13.3.

FIGURE 13.3 Breast self-examination. Regular performance of breast exams could save your life. (Source: From Rathus, S. A., J. S. Nevid, and L. Fichner-Rathus. *Human sexuality in a world of diversity.* Copyright © 1993 by Allyn & Bacon. Reprinted by permission.)

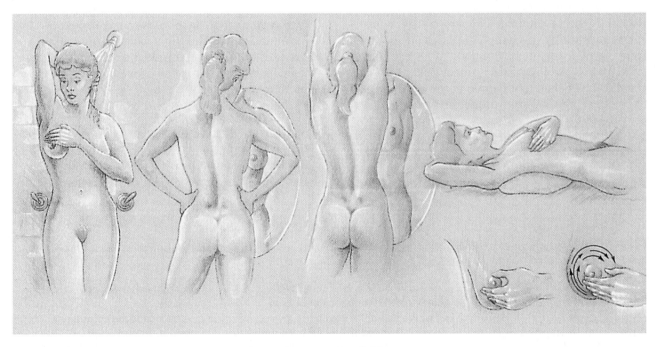

A ridge of firm tissue in the lower curve of each breast is normal. Then move in an inch, toward the nipple. Keep circling to examine every part of your breast, including the nipple. This requires at least three more circles. Now slowly repeat the procedure on your left breast. Place the pillow beneath your left shoulder, your left arm behind your head, and use the finger pads on your right hand.

After you examine your left breast fully, squeeze the nipple of each breast gently between your thumb and index finger. Any discharge, clear or bloody, should be reported to your doctor immediately.

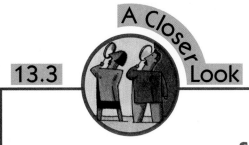

13.3 A Closer Look

Testicular Self-Examination

Cancer of the testes is one of the most common forms of cancer in men 15 to 34 years of age (1) (accounts for 12% of all deaths in this group). The key to surviving testicular cancer is early detection, so all young men should perform a monthly self-examination. This is best performed after a warm shower or bath when the scrotum (sack surrounding the testicles) is the most relaxed. The examination is performed by rolling each testicle between the thumb and fingers (see Figure 13.4). If you feel any lumps or nodules, you should see your doctor immediately. The lump you feel may not be cancer, but a medical exam is required to make a diagnosis.

6). Although the exact link between heredity and cancer remains unclear, cancers of the breast, stomach, colon, prostate, uterus, ovaries, and lungs appear to run in families. Whether these family patterns of increased cancer risk are due to genetics or the fact that people in the same family experience similar environmental risks remains uncertain.

Race Both the incidence of cancer and the cancer death rate are higher among Blacks than among Whites (5, 6). Over the last 40 years, cancer death among Blacks rose at approximately 50% versus a 10% increase for Whites (1). The explanation for the high death rate in Blacks is unclear, but it may be linked to the fact that cancers in Whites are often detected at an earlier, more treatable stage.

Radiation Up to 5% of all cancers may be caused by radiation exposure due to medical X-rays, occupational exposure through computer monitors, and environmental radiation (7). Further, many modern conveniences that emit elec-

FIGURE 13.4 Testicular self-examination. (Source: From Rathus, S. A., J. S. Nevid, and L. Fichner-Rathus. *Human sexuality in a world of diversity.* Copyright © 1993 by Allyn & Bacon. Reprinted by permission.)

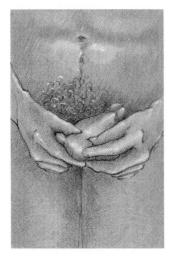

Self-examination is best performed shortly after a warm shower or bath, when the skin of the scrotum is most relaxed. The man should examine the scrotum for evidence of pea-sized lumps. Each testicle can be rolled gently between the thumb and the fingers. Lumps are generally found on the side or front of the testicle. The presence of a lump is not necessarily a sign of cancer, but it should be promptly reported to a physician for further evaluation. The American Cancer Society (1990) lists these warning signals:

1. A slight enlargement of one of the testicles.
2. A change in the consistency of a testicle.
3. A dull ache in the lower abdomen or groin. (Pain may be absent in cancer of the testes, however.)
4. Sensation of dragging and heaviness in a testicle.

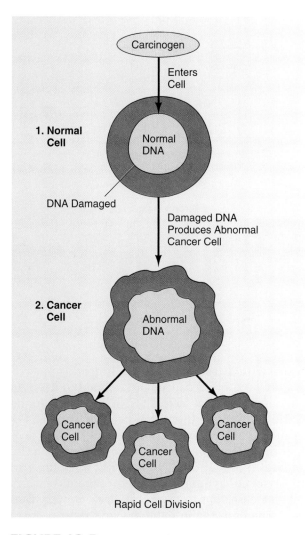

FIGURE 13.5 A normal cell can be transformed into a cancer cell by a carcinogen entering the cell and damaging the DNA.

tromagnetic fields, such as electric blankets, and low-frequency radio waves, such as those associated with cellular telephones, have been implicated in causing cancer.

Viruses It is clear that viruses are linked to many cancers (1, 7). Viruses can cause cancer by invading the cell and damaging DNA. Research has demonstrated that viruses play a role in several blood cancers (leukemias) as well as cancers of the lymphatic system (lymphomas). In addition, evidence suggests that viruses can cause liver, cervical, nose, and pharynx cancer.

Tobacco Tobacco use is the single largest cause of cancer deaths (approximately 25%) (5, 6, 8). Heavy smokers are 15 to 25 times more likely to die of cancer than nonsmokers (1, 7, 8). Although the major cancer risk of smoking is the increased chance of developing lung cancer, smoking also causes an increased risk of oral cancers (of the mouth, pharynx, larynx, and esophagus), as well as of pancreas and bladder cancer (7, 8). The average life expectancy for a chronic smoker is 7 years shorter than for a nonsmoker.

Even if you don't smoke, new evidence shows that second-hand tobacco smoke is also carcinogenic. Thus, you should avoid both active smoking and inhaling smoke from others. Cigarettes are not the only risk from tobacco; pipes, cigars, and smokeless tobacco also increase the risk of oral cancers.

Alcohol Heavy use of alcohol increases the risk for oral, esophagus, liver, and breast cancer (9). Combining drinking and smoking creates an even greater risk of cancer development. Even moderate drinking has been linked to an increased risk of breast cancer in women.

Occupational Carcinogens Factory workers and people living near factories may have an increased risk of cancer due to specific types of chemicals used or produced by the factory. Industrial chemicals known to be carcinogenic include benzene, nickel, chromate, asbestos, and vinyl chloride (7).

One of the most common occupational carcinogens is asbestos, a substance formerly used in the building and automobile industries. People who work with radioactive substances may also have increased risk for cancer. Working with coal tars, as in the mining professions, or working near air borne carcinogens such as in the auto painting business, is also dangerous. Many chemicals used to kill weeds (herbicides) and insects (pesticides) contain potential carcinogens and are found in excessive amounts in some water supplies.

Ultraviolet Light Exposure to the sun or to artificial tanning lights is a major contributor to an increased risk of skin cancer (1, 7). Ultraviolet radiation from these two sources is responsible for over 700,000 new cases of skin cancer each year. Tanning machines and sunlamps produce ultraviolet rays and present as much risk as do the sun's rays. Some tanning salons claim that their equipment emits ultraviolet light at different wavelengths than sunshine and is therefore less dangerous. This is not true! If a sunlamp causes you to tan or burn, it is just as dangerous as the sun.

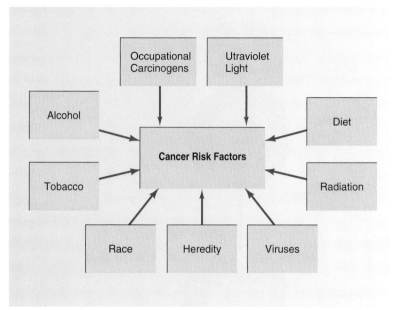

FIGURE 13.6 Cancer risk factors.

Diet According to the National Academy of Sciences, diet is implicated in 60% of the cancers in women and 40% of the cancers in men (10). A high-fat diet has been linked to breast, colon, and prostate cancer, and it contributes to obesity. Obesity increases the risk of colon, breast, and uterine cancer. In addition, salt-cured, smoked, and nitrite-cured foods have been linked to cancers of the esophagus and stomach.

Cancer Prevention

Recall from our earlier discussion of heart disease that we can control selected risk factors for CHD. Many cancers can be prevented in the same way—with lifestyle changes. Indeed, approximately 80% of all cancers are related to lifestyle and environmental factors (1, 7). According to the National Cancer Institute, people who lead a healthy lifestyle have only about one-third to one-half the rate of cancer deaths compared with the general population. Thus, with a change in lifestyle and avoidance of environmental factors that increase your risk, you can prevent many cancers. The first step in reducing your risk of cancer is to identify which cancer risk factors apply to you (see Laboratory 13.1) and then modify those aspects of your lifestyle that increase your chances of developing cancer. The following is a list of those cancer risk factors that can be modified.

Overexposure to sunlight increases your risk of skin cancer.

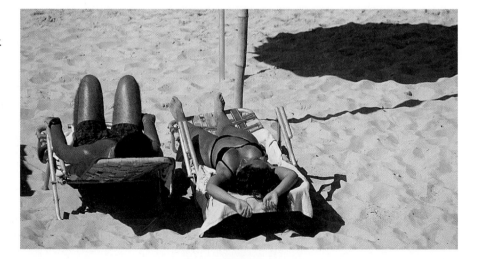

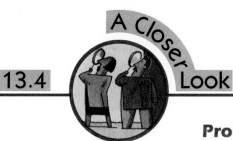

13.4

A Closer Look

Protect Your Skin from Ultraviolet Rays

A sunscreen lotion should be applied approximately 30 minutes prior to exposure, because the protective ingredients require several minutes to be absorbed. The sunscreen should have a sun protection factor (**SPF**) of at least 15. A sunscreen with an SPF of 15 provides you with 15 times greater protection than unprotected skin. The following guidelines can reduce your risk of developing skin cancer due to overexposure to ultraviolet rays.

1. Stay out of the sun between 10:00 A.M. and 2:00 P.M. This is when ultraviolet rays are the strongest.

2. If you use any skin preparation containing vitamin A (Retin A), stay out of the sun. Retin A skin lotions will increase your susceptibility to ultraviolet damage.

3. Avoid sunlamps and tanning booths. If sunlamps tan you, they damage your skin.

4. When exercising outdoors or during swimming, use a waterproof sunscreen and apply often and in adequate quantities.

5. Avoid sunburn by limiting your sun exposure.

Alcohol Oral cancer and cancers of the larynx, throat, esophagus, and liver occur more frequently among heavy drinkers of alcohol (7). Because even moderate alcohol consumption has been suggested as a cause of some cancers, it is wise to abstain from alcohol consumption or to at least decrease your consumption to a low level. Remember, combining alcohol and tobacco puts you at even greater risk.

Radiation Avoid overexposure to any source of radiation. Medical X-rays, low-frequency radio waves, and other sources of low-level radiation may not be avoidable and are not harmful unless encountered in excess.

Tobacco Both cigarette smoking and use of smokeless tobacco increase your risk of cancer. Cigarette smoking is responsible for 87% of all lung cancer cases, and use of chewing tobacco or snuff increases your risk of cancer of the mouth, larynx, throat, and esophagus (17, 8). Cancer risks can be greatly reduced by abstaining from all tobacco products. If you have never used any tobacco products, don't start. If you are using tobacco products, stop. Many of the ill-health effects of tobacco can be reversed if you quit using them.

Occupational Carcinogens Avoid all industrial pollutants and follow safety procedures in the work place. In particular, avoid exposure to industrial agents such as radon, dioxins, nickel, chromate, asbestos, and vinyl chloride. If you have questions concerning the carcinogenic risks of chemical exposure in your work place, contact the Environmental Protection Agency (EPA). The EPA can provide you with a complete list of cancer-causing chemicals and identify those used in your work place.

Ultraviolet Light Prolonged exposure to ultraviolet light from any source increases your risk of developing skin cancer (7). Limiting your sun exposure is an obvious way to avoid the carcinogenic effect of ultraviolet light. If you must be exposed to the sun for work or recreation, use a sunscreen to block the effects of the ultraviolet rays (see A Closer Look 13.4).

SPF Abbreviation for "sun protection factor." A sunscreen with an SPF of 15 provides you with 15 times more protection than unprotected skin.

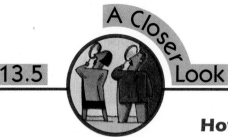

13.5

How Do Free Radicals Promote Cancer?

As we have seen, cell division is carefully controlled in healthy cells by molecules of DNA; cancer occurs when DNA is damaged and cells begin dividing out of control. Research suggests that free radical formation can promote cancer by damaging DNA. This occurs when free radicals are formed in large quantities and bind directly to the DNA. Radical binding to DNA alters normal DNA structure and function by promoting a rapid and uncontrolled rate of cell division resulting in cancer (see Figure 13.7).

FIGURE 13.7 Free radicals can promote cancer by damaging cellular DNA.

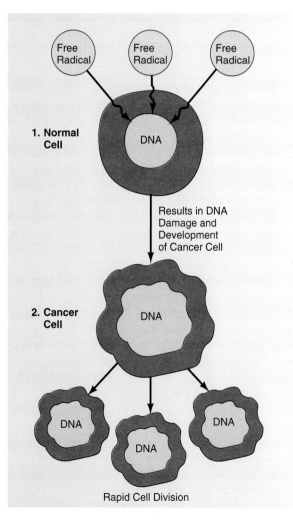

Remember, there is no such thing as a safe tan (11). A tan is damaging to your skin, whether you tan quickly or accumulate it slowly over time. Exposure to ultraviolet light is cumulative, and the exposure you get at age 20 may adversely affect you at age 40.

Although skin cancer is the most common cancer, many types of skin cancer are curable if treated early. Self-examination is the key to early detection. Self-examination should be performed once a month and should include the entire body, particularly those areas exposed to sun. When examining your skin, be alert for the following signs; if you have any of them, see a physician at once (11).

1. A sore that doesn't heal. Have it checked if it hasn't healed after 3 weeks and it bleeds or oozes.
2. A persistent reddish patch of skin. It may be painful or itch, or it may not bother you at all.
3. A shiny, waxy, scar-like spot. It may be yellow or white with irregular borders.
4. A mole that begins to enlarge, thicken, or change color.
5. A mole that bleeds or ulcerates.
6. A mole that has irregular rather than round borders.
7. A mole with irregular pigmentation; some areas may be light colored, whereas other areas may be black.

Foods High in Antioxidants May Reduce Your Risk of Cancer

Beta carotene (which the body converts to vitamin A), and vitamins C and E are antioxidant compounds that appear to reduce your risk of cancer and perhaps other diseases because they neutralize free radicals (10, 11, 20). Therefore, increasing your dietary intake of these vitamins is an important dietary goal. Food sources of beta carotene include apricots, asparagus, broccoli, carrots, peas, spinach, and tomatoes. Vitamin C is contained in a variety of foods, including asparagus, broccoli, cauliflower, grapefruit, oranges, peppers, red cabbage, tangerines, and tomatoes. Finally, vitamin E is contained in

vegetable oils, nuts, and seeds, and is present in low levels in a variety of other foods.

In addition to a healthy diet, should you use vitamin supplements to increase your intake of beta carotene and vitamins C and E? Nutritionists remain divided on this issue. Some researchers have suggested that it is safe to supplement your diet with up to 400 units of vitamin E and up to 500 mg of vitamin C (see ref. 12 for a review). Nonetheless, it is wise to consult your physician or a dietitian before deciding to use vitamin supplements.

Diet Diet is probably the most important factor in controlling your risk of cancer (10). Among the primary nutrients in foods that seem to have a protective effect are vitamins A, E, and C (11a). How do these particular nutrients reduce the risk for cancer? It seems that they protect against cell damage caused by free radicals. Recall that free radicals (sometimes called *oxygen radicals*) are molecules normally produced in cells. However, when produced in high quantities, free radicals can damage cells and promote the development of cancer (see A Closer Look 13.5). Recent research has shown that vitamins A, C, and E are all antioxidants (substances that are capable of absorbing free radicals and preventing cell damage) and may lower your risk of cancer by removing free radicals from the cells; these new findings have prompted many cancer experts to recommend a diet that is high in antioxidants (see Nutritional Links to Health and Fitness 13.1).

Consumption of a high-fiber, low-fat diet lowers your risk of colon and rectal cancers. The apparent advantage of a high-fiber diet is that fiber in food increases the frequency of bowel movements, decreasing the time that the colon and rectum are exposed to dietary carcinogens, thereby reducing the cancer risk. See Nutritional Links to

Health and Fitness 13.2 on page 296 for a complete dietary guideline for lowering the risk of cancer.

Exercise Reduces the Risk of Cancer
Studies have provided evidence that regular exercise may provide some protection against cancer (2, 13–16). The best evidence comes from studies demonstrating that people who engage in regular exercise have a lower incidence of colon cancer (16) (Figure 13.8 on page 296). In addition, some reports suggest that exercise training reduces the occurrence of breast and uterine cancer in women (15).

The primary debate about how exercise protects against cancer centers around the question, "Does exercise alter the immune system to reduce the formation of cancerous cells?" Tumors are normally formed in everyone from time to time, but the immune system functions to destroy the cancer cells before they increase in number. Therefore, a strong immune system acts to reduce the risk of cancer, whereas a weak immune system may increase your risk of cancer. Although numerous studies suggest that physically active individuals have an increased resistance to infection (17) and a decreased incidence of certain

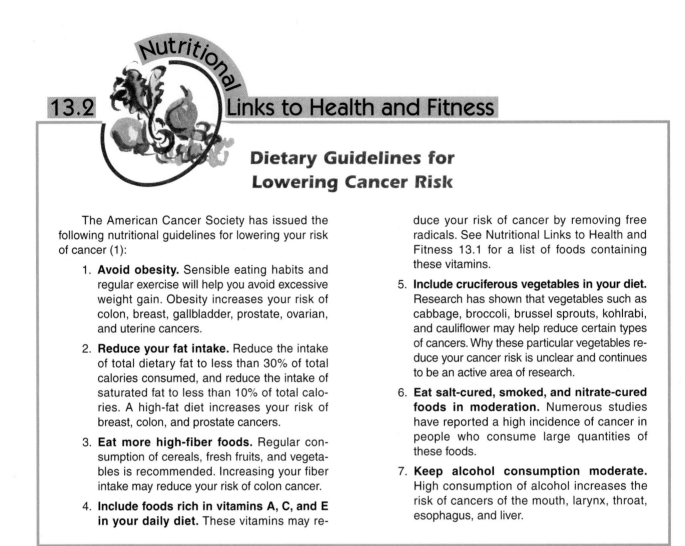

13.2 Nutritional Links to Health and Fitness

Dietary Guidelines for Lowering Cancer Risk

The American Cancer Society has issued the following nutritional guidelines for lowering your risk of cancer (1):

1. **Avoid obesity.** Sensible eating habits and regular exercise will help you avoid excessive weight gain. Obesity increases your risk of colon, breast, gallbladder, prostate, ovarian, and uterine cancers.

2. **Reduce your fat intake.** Reduce the intake of total dietary fat to less than 30% of total calories consumed, and reduce the intake of saturated fat to less than 10% of total calories. A high-fat diet increases your risk of breast, colon, and prostate cancers.

3. **Eat more high-fiber foods.** Regular consumption of cereals, fresh fruits, and vegetables is recommended. Increasing your fiber intake may reduce your risk of colon cancer.

4. **Include foods rich in vitamins A, C, and E in your daily diet.** These vitamins may re-

duce your risk of cancer by removing free radicals. See Nutritional Links to Health and Fitness 13.1 for a list of foods containing these vitamins.

5. **Include cruciferous vegetables in your diet.** Research has shown that vegetables such as cabbage, broccoli, brussel sprouts, kohlrabi, and cauliflower may help reduce certain types of cancers. Why these particular vegetables reduce your cancer risk is unclear and continues to be an active area of research.

6. **Eat salt-cured, smoked, and nitrate-cured foods in moderation.** Numerous studies have reported a high incidence of cancer in people who consume large quantities of these foods.

7. **Keep alcohol consumption moderate.** High consumption of alcohol increases the risk of cancers of the mouth, larynx, throat, esophagus, and liver.

FIGURE 13.8 Recent evidence shows that exercise can reduce your risk of cancer. Cancer death rate is expressed as number of deaths per 10,000 persons per year.

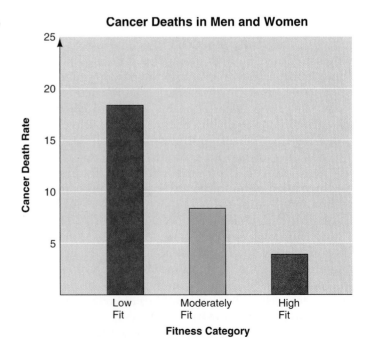

forms of cancer (2, 13–15), the scientific evidence that indicates that exercise positively alters the immune system is limited (18, 19). Therefore, it may be that factors other than adaptation of the immune system are responsible for the observation that exercise is associated with a reduced risk of cancer.

Summary

1. The diseases known as cancers are major killers, and the incidence of these diseases is increasing. Currently, cancer is the number two cause of death in the United States.

2. Cancer results from an abnormal growth of cells. This abnormal growth and division of cells forms a mass of mutated cells called a *tumor*. Tumors are classified as either benign (abnormal growth but not life threatening) or malignant (cancerous cells that are life threatening because they will eventually spread to other tissues and disrupt organ function).

3. Carcinogens are defined as cancer-causing agents.

4. Skin cancer is the most common type of cancer. Other common sites of cancer include the mouth, lung, colon, stomach, colon, liver, bone, prostate gland, and breast.

5. Normal cells become cancerous when DNA becomes damaged, which results in uncontrolled cell division.

6. Heredity, race, radiation, viruses, tobacco, alcohol, occupational carcinogens, ultraviolet light, and a high-fat diet are factors that increase your risk of developing cancer. Cancer risk can be lowered by reducing your exposure to radiation, tobacco, alcohol, ultraviolet light, and occupational carcinogens.

7. Approximately 80% of all cancers are related to lifestyle and environmental factors.

8. Diet is probably the most important factor in controlling your risk of cancer. Among the primary nutrients in foods that offer a protection from cancer are vitamins A, E, and C. These nutrients reduce the risk of cancer by removing free radicals.

9. Exercise has been shown to reduce the risk of certain types of cancers.

Study Questions

1. Define the following terms:
   cancer
   carcinogens
   tumor
2. What is the most common type of cancer?
3. How do normal cells become cancerous?
4. List nine cancer risk factors.
5. What is the sun protection factor?
6. Exercise has been shown to reduce the risk of which types of cancer?
7. What is an antioxidant? How do antioxidants reduce the risk of cancer?
8. What types of cancer are linked to tobacco use?
9. Name five occupational carcinogens.
10. Discuss the signs of skin cancer.
11. Outline the dietary guidelines for reducing your risk of cancer.

Suggested Reading

American Cancer Society. *1997 cancer facts and figures.* Atlanta, The American Cancer Society, 1997.

Bouchard, C., R. J. Shephard, T. Stephens, J. R. Sutton, and B. D. McPherson. *Exercise, fitness and health: A consensus of current knowledge.* Human Kinetics, Champaign, IL, 1990.

Donatelle, R., and L. Davis. *Brief second edition: Access to health.* Allyn and Bacon, Needham Heights, MA, 1996.

Leeds, M. *Nutrition for healthy living.* WCB-McGraw-Hill, Boston, MA, 1998.

Suggested Readings on the World Wide Web

American Institute for Cancer Research
(http://www.aicr.org/)
Links and articles about prevention, diagnosis, and coping with cancer.

American Cancer Society
(http://www.cancer.org/)
Facts and statistics about cancer.

Centers for Disease Control and Prevention
(http://www.cdc.gov/)
Facts and statistics on the incidence and control of disease in the United States.

References

1. American Cancer Society. *1997 cancer facts and figures.* Atlanta, The American Cancer Society, 1997.

2. Gerhardsson, M., S. E. Norell, H. Kiviranta, N. L. Pedersen, and A. Ahlbom. Sedentary jobs and colon cancer. *American Journal of Epidemiology* 123:775–780, 1986.

3. *The cancer process.* The American Institute for Cancer Research, November, 1991.

4. Robbins, S., and V. Kumar. *Basic pathology.* W. B. Saunders, Philadelphia, 1997.

5. American Cancer Society, Texas Division. *Cancer: Assessing your risk.* Dallas, 1982.

6. Greenwald, P. Assessment of risk factors for cancer. *Preventive Medicine* 9:260–263, 1980.

7. National Cancer Institute. Cancer rates and risks. U.S. Dept. of Health and Human services. NIH Publication No. 85-691, Bethesda, MD, 1985.

8. Fielding, J. Smoking: Health effects and controls. *New England Journal of Medicine* 313:491–497, 1985.

9. Rothman, K. The proportion of cancer attributable to alcohol consumption. *Preventive Medicine* 9:174–179, 1980.

10. Surgeon General's report on nutrition and health. Diane Publishing Co., 1994.

11. Donatelle, R., and L. Davis. *Access to health: Brief second edition.* Prentice-Hall, Englewood Cliffs, NJ, 1996.

11a. Kanter, M. Free radicals and exercise: Effects of nutritional antioxidant supplementation. *Exercise and Sport Science Reviews* 23:375–397, 1995.

12. Clarkson, P. Vitamins and trace minerials. Lamb, D., and M. Williams, eds. *Ergogenics.* Brown and Benchmark, Madison, WI, 1991, pp. 123–175.

13. Vena, J. E., S. Graham, M. Zielezny, J. Brasure, and M. K. Swanson. Occupational exercise and risk of cancer. *American Journal of Clinical Nutrition* 45:318–327, 1987.

14. Paffenbarger, R. S., R. T. Hyde, A. L. Wing, and C. C. Hsieh. Physical activity, all-cause mortality of college alumni. *New England Journal of Medicine* 314:605–613, 1986.

15. Frisch, R. E., G. Wyshak, N. L. Albright, et al. Lower prevalence of breast cancer and cancers of the reproductive system among former college athletes compared to non-athletes. *British Journal of Cancer* 52:885–891, 1985.

16. Blair, S., H. Kohl, R. Paffenbarger, D. Clark, K. Cooper, and L. Gibbons. Physical fitness and all-cause mortality: A prospective study of healthy men and women. *Journal of American Medical Association* 262:2395–2401, 1989.

17. Nash, M. Exercise and immunology. *Medicine and Science in Sports and Exercise* 26:125–127, 1994.

18. Woods, J., and M. Davis. Exercise, monocyte/macrophage function, and cancer. *Medicine and Science in Sports and Exercise* 26:147–157, 1994.

19. Shepard, R., S. Rhind, and P. Shek. The impact of exercise on the immune system: NK cells, interleukins 1 and 2, and related responses. *Exercise and Sport Sciences Reviews* 23:215–241, 1995.

20. Leeds, M. *Nutrition for healthy living.* WCB-McGraw-Hill, Boston, MA, 1998.

Determining Your Cancer Risk

NAME _____ DATE _____

The purpose of this laboratory is to increase your awareness of your risk of developing all forms of cancer. Complete the following questions by answering "yes" or "no."

Scoring

Answering "yes" to any of the questions means that you should modify your lifestyle to reduce your cancer risk. See text for details.

	yes	no
1. Do you consume a high-fat diet (e.g., >30% total calorie intake)?	_____	_____
2. Is your diet low in fiber?	_____	_____
3. Do you consume an excessive amount of alcohol?	_____	_____
4. Do you regularly eat smoked foods?	_____	_____
5. Are you exposed to environmental carcinogens?	_____	_____
6. Do you use tobacco products or breathe second-hand smoke?	_____	_____
7. Are you obese?	_____	_____
8. Do you have a family history of cancer?	_____	_____
9. Is your skin regularly exposed to excessive sunlight?	_____	_____
10. Do you have a fair complexion?	_____	_____

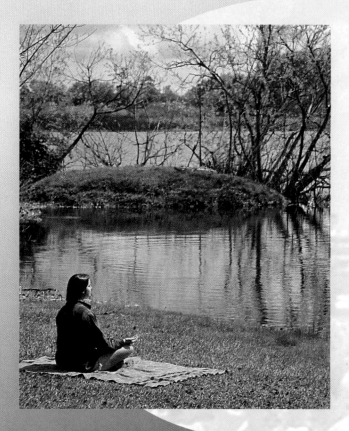

14

Stress Management and Modifying Unhealthy Behavior

Learning
Objectives

After reading this chapter, you should be able to

1 Discuss the terms *stress* and *stressors.*

2 Outline the steps involved in stress management.

3 List several common relaxation techniques used to manage stress.

4 Outline the general model for behavior modification.

5 Provide an example of how behavior modification can be used to modify unhealthy behavior.

6 Identify the most common types of accidents.

7 Outline steps to reduce your risk of accidents.

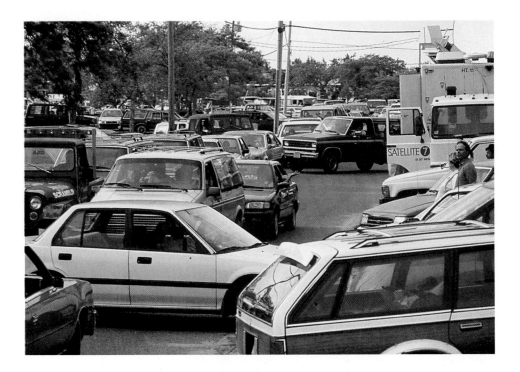

Automobile accidents are one of many forms of stress.

Although many behaviors affect your health, the five that are most important for promotion of good health (1–4) are: regular exercise, good nutrition, weight control, stress management, and modification of unhealthy behaviors that increase your risk of disease or increase your risk of an accident. Earlier chapters have focused on improving health through physical fitness, proper diet/weight control, and actively reducing the risk of cancer and heart disease. This chapter expands on these strategies by introducing the concepts of stress reduction and behavior modification aimed at reducing your risk of disease and accidents. Let's begin our discussion with an overview of stress management.

Stress Management

Studies suggest that 10% to 15% of U.S. adults may be functioning at less than optimal levels because of stress-related anxiety and depression (4). Indeed, millions of people take medication for stress-related illnesses. Stress-related problems result in annual losses of billions of dollars to both businesses and government due to employee absenteeism and health care costs. Therefore, stress

is a major health problem in the United States that affects individual lives and the economy as a whole. In the following sections, we will discuss several key aspects of stress management.

Stress: An Overview

Stress is a physiological and mental response to something in our environment that causes us to become uncomfortable. The factor that produces stress is called a **stressor.** Stressors can be

FIGURE 14.1 The health effects of chronic stress.

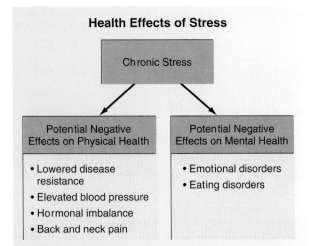

Health Effects of Stress

Chronic Stress

Potential Negative Effects on Physical Health

- Lowered disease resistance
- Elevated blood pressure
- Hormonal imbalance
- Back and neck pain

Potential Negative Effects on Mental Health

- Emotional disorders
- Eating disorders

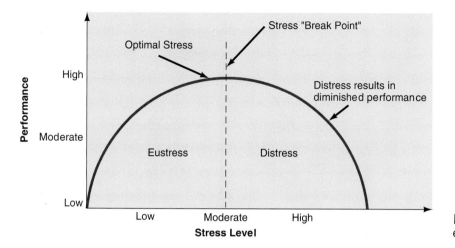

FIGURE 14.2 The concepts of eustress and distress.

physical in nature (such as an injury) or mental (such as emotional distress resulting from a personal relationship). Regardless of the nature of the stressor, the physiological and mental responses to stress usually include the feelings of strain, tension, and anxiety.

From a medical standpoint, stress can impact both emotional and physical health. Chronic (persistent) stress has been linked to elevated blood pressure, hormonal imbalances, reduced resistance to disease, eating disorders, and emotional disorders (1–4) (see Figure 14.1).

There are many sources of stress in everyday life. Driving in heavy traffic, being involved in an automobile accident, encountering emotional conflicts at work or school, and experiencing personal financial problems are just a few. Let's continue our discussion of stress by examining your stress profile.

Assessment of Stress

Stress can be acute (e.g. the death of a loved one), cumulative (such as a series of events leading to a divorce), or chronic (such as daily job-related stress). Although it is clear that chronic or extreme stress is unhealthy, some degree of stress is required to maximize performance. For instance, athletes and business professionals often perform better when faced with mild-to-moderate stress. A stress level that results in improved performance is called **eustress** or positive stress. Although some level of stress is desirable, each of us has a breaking point in terms of stress. This idea is illustrated in Figure 14.2. When we surpass the stress level needed to optimize performance (optimal stress), we reach our stress break point and

distress (negative stress) results. Distress promotes a decline in performance, and chronic distress can increase the risk of disease.

Different people may react differently to the same stressful situation. For example, a violent movie may evoke anger in one person and no emotion at all in another. This difference in "stress perception" is due to personality differences. When it comes to stress, individuals can be classified into one of three personality categories: type A, type B, and type C (Figure 14.3 on page 304). Type A individuals are highly motivated, time-conscious, hard driving, sometimes hostile, and impatient. They have a heightened response to stress. Because stress is a risk factor for heart disease, type A people exhibit this risk (4). In contrast, type B individuals are easygoing, nonaggressive, and patient. Type B personalities do not generally respond greatly to stress and are considered to be at low risk (from a stress perspective) for heart disease. People with type C personalities have many of the qualities of type A people. They are confident, highly motivated, and competitive. However, these unique individuals use their personality traits to their advantage by maintaining a constant level of emotional control and channeling their ambition into creative directions. Interestingly, although type C person-

stress A physiological and mental response to something in the environment that causes people to become uncomfortable.

stressor A factor that produces stress.

eustress A stress level that results in improved performance.

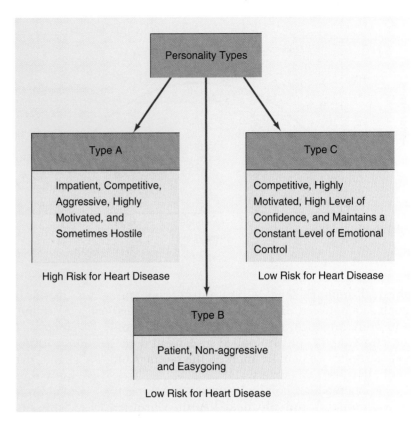

FIGURE 14.3 Personality types.

alities are highly driven, they experience the same low stress-related risk for heart disease as type B personalities.

The first step in learning to deal with stress is to examine your stress level. The most convenient way to do this is to complete a questionnaire designed to evaluate your stress level. Laboratory 14.1 is designed to accomplish this goal. If the results suggest that you are under stress, you should begin stress reduction techniques.

Steps in Stress Management

Now that you have identified your stress level, it is time to deal with stress by using techniques known collectively as "stress management." Although there are no magic formulas or nutritional supplements capable of eliminating stress (see Nutritional Links to Health and Fitness 14.1), there are two general steps to managing stress (4, 5): Reduce the amount of stress in your life, and learn to cope with stress by improving your ability to relax. Let's discuss each of these steps individually.

Stress Reduction Reducing sources of stress is the ideal means of lowering the impact of

stress on your life. The first step in stress reduction is to recognize those factors that promote daily stress. After identification of these factors, you should eliminate activities that result in daily stress. While it may not be possible to avoid all sources of stress, many "unnecessary" forms of stress can be eliminated.

A classic example of stress that can often be avoided is overcommitment, a frequent cause of stress in college students. Plan your time carefully and prioritize your activities. It may not be possible to do everything that you want to do during a given day or week. Plan a daily schedule that permits doing the things you need to accomplish without being overwhelmed with less important activities. A Closer Look 14.1 on page 306 discusses the key elements of time management.

Coping with Stress: Relaxation Techniques Because it is impossible to eliminate all forms of stress from daily life, it is necessary to use stress management techniques to reduce the potentially harmful effects of stress. Most of these techniques are designed to produce relaxation, which reduces the stress level. The following are some of the more common approaches used in stress management.

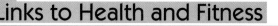

14.1 Links to Health and Fitness

Can Nutritional Supplements Reduce Emotional Stress?

Because vitamins are good for us, many people feel that the more we get, the better we feel. Because of this prevailing public attitude, many manufacturers have taken advantage of this belief by marketing products that are advertised as "magic bullets" to reduce stress. The fact is that there are no nutritional products that have been proven to reduce emotional stress. Further, because huge amounts of any vitamin could pose health risks, consult your physician or dietitian before deciding to take any nutritional supplements. See ref. 6 for a complete review of vitamins and minerals.

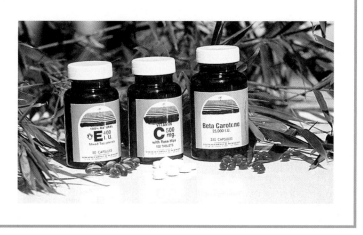

Numerous nutritional products are advertised to reduce stress; however, none of these products have proven to be effective.

Progressive relaxation. Progressive relaxation is a stress reduction technique for reducing muscular tension using exercises designed to promote relaxation. In essence, the technique is practiced as follows. While sitting quietly or lying down, contract and then relax various muscle groups one at a time, beginning with your feet and then moving up the body to the hands and neck, until a complete state of muscle relaxation is achieved. The details of this technique are outlined in A Closer Look 14.2 on page 307.

The proponents of progressive relaxation techniques for reducing stress argue that relaxing the muscles in this manner will also relax the mind and therefore relieve stress. The theory behind this concept is that an anxious (stressed) mind cannot exist in a relaxed body.

Breathing exercises. A simple means of achieving relaxation is by performing **breathing exercises.** A sample exercise designed to reduce stress is performed as follows (4):

1. Assume a comfortable position, sitting or lying down, with eyes closed.
2. Begin inhaling and exhaling slowly. Count from one to three during each inhalation and each exhalation to maintain a slow and regular breathing pattern.
3. Now combine stretching and breathing to provide greater relaxation and stress reduction. For example, stretch your arms toward the ceiling as you inhale, then lower your arms during exhalation.

breathing exercises A simple means of achieving relaxation.

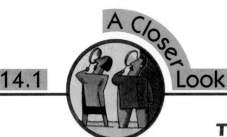

Time Management

Use the following guidelines to improve your time management skills and increase your productivity:

Establish goals. Establish a list of goals that you hope to accomplish. Identify your immediate and long-term goals and rank your goals according to priority. By establishing goals and prioritizing them, you can focus your efforts on those projects that are the most important to you.

Use a daily planner. Plan your day by using a daily planner. Chart your daily schedule, hour by hour, and place priority on your most important goals.

Evaluate your time management skills regularly. At the completion of your day, take 5 to 10 minutes to evaluate your time management. Note the time that was wasted and make plans to correct these mistakes for the following day.

Learn to say "no." Say "no" to those activities that prevent you from achieving your goals. Before you accept a new responsibility, complete your current task or eliminate an unnecessary project. Although saying "no" is often difficult, it is critical in proper time management.

Delegate responsibility. Most of us like to feel in control, and this makes delegation of responsibilities to others difficult. Nonetheless, if you become overloaded when working on a group project, don't be afraid to ask for assistance. Delegating responsibility to others is an easy way to reduce your work load and lower stress.

Eliminate distractions. Interruptions and distractions can rob precious time from your day. Identify those factors that distract you and eliminate them if possible.

Schedule time for you. Find time each day to relax and do something that you enjoy. Remember that taking an occasional break from your work is not wasting time and will improve your overall productivity by helping to energize yourself.

Reward yourself when you complete a goal. One of the simple pleasures in life is to reward yourself after you complete a goal. The reward can come in many forms: a new pair of shoes, a movie, a few days of relaxation, and so on. The importance of rewarding yourself cannot be overemphasized. People perform better when rewarded for a job well done, and a reward is an excellent means of providing encouragement (even for yourself) for future good work.

Try this exercise for 5 to 15 minutes in a quiet room. Although breathing exercises may not reduce all stress, they have been shown to be a simple means of stress reduction.

Rest and sleep. One of the most effective means of reducing stress and tension is to get an adequate amount of rest and sleep. How much sleep do you need? It appears that individual needs vary greatly; however, a good rule of thumb is 7 to 9 hours of restful sleep per night (see A Closer Look 14.3 on page 308). Further, because of the body's natural hormonal rhythms, it is recommended that you go to bed at approximately the same time every night.

In addition to a good night's sleep, 15 to 30 minutes of rest per day is useful in stress reduc-tion. This can be achieved as simply as putting your feet up on a desk or table and closing your eyes. A well-rested body is the best protection against stress and fatigue.

Exercise. Although prolonged or high-intensity exercise can impose both mental and physical stress, research has shown that light-to-moderate exercise can reduce many types of stress. The recommended types of exercise for optimal stress reduction are low- to moderate-intensity aerobic exercises (such as running, swimming, and cycling). The guidelines for this type of exercise prescription were presented in Chapter 4.

How good is exercise at reducing stress? Studies have shown that exercise is a very effective form of stress reduction (7–9). Figure 14.4 on

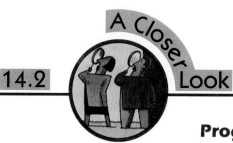

A Closer Look

14.2

Progressive Relaxation Training

There are many types of progressive relaxation training methods, and over 200 different exercises have been described. In essence, the technique involves contracting and relaxing muscle groups, starting in your lower body and moving toward your upper body. The following technique is one of the many forms that is easy to learn and use (4):

1. The first step is to assume a relaxed position (either sitting or lying down). Extend your legs, put your arms at your sides, and close your eyes. Let your muscles relax and your body go limp.
2. Take a few slow, deep breaths and concentrate on relaxing muscular tension.
3. Contract the following muscle groups in the order that they are presented. For each muscle group, contract the muscle as hard as possible, and hold the contraction for 5 seconds. Release the contraction and take a deep breath. Repeat this procedure two or more times until the muscle group is relaxed. Try to limit your contraction to the isolated body parts described here:
   a. Curl the toes on your right foot. Repeat this action with your left foot.
   b. Bend your right foot toward your head as far as possible. Repeat this action with your left foot.
   c. Extend your right foot downward (point your toes) as far as possible. Repeat this action with your left foot.
   d. Contract your upper leg (thigh). Repeat this action with your left leg.
   e. Contract your stomach muscles by attempting to curl your upper body (like a sit-up without performing the sit-up).
   f. Contract your shoulders by moving your shoulders as far forward as possible (keep your head and arms in place).
   g. Contract your shoulders by moving your shoulders as far backward as possible (keep your head and arms in place).
   h. Spread the fingers on your right hand as far as possible. Repeat this action with the left hand.
   i. Contract the muscles in your forearm by making a fist with your right hand. Repeat this action with your left hand.
   j. Contract the muscles in the front of your neck by bringing your head forward (chin to chest) as far as possible.
   k. Contract the muscles in the back of your neck by moving your head backward (push your head toward your back).
   l. Open your mouth as wide as possible.
   m. Wrinkle your forehead.

With practice, you will improve your ability to isolate the muscle groups described, and your ability to relax using this technique will also improve. As you become more comfortable with progressive relaxation, feel free to incorporate your own exercises into this routine.

---

page 308 compares the effects of a 30-minute bout of light-to-moderate exercise (running) to three other common forms of stress reduction, rest, reading, and meditation. In this study, meditation provided the greatest stress reduction, with exercise finishing a close second (9).

Why does regular exercise reduce stress? Several possibilities exist. One theory is that exercise causes the brain to release several naturally produced tranquilizers, called *endorphins,* which reduce stress levels (10). Endorphins work by blocking the effects of stress-related chemicals in the brain. Another theory is that exercise may be a diversion that frees your mind from worry or other stressful thoughts. Another possibility is that regular exercise results in an improvement in physical fitness and self-image, which increases your resistance to stress. A final possibility is that all of these factors may be involved in the beneficial effects of exercise on stress management. The next time you feel stressed, try exercise; you will feel and look better as a result.

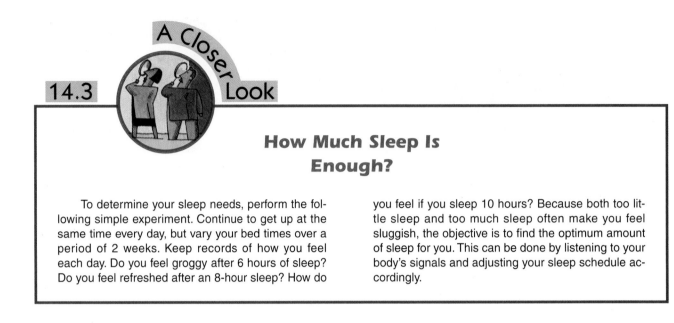

How Much Sleep Is Enough?

To determine your sleep needs, perform the following simple experiment. Continue to get up at the same time every day, but vary your bed times over a period of 2 weeks. Keep records of how you feel each day. Do you feel groggy after 6 hours of sleep? Do you feel refreshed after an 8-hour sleep? How do you feel if you sleep 10 hours? Because both too little sleep and too much sleep often make you feel sluggish, the objective is to find the optimum amount of sleep for you. This can be done by listening to your body's signals and adjusting your sleep schedule accordingly.

Meditation. **Meditation** has been practiced for ages in an effort to produce relaxation and achieve inner peace. There are many types of meditation, and there is no scientific evidence that one form is superior to another. Most types of meditation have the same common elements: sitting quietly for 15 to 20 minutes twice a day, concentrating on a single word or image, and breathing slowly and regularly. The goal of meditation is to reduce stress by achieving a complete state of physical and mental relaxation. Although beginning a successful program of meditation may require initial instruction from an experienced individual, the following is a brief overview of how meditation is practiced (4):

1. To begin, you must choose a word or sound, called a *mantra,* to be repeated during the meditation. The idea of using a mantra is that this word or sound should become your symbol of complete relaxation. Choose a mantra that has little emotional significance for you, such as the word *red.*

2. To begin meditation, find a quiet area and sit comfortably with your eyes closed. Take several deep breaths and concentrate on relaxation; let your body go limp.

3. Concentrate on your mantra. This means that you should not hear or think about anything but your mantra. Repeat your mantra over

FIGURE 14.4 Exercise and stress reduction.

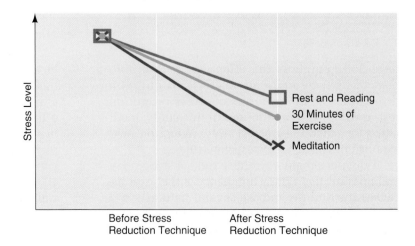

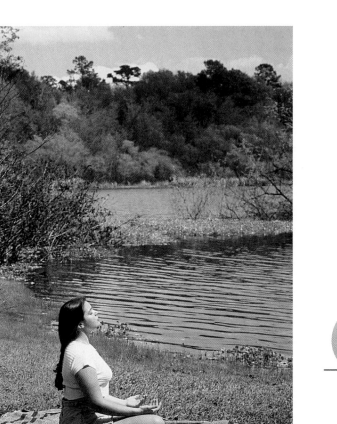

Assuming a relaxed position is important in progressive relaxation techniques.

ing your relaxing scene for the mantra. If you fail to reach a complete state of relaxation after your first several sessions, don't be discouraged. Achieving complete relaxation with this technique may require numerous practice sessions.

In summary, there are many ways to successfully manage stress. The key is to find the technique that is best for you and stick with it. Regular exercise may be the only type of stress management you require. However, if exercise alone is not sufficient, try one of the other forms of stress management as well. Remember, regardless of your personality type or your lifestyle, you can successfully manage stress by applying one or more of the previously discussed techniques.

Modifying Unhealthy Behavior

A healthy lifestyle is achieved by eliminating unhealthy behavior; this requires behavior modification. Behavior modification is the process of changing an undesirable behavior to a more desirable behavior. In the next two sections, we will discuss behavior modification and provide specific examples of how unhealthy behavior can be eliminated.

Model for Changing Behavior

The general plan to modify behavior is similar for all types of behavior modification (see Table 14.1 on page 310). A logical starting point in eliminating unhealthy behavior is to analyze your current behavior and identify problem areas. Laboratory 14.1 is designed to assist you.

The desire to change is the key point in any behavior modification plan. Without a personal

and over again in your mind and relax. Avoid distracting thoughts and focus only on the mantra.

4. After 15 to 20 minutes of concentration on the mantra, open your eyes and begin to move your thoughts away from the mantra. End the session by making a fist with both hands and saying to yourself that you are alert and refreshed.

Visualization. **Visualization** (sometimes called imagery) uses mental pictures to reduce stress. The idea is to create appealing mental images (such as a quiet mountain setting) that promote relaxation and reduce stress. Visualization is similar to meditation except that instead of using a mantra, you substitute a relaxing scene.

To practice visualization, simply follow the instructions presented for meditation, substitut-

meditation A method of relaxation that has been practiced for ages in an effort to produce relaxation and achieve inner peace. There are many types of meditation, and there is no scientific evidence that one form is superior to another.

visualization; also called *imagery* A relaxation technique that uses mental pictures to reduce stress. The idea is to create appealing mental images that promote relaxation and reduce stress.

Table 14.1

General Steps in Behavior Modification

Step No.	Action
1	Identify problem.
2	Desire change.
3	Analyze history of problem (past and current).
4	Establish short-term goals (written).
5	Establish long-term goals (written).
6	Sign contract (with friends).
7	Identify strategy for change.
8	Start strategy and learn new coping skills to deal with problem.
9	Evaluate your progress in making behavioral changes. Provide friends with progress reports.
10	Plan long-term maintenance for behavior change.

desire to make lifestyle changes, any behavior modification plan is doomed to fail.

After identifying the problem and establishing a desire to change a specific behavior, the next move is to analyze the history of the problem. The objective here is to learn what factors contribute to the development of the behavior to be modified. Learning the cause is useful when developing a strategy for change.

The next two steps (steps 4 and 5 in Table 14.1) in the behavior modification plan are the development of both short- and long-term goals for behavior change. Short-term goals establish the need for a rapid change in behavior. Long-term goals provide the incentive required to maintain behavior changes. The importance of goal setting in behavior modification cannot be overemphasized. A behavior modification plan without goals is like a race without a finish line.

The subsequent stage in the behavior modification plan is to sign a behavior modification contract in the presence of friends (see Laboratory 14.2). The purpose of signing a formal contract is to confirm in writing your commitment to a behavior change. Having friends present during the signing of the contract is important. They provide moral support and encouragement during the difficult early periods of behavior change.

The final four steps (steps 7–10) incorporate the development of a strategy for behavior change,

the learning of new coping skills, evaluation of your progress, and the planning of long-term maintenance for behavior change.

Many people who have had previous difficulty in changing behavior develop the attitude that some bad habits cannot be changed. This is not true! Unhealthy behaviors are learned; therefore, they can be unlearned.

Specific Behavior Modification Goals

Let's extend our behavior modification model by illustrating how these plans can be applied specifically to smoking cessation and weight loss.

Smoking Cessation As mentioned earlier, cigarette smoking is a serious health risk that increases the risk of cancer and heart disease. Research shows that smoking is the largest avoidable cause of death in the United States (11). Although millions of people have quit smoking, the number of smokers has increased since the late 1960s because of an increase in young smokers, particularly young women.

The first step in smoking cessation is the desire to stop. After expressing this desire and analyzing smoking behavior (see A Closer Look 14.4), the individual can develop a three-phase plan to stop smoking that incorporates steps 4 through 10 of the general steps of the behavior modification model. Phase one is often termed the *preparation phase*. In this phase, smokers develop the confidence to stop smoking by establishing both short-term and long-term goals, signing a written contract, and developing a plan to stop smoking.

The second phase of smoking cessation is commonly termed *cessation*. On the cessation date established in the *stop smoking contract*, the individual stops smoking. Quitting smoking "cold turkey" has been shown to be more effective than a gradual slow-down (2). After a smoking cessation program has begun, it is important that the individual get strong peer support, especially during the first few days and weeks.

The final phase of smoking cessation is termed the *maintenance phase*. The obvious objective of the maintenance phase is to ensure that the individual does not start smoking again. There are several strategies to assist in this process. Continued peer and family support for the individual's decision to stop smoking is critical, and its importance cannot be overemphasized. A second strategy is to avoid social circumstances that accept or encour-

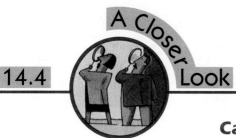

Causes of Smoking Behavior

Before beginning a smoking cessation effort, it is useful to ask the question, "Why do I smoke?" Three explanations have been proposed to explain smoking behavior:

1. social learning
2. nicotine addiction
3. opponent process

The social learning theory of smoking argues that smokers develop the habit of smoking from peers and continue the habit because of social reinforcement. Positive support from friends who smoke and the social interaction that centers around smoking make this habit difficult to break.

A second potential explanation for smoking

behavior is that the smoker develops an addiction to nicotine. This theory is supported by the fact that most smokers can attest to the sensation of a "smoker's high" and that smoking cessation often leaves the individual with withdrawal symptoms and a physical craving for nicotine.

The theory of the *opponent process* argues that smoking results from two opposing processes, one pleasant and one unpleasant. Social reinforcement and the smoker's high interact to cause a pleasant emotion, whereas attempts to stop smoking result in unpleasant withdrawal symptoms that can be eliminated by smoking. Therefore, the pleasant sensation of smoking and the unpleasant sensation of not smoking combine to encourage regular smoking behavior.

---

age smoking. For example, if going to a bar encourages smoking, then the individual should avoid bars. Finally, self-education about the health hazards of smoking provides a continuous incentive to maintain a smokeless life.

Weight Control In Chapter 8 we discussed the general principles of losing weight. Unfortunately, losing weight and maintaining the weight loss is difficult for many people. Clearly, the application of behavior modification principles is essential in the weight loss process. Although there is no single weight loss program that works for all people, the following eight components are common ingredients of most successful efforts:

1. The individual desires to lose weight.
2. The program begins with a 2-week dietary diary that includes the kind and amount of food eaten and the environmental and social circumstances.
3. Short- and long-term weight loss goals are established.
4. The individual signs a weight loss contract with friends.

5. The new dietary plan includes a balanced diet that results in a negative caloric balance and a fat deficit so that a loss of fat will result. Further, the addition of a regular exercise program is a key factor in any weight loss plan (see Chapter 8 for details).
6. New coping skills for overeating include avoiding those environments or social settings that promote it (such as parties).
7. The individual evaluates weight loss progress on a weekly basis and gets positive feedback from a support group (such as spouse, friends, or relatives).
8. After obtaining weight loss goals, the individual makes a plan for long-term behavioral changes that maintain the desired weight.

In summary, weight control is a specific application of general behavior modification principles. Indeed, these eight components incorporate most of the general behavior modification principles outlined in Table 14.1. Remember that the key elements in a weight control program are the desire to lose weight, establishment of goals,

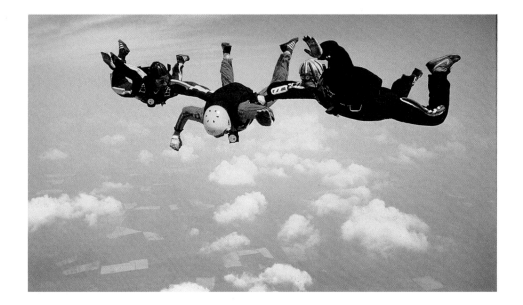

Skydiving is a high-risk activity.

development of a plan, and positive feedback from peer/family support.

Accident Prevention

In the United States, accidents are the number one killer of people under the age of 35, and they account for 50% of all childhood deaths (1, 2). Although accidents come in many forms, the most common types of accidents are from automobile accidents, falls, poisonings, drownings, and fires. While most accidents may seem to be a matter of chance, this is not the case! By behavior modification, you have control over many factors that increase your accident risk and can lower them. Let's examine the most common risk factors for accidents.

Risk Factors for Accidents One of the most important accident risk factors is an unsafe attitude, which promotes risk-taking behaviors. For example, people who are overly confident in their driving skills may speed on a winding or wet road and increase their chances of having an automobile accident. Similarly, people who are overconfident in their job skills may take unnecessary risks at work.

Some people crave excitement or the sensation of danger (2). This type of thrill-seeking attitude increases the risk of accidents. These people often engage in high-risk physical activities such as skydiving, auto racing, or rock climbing, which increase their risk of injury due to accidents.

Stress also increases your risk of accidents (1, 2). During periods of emotional or physical stress, you tend to be less careful. If you find yourself having a series of small mishaps or "near misses" when performing routine activities (such as yardwork, house cleaning, or sports activities), this may be an index that you should reduce your stress level by rest and the use of stress management techniques.

As we have seen, use of alcohol and other drugs may increase your risk of accidents. Drug use does this by altering your judgment and by decreasing both reaction speed and motor coordination. Alcohol is involved in nearly one-half of all auto accidents and plays a major role in many boating accidents. Similarly, cocaine and marijuana use are associated with a wide range of accidents, including falls, drownings, fires, and automobile accidents.

A number of environmental factors can increase your risk of accident. For example, storing combustible materials close to a heater and a lack of properly operating smoke detectors both increase your risk of injury due to fire. Other factors, such as failing to properly maintain ladders or steps around your home or work place, may also increase your risk of accidental injury.

Reducing Your Risk of Accidents There are a number of steps that you can take to reduce your risk of injury. The key is to increase your awareness of the risk factors. Table 14.2 summarizes key steps that can reduce your risk of injury due to automobile accidents, fire, falls, drowning, and poisoning. Take time to study each of these recommendations and alter your lifestyle to reduce your injury risk.

Table 14.2

Reducing Your Risk of Injury

Bicycle or motorcycle accidents
•On a bike or motorcycle, always wear a helmet and use reflectors and protective clothing.
•Ride with the traffic.
•Obey the rules of the road (e.g., use turn signals) and ride defensively.

Automobile accidents
•Never drive while or after using drugs or alcohol.
•Do not drive when you are overly tired or sleepy.
•Maintain your motor vehicle in good mechanical condition.
•Obey the rules of the road and drive defensively.
•If you need assistance, stay in your car and wait for help.
•Always wear your seat belt.
•Always drive within the legal speed limit.
•Do not drive when emotionally upset.

Falls
•Use handrails when going up and down stairs.
•Do not attempt to climb ladders or stairs when ill or physically impaired due to drug use.
•Maintain ladders and steps in good working condition.
•Never run up or down stairs.
•Make sure stairways are well lit.

Poisoning
•Properly mark all drugs.
•Never take more of any drug than is recommended.
•Keep all drugs out of the reach of children.
•Use only nontoxic cleaning materials.
•Increase your knowledge of poisons.
•Do not take medication in the dark.
•Discard old or expired prescriptions.
•Do not combine drugs.
•Keep the poison control center telephone number near your phone.

Fire
•Reduce the risk of fire in your home or workplace by storing combustible materials in a safe place.
•Maintain smoke detectors, fire extinguishers, and sprinkler systems in proper working condition.
•Know how to properly use a fire extinguisher.
•Practice safe evacuation procedures from your home and workplace.

Drowning
•Learn to swim, and learn proper water safety procedures.
•Do not swim alone or in the dark.
•Dive only in designated areas.
•Do not swim immediately after eating or when tired.
•Do not swim when using drugs of any kind.
•Avoid swimming in dangerous areas, such as rivers with strong currents.
•Learn cardiopulmonary resuscitation.

Summary

1. The five key behaviors that promote a healthy lifestyle are health-related physical fitness, good nutrition, weight control, stress management, and modification of unhealthy behaviors.

2. *Stress* is defined as a physiological and mental response to something in our environment that makes us feel uncomfortable. A factor that produces stress is called a *stressor.*

3. Two steps in stress management are to reduce stress in your life and to learn to cope with stress by improving your ability to relax.

4. Common relaxation techniques to reduce stress include progressive relaxation, visualization, meditation, breathing exercises, rest and sleep, and exercise.

5. Behavior modification is the elimination of an undesirable behavior. The general model of behavior modification can be applied to achieve any desired health-related behavior.

6. The five most common accidents are automobile accidents, fires, drownings, poisonings, and falls.

7. Risk factors for accidents include unsafe attitudes, stress, drug use, and an unsafe environment.

Study Questions

1. Define *stress.* What is a *stressor*?

2. Why is stress management important to health?

3. List the steps in stress management. Identify some common stress management (relaxation) techniques.

4. Define *behavior modification.* What are the steps involved in behavior modification?

5. Outline a plan to use behavior modification to eliminate a specific unhealthy behavior.

6. Discuss the concept of eustress.

7. Explain how exercise is useful in reducing stress.

8. List the key guidelines for the development of a time management program.

9. List the steps to reduce your risks of injury due to automobile accidents, falls, fires, water accidents, and poisonings.

Suggested Reading

Donatelle, R., and L. Davis. *Brief second edition: access to health.* Allyn and Bacon, Needham Heights, MA, 1996.

Howley, E., and B. D. Franks. *Health fitness: Instructors handbook.* Human Kinetics, Champaign, IL, 1997.

Margen, S., et al, eds. *The wellness encyclopedia.* Houghton Mifflin, Boston, 1992.

Suggested Readings on the World Wide Web

Healthy Way: Stress Management (http://www.bc.sympatico.ca/healthyway/LIST/B4-C05_all1.html)
Links to several sites with information on assessing and managing stress levels.

Stress Management: Links (http://www.siu.edu/departments/bushea/stress.html)
Links to sites with information on stress management. Create your own relaxation tape!

References

1. Donatelle, R., and L. Davis. *Brief second edition: access to health.* Allyn and Bacon, Needham Heights, MA, 1996.

2. Hales, D. *An invitation to health.* Benjamin Cummings, Redwood City, CA, 1992.

3. Margen, S., et al, eds. *The wellness encyclopedia.* Houghton Mifflin, Boston, 1992.

4. Williams, M. *Lifetime fitness and wellness.* Wm. C. Brown, Dubuque, IA, 1996.

5. Howley, E., and B. D. Franks. *Health fitness: Instructors handbook.* Human Kinetics, Champaign, IL, 1997.

6. Clarkson, P. Vitamins and trace minerals. In: Lamb D., and M. Williams, eds. *Ergogenics.* Brown and Benchmark, Madison, WI, 1991, pp. 123–175.

7. Raglin, J., and W. Morgan. Influence of exercise and quiet rest on state anxiety and blood pressure. *Medicine and Science in Sports and Exercise* 19:456–463, 1987.

8. Berger, B., and D. Owen. Stress reduction and mood enhancement in four exercise modes: Swimming, body conditioning, hatha yoga, and fencing. *Research Quarterly for Exercise and Sport* 59:148–159, 1988.

9. Bahrke, M., and W. Morgan. Anxiety reduction following exercise and meditation. *Cognitive Therapy and Research* 2:323–333, 1978.

10. Farrell, P. Enkephalins, catecholamines, and psychological mood alterations: Effects of prolonged exercise. *Medicine and Science in Sports and Exercise* 19:347–353, 1987.

11. Fielding, J. Smoking: Health effects and controls. *New England Journal of Medicine* 313:491–497, 1985.

Stress Index Questionnaire

NAME _____ DATE _____

Directions

The purpose of this stress index questionnaire is to increase your awareness of stress in your life. Answer "yes" or "no" to each of the stress index questions. Circle your answer.

Yes	No	1. I have frequent arguments.
Yes	No	2. I often get upset at work.
Yes	No	3. I often have neck and/or shoulder pains due to anxiety/stress.
Yes	No	4. I often get upset when I stand in long lines.
Yes	No	5. I often get angry when I listen to the local, national, or world news or read the newspaper.
Yes	No	6. I do not have a sufficient amount of money for my needs.
Yes	No	7. I often get upset when driving.
Yes	No	8. At the end of a workday I often feel stress-related fatigue.
Yes	No	9. I have at least one constant source of stress/anxiety in my life (e.g., conflict with boss, neighbor, mother-in-law, etc.).
Yes	No	10. I often have stress-related headaches.
Yes	No	11. I do not practice stress management techniques.
Yes	No	12. I rarely take time for myself.
Yes	No	13. I have difficulty in keeping my feelings of anger and hostility under control.
Yes	No	14. I have difficulty in managing time wisely.
Yes	No	15. I often have difficulty sleeping.
Yes	No	16. I am generally in a hurry.
Yes	No	17. I usually feel that there is not enough time in the day to accomplish what I need to do.
Yes	No	18. I often feel that I am being mistreated by friends or associates.
Yes	No	19. I do not regularly perform physical activity.
Yes	No	20. I rarely get 7 to 9 hours of sleep per night.

Scoring and Interpretation

Answering "yes" to any of the questions means that you need to use some form of stress management techniques (see text for details). Add your "yes" answers and use the following scale to evaluate the level of stress in your life.

Number of "Yes" Answers	Stress Category	
	6–20	High stress
	3–5	Average stress
	0–2	Low stress

Behavior Modification Contract

NAME _____ DATE _____

Directions

Complete the following behavior modification contract, using friends or peers as witnesses. See the reverse of this sheet for an example of a completed contract.

Behavior Modification Contract

1. I _____ (name) agree to make the following behavioral change(s):

   _____

   _____

   _____

   _____ beginning on _____ (date).

2. My short-term goal(s) are to

   _____

   _____ by _____ (date).

3. My long-term goal(s) are to

   _____

   _____

4. I will assess my progress on the desired behavioral change on a regular basis:

   _____ (note how often).

   Further, I will report my progress to at least two friends and/or peers on a regular basis.

Signed: _____ Date: _____

Witness: _____ Witness: _____

Illustration of Behavior Modification Contract for Smoking Cessation

Behavior Modification Contract

1. I _____ John Doe _____ (name) agree to make the following behavioral change(s):

   Stop smoking _____

   _____

   _____

   _____ beginning on _ May 20, 1996 _ (date).

2. My short-term goal(s) are to

   Stop smoking _____

   _____ by _ 5/20/1996 _ (date).

3. My long-term goal(s) are to

   Remain smoke free during the rest of my life _____

   _____

4. I will assess my progress on the desired behavioral change on a regular basis:

   _____ weekly _____ (note how often).

   Further, I will report my progress to at least two friends and/or peers on a regular basis.

   Signed: _____ John Doe _____ Date: _ April 1, 1996 _

   Witness: _____ Jane Doe _____ Witness: _____ William Jones _____

15

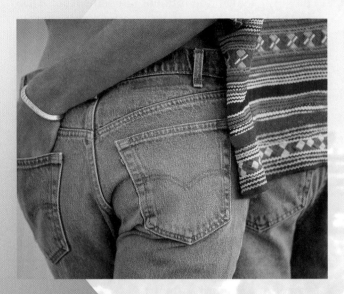

Sexually Transmitted Diseases and Drug Abuse

Learning Objectives

After reading this chapter, you should be able to

1 List the most common sexually transmitted diseases in the United States.

2 Identify the guidelines to reduce your risk of acquiring sexually transmitted diseases.

3 Discuss the incidence of sexually transmitted diseases in the United States.

4 Outline the acute physiological effects of alcohol, marijuana, and cocaine use.

5 List several guidelines that can be used to maintain control over alcohol and drug abuse.

6 Discuss the long-term health consequences of alcohol, marijuana, and cocaine use.

Throughout this book, we have discussed factors that influence your health and well-being. Two important factors that can negatively impact health and wellness are sexually transmitted diseases and drug abuse. This chapter discusses these health threats, with an emphasis on ways to reduce your risk of each.

Sexually Transmitted Diseases

Every year twelve million people in the United States are infected by one or more **sexually transmitted diseases** (STDs) (1). STDs are generally spread through sexual contact. More than 20 different STDs have been identified. Current estimates are that one in four people in the United States will contract at least one STD in their lifetime. The most common STDs include acquired immunodeficiency syndrome (AIDS), chlamydia, gonorrhea, pelvic inflammatory disease, genital warts, herpes, and syphilis (2).

AIDS

AIDS is a fatal disease that develops from infection by the human immunodeficiency virus (HIV). Current estimates are that approximately one million people in the United States are infected with HIV, with the number growing every day (3–7). Also, the number of deaths from AIDS in the United States is increasing every year. In fact, a recent study shows that AIDS is the leading cause of death in American men aged 25 to 44 and the fourth leading cause of death in women in the same age group (8).

Many people infected with HIV are unaware that they carry the virus because symptoms may not appear for months or even years after infection. Evidence now suggests that in many cases the virus may remain dormant in the body for 5 to 10 years before creating health problems (2, 5). After this incubation period, the virus begins to multiply and eventually damages the immune system. Because an impaired immune system is incapable of preventing infections and cancer, the body becomes vulnerable to a variety of diseases. When disease symptoms appear due to the HIV infection, the individual has developed AIDS. The number of AIDS deaths in the United States has grown at a rapid rate (Figure 15.1).

Early symptoms of AIDS include constant fatigue, fever, weight loss, swollen lymph glands, and sore throats. Symptoms developing later include night sweats, chronic infections, skin disorders, and ulcers of the membranes lining the nose, mouth, and other body cavities.

HIV can be transmitted by any exchange of body fluids (such as blood, semen, and vaginal secretions). Common methods of transmission include sexual intercourse and using a hypodermic needle previously used by an HIV-infected person. At present, taking measures to prevent AIDS is your only protection, because there is no known cure for this disease.

Chlamydia

Chlamydia is one of the common STDs among heterosexual people worldwide (2). The disease is caused by a bacterial infection within the reproductive organs and is spread through vaginal, anal, and oral sex. The Centers for Disease Control in Atlanta, Georgia, estimate that over three million new cases of chlamydia occur each year in the United States (9). Equally alarming is the estimate that about 20% of all college students may have chlamydia (1).

Symptoms of chlamydia vary among individuals. Over 70% of the women infected do not develop symptoms and are unaware that they have the disease. Apparent symptoms in women include a yellowish vaginal discharge and an occa-

FIGURE 15.1 The growth of AIDS in the United States.

sional bleeding between menstrual periods. In men, early symptoms include painful urination and a watery discharge from the penis.

Fortunately, chlamydia can be cured by administration of antibiotics. If untreated, however, chlamydia can result in male and female infertility. Further, untreated chlamydia in women can lead to **pelvic inflammatory disease,** an inflammatory infection of the lining of the abdominal and pelvic cavity. Common symptoms of pelvic inflammatory disease include pain in the lower abdominal cavity, fever, and menstrual irregularities. If you suspect that you have been infected by chlamydia or any other STD, see your physician at once.

Gonorrhea

Gonorrhea is another common STD, and it is estimated that about two million new cases of gonorrhea will be reported in the United States each year (9). The infection can be transmitted through vaginal, anal, and oral sex. Similar to chlamydia, gonorrhea is caused by a bacterial infection and is curable by treatment with antibiotics. Untreated gonorrhea may spread to the prostate, testicles, kidney, and bladder and can result in sterility in both men and women (2, 10).

Over 80% of men develop symptoms within 2 to 10 days after contact with an infected person. Typical symptoms include a milky discharge from the penis and painful urination (10).

In contrast, only 20% of women infected with gonorrhea develop symptoms. When symptoms are present, they include painful urination and an occasional fever (10). The lack of symptoms in women poses a serious problem because the woman is unaware that she has been infected and may continue to spread the disease to sex partners.

Venereal Warts

Venereal warts (also known as *genital warts*) are caused by a small group of viruses called *human papilloma viruses* (1, 2, 10). Infection generally occurs through sexual contact with an infected individual; after exposure, the virus penetrates the skin or mucous membranes of the genitals or anus, and warts appear within 6 to 8 weeks (1, 2, 10).

On dry skin (such as the penis), warts may develop as a series of small itchy bumps on the genitals and may range in size from the size of a pencil eraser to the size of a pinhead. Men can detect these warts by routinely examining their genitals for suspicious growths. If, however, the warts are inside the reproductive tract, symptoms may be absent. In women, these warts are often first detected by a physician during a routine Pap test. Similarly, venereal warts of the rectum must be diagnosed by a physician.

Treatment for venereal warts may take several forms. Warts can be painted with several different types of medication, which results in the warts drying up within a few days. Also, the warts can be removed by cryosurgery (freezing them), laser surgery, or excision surgery.

Do venereal warts present a serious health threat? In some cases, no. Many venereal warts will disappear on their own without treatment. The greatest risk from venereal warts is that untreated warts in women increases the risk of uterine and cervical cancer. Exactly how venereal warts result in cancer is unclear. What is known is that within 5 years after infection, about 30% of all untreated warts result in a precancerous growth. If this precancerous growth remains untreated, 70% will lead to a malignant cancer (2, 10).

sexually transmitted diseases (STDs) A group of more than 20 diseases that are generally spread through sexual contact.

AIDS A fatal disease that develops from infection by the human immunodeficiency virus, or HIV.

chlamydia The most common sexually transmitted disease among heterosexuals in the United States. The disease is caused by a bacterial infection within the reproductive organs and is spread through vaginal, anal, and oral sex.

pelvic inflammatory disease An inflammatory infection of the lining of the abdominal and pelvic cavities. Common symptoms of pelvic inflammatory disease include pain in the lower abdominal cavity, fever, and menstrual irregularities.

gonorrhea A common sexually transmitted disease. The infection can be transmitted through vaginal, anal, and oral sex. Gonorrhea is caused by a bacterial infection and is curable by antibiotics.

venereal warts; also known as *genital warts* Warts caused by a small group of viruses called *human papilloma viruses.* Infection generally occurs through sexual contact with an infected individual; after exposure, the virus penetrates the skin or mucous membranes of the genitals or anus, and warts appear within 6 to 8 weeks.

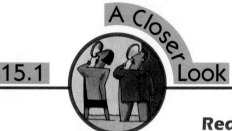

A Closer Look

Reducing Your Risk of Sexually Transmitted Diseases

Sexually transmitted diseases are usually spread through sexual contact. Sexual intercourse, oral genital contact, hand-to-genital contact, and anal intercourse are common modes of transmission. Remember, no one is immune to STDs. Adherence to the following guidelines will reduce your risk of contracting them (1, 5, 11).

1. Avoidance of sexual contact with an infected person is the only absolute means of preventing STDs. Maintaining a monogamous relationship with a healthy partner is a proven way to avoid an STD.
2. Avoid casual sexual partners. If you have more than one sexual partner, do not be afraid to ask intimate sexual questions about your partner's history. Do not have sexual intercourse with anyone that is at high risk for STD infection (such as intravenous drug users or prostitutes).
3. Avoid using drugs or alcohol; these products may dull your senses and reduce your ability

to make sound decisions regarding sexual activity.
4. Always practice safe sex. Safe sex means properly using a good-quality latex condom.
5. Never share hypodermic needles with anyone; HIV is often spread through the use of common hypodermic needles. Further, never share any devices through which blood exchange may occur (such as razors, ear-piercing instruments, or tattoo instruments).
6. Avoid oral sex or any activity in which body fluids can penetrate through the skin.
7. If possible, wash your hands and genitals before and after sexual encounters. Urinate after sexual intercourse. Collectively, these practices reduce your risk of infection by an STD.
8. If you become concerned about the possibility of having contracted an STD, stop any sexual activity and contact your physician at once. STDs can be detected only by blood tests or examination of genital fluid.

Herpes

Herpes is a general term for a family of diseases that are also caused by viral infections. Herpes is highly contagious and can be transmitted through any form of sexual contact (such as hand-to-genital contact, oral sex, or intercourse). Over half a million new cases of herpes were reported in the United States during 1993 (9). Symptoms of herpes vary from sores (blisters) on the mouth, rectum, and genitals, to fever and swollen glands. Interestingly, symptoms may disappear and then reappear without warning.

At present, there is no cure for herpes, but newly developed drugs show promise. Although treatment with cold sore medication reduces the pain and irritation of the sore, remember that rubbing anything on the herpes blister increases the

chance of spreading herpes-laden fluids to other body parts or to other people.

Syphilis

Syphilis is a well-known STD that can be transmitted through direct sexual contact. Each year about 300,000 new cases of syphilis are reported in the United States (9). Similar to chlamydia and gonorrhea, syphilis is caused by a bacterial infection and can be cured by antibiotics (2, 10).

The symptoms of untreated syphilis vary because the disease generally progresses through several distinct stages. Early symptoms of syphilis generally include a painless sore (called a *chancre*) located at the initial site of infection (such as the penis, vaginal walls, or mouth). The size of

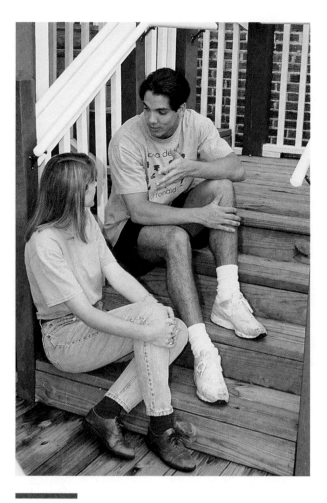

Maintaining a monogamous relationship is a good strategy for reducing your risk of infection from a sexually transmitted disease.

the chancre may vary, but it is often about the size of a dime. In both men and women, this chancre will completely disappear in 3 to 6 weeks.

Within 1 to 12 months after the disappearance of the chancre, secondary symptoms appear. These include a skin rash or white patches on the mucous membranes of the mouth, throat, or genitals. Hair loss may occur, lymph glands may become swollen, and infectious sores may develop around the mouth or genitals. After the appearance of these secondary symptoms, the disease may once again "go into hiding," and all symptoms may disappear.

Although the individual may be without symptoms for several years, the syphilis infection is slowly spreading to organs throughout the body. Late stages of untreated syphilis may result in heart damage, blindness, deafness, paralysis, and mental disorders.

Reducing Your Risk for Sexually Transmitted Diseases

There is no cure for AIDS or herpes, and although treatment methods exist for many other STDs, prevention is clearly the best approach. The key to prevention of STDs is education and responsible action. Complete abstinence from sexual activity is the only certain way to prevent STDs; however, if you engage in sexual activity, following the guidelines presented in A Closer Look 15.1 will greatly reduce your risk of developing one of these diseases.

Drug Abuse

Alcohol abuse and the use of illegal drugs are two of the biggest problems in the United States today. Millions of Americans abuse alcohol and use illegal (recreational) drugs such as cocaine or marijuana (1). Unfortunately, alcohol or recreational drug abuse can lead to drug addiction (also called **chemical dependency**). Further, abuse of alcohol or recreational drugs increases your risk of accidents and may damage your health. Let's discuss the three most common forms of drug abuse in the United States: alcohol, marijuana, and cocaine.

Alcohol

Alcohol is the most widely used recreational drug in U.S. society and is the most popular drug on college campuses—used twice as much as marijuana and five times as much as cocaine (11). It is estimated that over 85% of college students

herpes A general term for a family of diseases that are also caused by viral infections. Herpes is highly contagious and can be transmitted through any form of sexual contact (e.g., hand-to-genital contact, oral sex, or intercourse).

syphilis A sexually transmitted disease that can be transmitted through direct sexual contact. Syphilis is caused by a bacterial infection and can be cured by antibiotics.

chemical dependency A term for drug addiction.

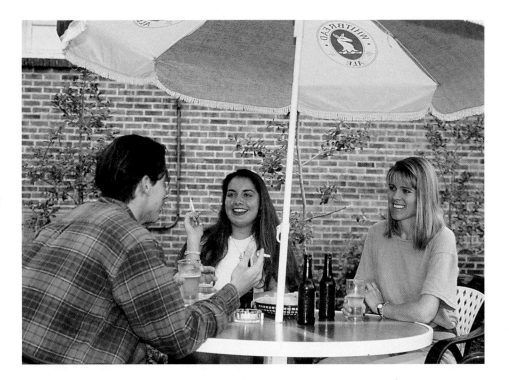

Social drinking is popular among college students.

in the United States use alcohol and, unfortunately, some 20% to 28% abuse it (11).

Although many people consume alcohol to "get high," in reality, alcohol is a central nervous system depressant that slows down the function of the brain; this results in impaired vision, slowed reaction time, and impaired motor coordination. Overconsumption of alcohol also impairs mental judgment, which may decrease the fear of danger. This can result in increased risk-taking behaviors, which elevates your chance of accidents (such as driving too fast) and increases your risk of using bad judgment in social or sexual behavior.

Chronic abuse of alcohol over a period of years can result in liver disease (cirrhosis), damage to the nervous system, and an increased risk of certain cancers (10). Development of liver disease due to years of drinking may eventually result in total liver failure and death. The damage to the nervous system that results from alcohol abuse is localized to the left side of the brain, which is responsible for written and spoken language, logic, and mathematical skills. The degree of brain damage that occurs appears to be directly related to the amount of alcohol consumed. Further, repeated irritation of the gastrointestinal system by alcohol has been linked to cancers of the esophagus, stomach, mouth, tongue, and liver.

Another and often overlooked problem with chronic consumption of alcohol is malnutrition (see Nutritional Links to Health and Fitness 15.1).

Addiction to alcohol is usually a slowly developing disease that can happen to anyone. Research into the cause of alcoholism has revealed that addiction to alcohol may have hereditary, psychological, and environmental components. Unfortunately, the details of how and why alcoholism begins are still somewhat a mystery.

If you feel that you are drinking too much, seek professional help from your physician or organizations such as Alcoholics Anonymous (see Laboratory 15.1). Using the following guidelines will assist you in maintaining control over your drinking habits (1, 11):

1. Know your limits and stay within them. If you are at a party and feel that you are drinking too much, learn to say "no," and begin drinking a nonalcoholic beverage.

2. When drinking, stick to the rule of 1 ounce of alcohol per hour. This will reduce your possibility of becoming physically or mentally impaired by alcohol abuse.

3. Wine, beer, and diluted mixed drinks are less intoxicating than straight liquor. Stick to these drinks instead of the higher-alcohol beverages.

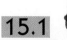

15.1 Nutritional Links to Health and Fitness

Alcohol Abuse and Undernutrition

A common problem associated with chronic alcohol abuse is undernutrition. This occurs due to alcohol's repeated irritation of the gastrointestinal system; the combination of chronic consumption of alcohol and gastric irritation often impairs appetite, which reduces the intake of essential nutrients. The end result is a state of undernutrition, which, in extreme cases, can promote a loss of muscle mass and abnormal functioning of many body organs. The cure for this alcohol-related problem is to seek professional help for alcoholism. In many cases, cessation of alcohol abuse eliminates the alcohol-induced reduction in appetite, and the individual returns to normal eating habits. In severe cases of alcohol-related undernutrition, the nutritional advice of a physician and nutritionist is required.

4. Eating and drinking at the same time will slow down the rate of alcohol absorption and reduce your chance of becoming impaired. Never drink on an empty stomach.

5. When leaving a party or bar after drinking, if you have any doubts about your ability to drive, call a cab or have someone else drive you home. The best course is to never drink and drive.

Marijuana

Use of **marijuana** became popular in the United States in the 1960s and it remains the most popular illegal drug among college students (1, 12). As ingested or smoked, marijuana is a plant mixture (stems, leaves, or seeds) from either the *Cannabis sativa* or *Cannabis indica* (hemp) plants. The active chemical in marijuana which produces physical effects is tetrahydrocannabinol (THC); the higher the THC concentration in the marijuana, the greater the effect. The THC content in marijuana varies between 0.5% and 3.0% and the average percentage of THC in marijuana sold in the United States is about 1.0% (12).

Marijuana can be used in many forms. It can be brewed and drunk as a tea, or it can be baked into cookies or brownies. However, marijuana is most often smoked in pipes or by rolling the marijuana into cigarettes. Effects are generally felt within 15 to 30 minutes and usually disappear within 2 to 3 hours.

Marijuana is classified as a stimulant, with the immediate effects being an increased heart rate and blood pressure, blood-shot eyes, and dry mouth and throat. Use of marijuana impairs motor coordination and may increase your risk of accidents. Further, acute use of marijuana alters the normal function of memory centers in the brain. This memory loss resembles that observed in normal aging. However, whether these changes in function place long-term marijuana users at risk for early mental disorders is not clear.

Long-term use of marijuana presents several dangers. First, consistent users of marijuana may become psychologically dependent on its use. Further, regular smoking of marijuana causes lung damage similar to that of tobacco smoking (12). The effects of long-term marijuana use on the heart is not well known; however, many

marijuana A plant mixture (stems, leaves, or seeds) from either the *Cannabis sativa* or *Cannabis indica* (hemp) plants. The active chemical in marijuana that produces physical effects is tetrahydrocannabinol (THC); the higher the THC concentration in marijuana, the greater the effect.

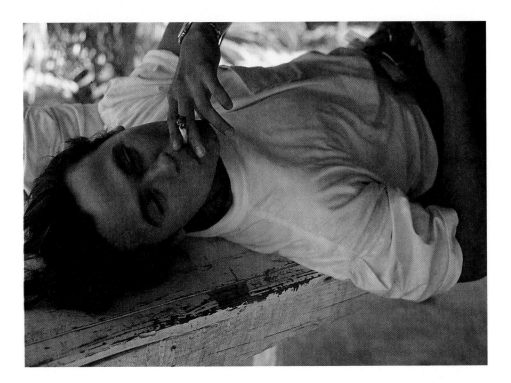

Smoking marijuana may increase your risk of accidents and health damage.

investigators believe that marijuana increases the workload on the heart, which may eventually result in damage.

Cocaine

The use of **cocaine** (coke) in the United States increased dramatically during the 1980s, and current estimates are that approximately five million Americans use the drug (1). Further, a recent survey suggests that as many as 6% of college students have also experimented with cocaine (1). This makes cocaine the third most widely used drug by college students.

Cocaine is a powerful stimulant derived from the leaves of the South American coca shrub, which grows primarily in the Andes Mountains. Cocaine is extracted from the coca leaves by using a multistep process to produce a white powder (similar to sugar in appearance). Varying the extraction process can produce several different

forms of cocaine, such as crack cocaine, rock cocaine, or freebase cocaine.

Cocaine can be used in several ways. Common uses include snorting (sniffing cocaine into the nose), smoking, and intravenous injections. All routes of administration result in a rapid and short-lived high (effects generally last from 5 to 20 minutes). Cocaine is a highly addictive drug; when the cocaine high disappears, the user wants more. Spending over $1000 per day for cocaine is not uncommon for an addict. As a result of the addiction, cocaine addicts often suffer psychological damage, which eventually contributes to loss of jobs and financial ruin.

The immediate physiological effects of cocaine are varied. The drug is both an anesthetic and a central nervous system stimulant. Cocaine use increases heart rate and blood pressure. Other effects include a feeling of euphoria and heightened self-confidence. In large doses, cocaine is extremely dangerous, and numerous deaths have resulted from overdoses. Further, long-term cocaine use may damage the heart, the brain, and the respiratory system.

Treatment for cocaine addiction requires professional help. To assist cocaine addicts, the National Institute for Drug Abuse has established toll-free hotlines (1-800-COCAINE). If you or anyone you know uses cocaine, seek professional

cocaine Cocaine is a powerful stimulant derived from the leaves of the South American coca shrub, which grows primarily in the Andes mountains. Cocaine is extracted from the coca leaves using a multistep process to produce a white powder.

help at once. Cocaine addiction is a serious problem that requires immediate attention.

Say "No" to Drugs

Avoiding drug use requires self discipline and control. Several steps can protect you from the temptation to use drugs (1, 11):

1. *Increase your self-esteem.* Take pride in yourself and your achievements; this will boost your confidence and improve your ability to say "no" to drugs.

2. *Learn how to cope with stress.* When stressed, use one or more of the stress management techniques discussed in Chapter 14 (such as exercise or progressive relaxation).

3. *Develop numerous interests.* Develop interest in hobbies or sports that provide you with pleasure.

4. *Practice assertiveness.* Becoming assertive is an important key to learning to say "no" to drugs.

Summary

1. Some of the most common sexually transmitted diseases include AIDS, chlamydia, gonorrhea, pelvic inflammatory disease, venereal warts, herpes, and syphilis.

2. All sexually transmitted diseases require medical treatment. Successful treatments for chlamydia, gonorrhea, pelvic inflammatory disease, venereal warts, and syphilis are available. At present, there are no cures for AIDS or herpes.

3. Most sexually transmitted diseases can be avoided by following "safe sex" guidelines.

4. Alcohol, marijuana, and cocaine are the most widely used and abused drugs in the United States.

5. Use of alcohol, marijuana, and cocaine increases your risk of accidents, and prolonged use of these substances may result in addiction and health damage.

6. Alcohol is the most common recreational drug used in U.S. society.

7. Chronic abuse of alcohol can result in liver disease, damage to the nervous system, and increased risk of certain cancers.

8. Long-term use of marijuana may result in psychological dependence and may increase your risk of cardiopulmonary diseases (similar to tobacco smoking).

9. Cocaine is a highly addictive drug and, when taken in large doses, can be lethal.

Study Questions

1. Outline the guidelines to reduce your risk of being infected by a sexually transmitted disease.

2. Name the seven most common STDs in the United States.

3. Which of the most common STDs are currently incurable?

4. Discuss the relationship between venereal warts and uterine or cervical cancer.

5. Discuss the short-term and long-term effects of alcohol use.

6. What is the most widely used recreational drug in America?

7. List four steps that can reduce your temptation to use drugs.

8. Discuss the short-term and long-term use of marijuana and cocaine.

Suggested Reading

Donatelle, R., and L. Davis. *Brief second edition: access to health.* Prentice-Hall, Englewood Cliffs, NJ, 1993.

Margen, S., et al., eds. *The wellness encyclopedia.* Houghton Mifflin, Boston, 1992.

Nevid, J. *201 things you should know about AIDS.* Allyn and Bacon, Boston, 1993.

Suggested Readings on the World Wide Web
Centers for Disease Control and Prevention (http://www.cdc.gov/)
Facts and statistics on the incidence and control of disease in the United States.

Sympatico: Health Links Reviews: Sex and Sexuality (http://www.ns.sympatico.ca/healthyway) Articles about prevention, treatment, and incidence of sexually transmitted diseases.

National Clearing House for Alcohol and Drug Information (http://www.healthorg/) Provides electronic data and information on alcohol and substance abuse issues.

References

1. Donatelle, R., and L. Davis. *Brief second edition: access to health.* Allyn and Bacon, Needham Heights, MA, 1996.

2. Daniels, D., R. Hillman, S. Barton, and D. Goldmeir. *Sexually transmitted disease and AIDS.* Springer-Verlag, London, 1993.

3. *HIV/AIDS surveillance report.* Centers for Disease Control, Atlanta, 9:(1), 1997.

4. AIDS. Statistics from the Centers for Disease Control and Prevention. 7:1691–1693, 1993.

5. Nevid, J. *201 things you should know about AIDS.* Allyn and Bacon, Boston, 1993.

6. Rosenberg, P., and M. Gail. Uncertainty in estimates of HIV prevalence derived by back calculation. *Annals of Epidemiology* 1:105–115, 1990.

7. Biggar, R., and P. Rosenberg. HIV infection/AIDS in the U.S. during the 1990's. *Clinical Infectious Diseases* 17(Suppl.):S219–S223, 1993.

8. Hamm, R., H. Donnell, and W. Watkins. An update on the epidemiology of AIDS in Missouri. *Missouri Medicine* 91:132–136, 1994.

9. Incidence of sexually transmitted diseases in the U.S. Centers for Disease Control and Prevention. Atlanta, 1996.

10. Robbins, S., and M. Angell. *Basic pathology.* W. B. Saunders, Philadelphia, 1997.

11. Hales, D. *An invitation to health.* Benjamin Cummings, Redwood City, CA, 1992.

12. Liska, K. *Drugs and the human body.* Prentice-Hall, Englewood Cliffs, NJ, 1997.

Alcohol Abuse Inventory

NAME _____ DATE _____

This laboratory is designed to increase your awareness of your drinking habits. For this inventory to provide a valid assessment of your drinking behaviors, you must provide an honest answer to each question. After answering the questions, use the scoring information to determine your alcohol consumption status.

Directions

Answer "yes" or "no" to the following questions regarding your use of alcohol.

1. Do you often drink alone?

2. When drinking, do you often worry about running out of alcoholic beverages?

3. Do you drink alcohol on a daily basis?

4. When stressed, do you immediately drink alcohol to reduce your stress levels?

5. Do you crave alcohol at any time of the day?

6. Do you have trouble saying "no" to drinking at a party?

7. Do you sometimes have trouble remembering what you did the night before?

8. Does your drinking impair your school or job performance?

9. Does your drinking impair your ability to use good judgment or cause you to have accidents?

10. Do you ever lie about how much you drink to friends or family?

Scoring

Answering "yes" to one of the questions above is a suggestion that you may be drinking too much. Answering "yes" to two questions is a clear warning sign that you may have or are in the process of developing an alcohol abuse problem. Answering "yes" to three or more questions indicate that you have a serious alcohol abuse problem and that you should seek professional help.

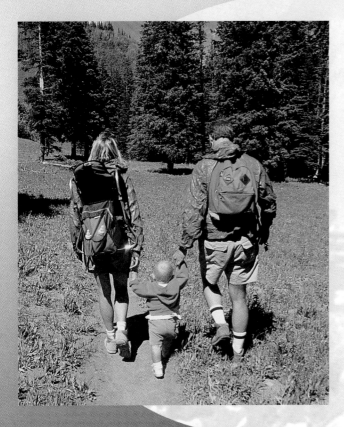

16

Lifetime Fitness

After studying this chapter, you should be able to

1 Identify several factors that will assist you in maintaining a regular exercise program.

2 List key considerations in choosing a fitness facility.

3 Discuss the term *fitness expert*.

4 Discuss several common exercise misconceptions.

5 Identify factors to consider when purchasing exercise equipment.

6 List several precautions for the use of hot tubs, saunas, and steambaths.

Exercise must be performed regularly throughout your life to achieve the benefits of physical fitness, wellness, and disease prevention. Fitness cannot be stored! If you stop exercising, you begin to lose fitness.

This chapter suggests strategies for the maintenance of a lifetime fitness program. We will also consider key factors in choosing an exercise facility or health club and will discuss issues important to being an informed fitness consumer.

Exercise Adherence: Lifetime Fitness

Studies have shown that over 60% of adults who start an exercise program quit within the first month (1). In contrast, people who start an exercise program and continue to exercise regularly for at least 6 months have an excellent chance of maintaining a regular exercise routine for years to come (1). Thus, the first 6 months of your exercise program are critical in determining your lifetime adherence to exercise. The significance of exercising regularly for several months is probably linked to the fact that 2 to 6 months of training are generally required to bring about significant improvements in both fitness and body composition (i.e., fat loss). This positive feedback, once achieved, provides a strong incentive to continue exercising.

Beginning a lifetime exercise program requires a strong personal commitment to physical fitness and application of the principles of behavior modification to change from a sedentary to an active lifestyle. In the next sections, we discuss several factors that will assist you in maintaining a lifetime commitment to physical activity.

Goal Setting for Active Lifestyles

Although the first step in beginning a successful exercise program is desiring to be physically fit, the second step is the establishment of both short- and long-term fitness goals (goal setting was introduced in Chapter 1 and discussed in detail in Chapter 3). Your goals should be based on your personal needs and desire for fitness, and they should be realistic. Goal setting provides a target to shoot for and adds an incentive to con-

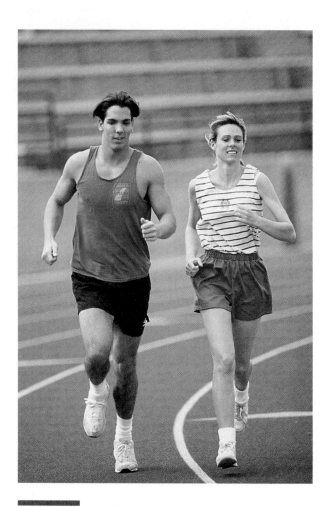

A strong personal commitment to exercise is required to adhere to a lifetime program of physical fitness.

tinue regular exercise habits. Goals can be either maintenance goals or improvement goals. For example, a realistic short-term improvement goal for cardiorespiratory fitness might be to decrease your 1.5-mile run time from 15 minutes to 14 minutes during your first 6 months of training. In contrast, a short-term maintenance goal might be to average running 20 miles per week during the first year of training. A key point to remember about fitness goals is that they should be modified from time to time to accommodate any changes in your fitness needs and to allow you to correct any unrealistic goals that you may have set.

Selecting Activities

Exercise should be fun! You should choose exercise activities that you enjoy. However, not all enjoyable physical activities will promote im-

Table 16.1

Fitness Evaluation of Various Activities and Sports

Sport/Activity	Fitness Ranking				
		Muscular Strength and Endurance			
	Cardiorespiratory Endurance	Upper Body	Lower Body	Flexibility	Caloric Expenditure (calories/min)
Aerobic dance	Good	Good	Good	Fair	5–10
Badminton	Fair	Fair	Good	Fair	5–10
Baseball	Poor	Fair	Fair	Fair	4–6
Basketball	Good	Fair	Good	Fair	10–12
Bowling	Poor	Fair	Poor	Fair	3–4
Canoeing	Fair	Good	Poor	Fair	4–10
Football (flag/touch)	Fair	Fair	Good	Fair	5–10
Golf (walking)	Poor	Fair	Good/fair	Fair	2–4
Gymnastics	Poor	Excellent	Excellent	Excellent	3–4
Handball	Good	Good/fair	Good	Fair	7–12
Karate	Fair	Good	Good	Excellent	7–10
Racquetball	Good/fair	Good/fair	Good	Fair	6–12
Running	Excellent	Fair	Good	Fair	8–15
Skating (ice)	Good/fair	Poor	Good/fair	Good/fair	5–10
Skating (roller)	Good/fair	Poor	Good/fair	Fair	5–10
Skiing (alpine)	Fair	Fair	Good	Fair	5–10
Skiing (nordic)	Excellent/good	Good	Good	Fair	7–15
Soccer	Good	Fair	Good	Good/fair	7–17
Tennis	Good/fair	Good/fair	Good	Fair	5–12
Volleyball	Fair	Fair	Good/fair	Fair	4–8
Waterskiing	Poor	Good	Good	Fair	4–7
Weight training	Poor	Excellent	Excellent	Fair	4–6

Source: From Getchell, B. *Physical fitness: A way of life.* Copyright © 1992. Reprinted by permission of Allyn & Bacon.

provement in health-related physical fitness. Which sport activities provide the best training effect to improve physical fitness? Table 16.1 evaluates the fitness potential of a variety of popular sports and activities. Note that no one activity is rated as being excellent in promoting all aspects of fitness. To achieve total physical fitness, you should participate in several.

Another key consideration is the availability and convenience of the activity. Regardless of how much you enjoy a particular activity, if it is not convenient, your chances of regular participa-

tion are greatly decreased. For example, suppose you enjoy swimming but the pool closest to your home or school is 10 miles away, and to make matters worse, the pool hours of operation conflict with your daily schedule. In combination, these two factors decrease your chances of using swimming as your primary mode of regular exercise. The solution to this problem is simple. Continue to swim when you have the opportunity but choose another convenient activity that you enjoy as your regular exercise mode. Remember, selecting a convenient and enjoyable activity will greatly increase your chances of maintaining a regular exercise program.

Planning Exercise Sessions

Exercise sessions should be systematic and workouts carefully planned (2, 3). This is particularly true during the first several weeks of an exercise program. To achieve your objectives, you must train on a regular basis.

Choosing a regular time to exercise helps to make it a habit. Some fitness instructors suggest that morning exercise is superior to exercise at other times of the day; however, there is no scientific evidence to support the notion that there is an optimal time of day to exercise. This is fortunate because individual preferences for a daily exercise time will vary. Some people prefer to exercise in the morning hours, whereas others may prefer a noon workout. Choose a time that works for you; the key to exercising regularly is to choose a convenient time to work out and stick with it.

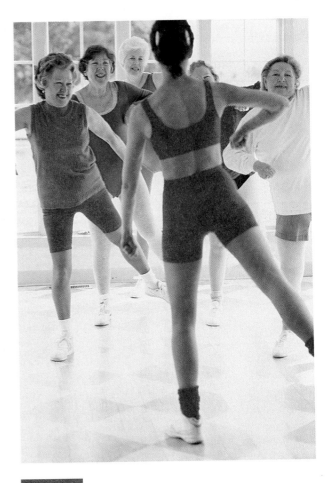

Aging may change your physical activity needs over the course of a lifetime.

Exercising with friends makes workouts more fun.

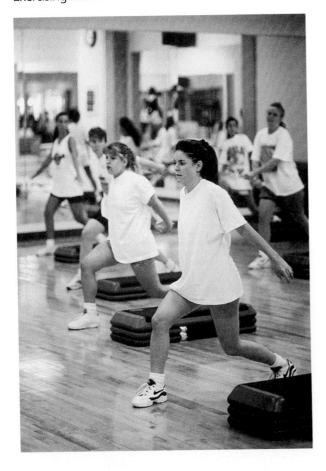

Monitoring Progress

Monitoring your exercise progress is an important factor in providing feedback and motivation to continue. You can monitor your progress in at least two ways. First, maintain a training log to provide feedback in terms of the amount of exercise performed. For example, a daily training log can assist you in monitoring the number of miles run, the amount of weight lifted, total calories expended during exercise, any changes in body weight, and so on. A number of commercially available training diaries and computer programs are available.

A second means of monitoring your fitness progress is through periodic fitness testing (see Chapter 2). Fitness testing provides positive feedback when fitness levels are improving. This type of information is a useful motivational tool and should be a part of every fitness program.

Social Support

Social support is another key factor in many successful exercise programs. Enjoying interaction with friends or colleagues during exercise or in the locker room before or after a workout is an important part of making exercise fun. Beginning an exercise program with a friend is an excellent way to start exercising on a regular basis, provided that both individuals share the same commitment to improving personal fitness.

Peers as Role Models

Your personal commitment to exercise can be positively influenced by peers who serve as good role models for the benefits of exercise. Most of us know individuals who exercise regularly and look terrific as a result of proper training and diet. These role models can be motivational to people who are beginning an exercise program.

Aging and Changing Physical Activity Needs

As we age, our needs and interest in physical activity often change. It is thus important to modify your fitness program throughout your life. For instance, while some people engage in a single game activity such as basketball over the course of several years, many people lose interest in repeating the same daily activity. When this occurs, it becomes important to find other activities that interest you. Many physical activity options exist, so individuals should remain flexible in their exercise habits and be willing to modify their programs as the need arises. Maintaining enthusiasm for exercise is the foundation of lifetime fitness.

Health Clubs: Choosing a Fitness Facility

Although it is not necessary to join a club, spa, or fitness salon to become physically fit, many people prefer exercising in the social atmosphere that a club may provide. However, before joining a fitness facility, there are several factors to consider (6):

1. Investigate programs offered throughout your community before deciding to join a health club. For example, many good and inexpensive programs are offered through your local YMCA or through a college or university.

2. When considering a club, check the club's reputation with the local Better Business Bureau before joining. Inquire about how long

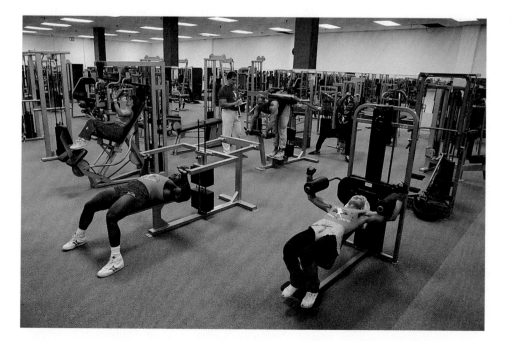

Examine the features of a health club carefully before joining.

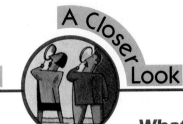

A Closer Look

16.1

What Is a Fitness Expert?

At present, there is no standard definition of a *fitness expert.* However, someone can be generally considered a fitness expert who has earned an advanced degree (such as an M.S. or Ph.D.) in exercise science, kinesiology, or exercise physiology from a reputable university. While individuals with bachelor's degrees in exercise science may have sufficient background to answer many fitness questions, the more advanced the degree earned, the more knowledgeable the individual should be about exercise and fitness. Exercise scientists who are actively performing research in exercise physiology and

are active in professional organizations (e.g., American Physiological Society, American College of Sports Medicine) are generally the best sources of valid information. Finally, physicians with postgraduate training in exercise physiology or a strong personal interest in preventive medicine are also good sources of scientifically based fitness information.

If you do not have a local fitness expert available, contact the American College of Sports Medicine (P.O. Box 1440, Indianapolis, IN 46206-1440) for the name of a fitness expert who can answer your questions.

they have been in business and if a large number of clients have registered complaints. Further, if you have access to an independent fitness expert (see A Closer Look 16.1), ask his or her advice about local fitness facilities.

3. Before joining any facility, arrange to make several trial visits. This will provide you with answers as to whether the locker room facilities are well maintained and clean, the exercise machines are in good working order, the club employees are well trained (see A Closer Look 16.1) and eager to answer your fitness-related questions, and the facility is overcrowded during the hours that you plan to use the club.

4. If you must sign a contract to join the club, examine the membership contract carefully. Resist signing a long-term contract; choose a "pay as you go" option if possible. If you sign a contract, read the fine print carefully. Be wary of contract clauses that waive the club's liability for injury to you or waive your right to defend yourself in court.

5. Avoid clubs that advertise overnight fitness or quick weight loss success. After reading the first eight chapters of this text you are already well aware that these types of claims must be false.

Diet and Fitness Products: Consumer Issues

The fitness boom in the United States has brought an explosion of fitness and diet books and magazines as well as huge numbers of companies that produce exercise equipment. Although some fitness books and magazines are written by experts, many are written by individuals with little formal training in exercise physiology. Unfortunately, books and articles written by nonexperts often convey misinformation, and some have created many exercise myths. Further, many exercise products are not useful in promoting physical fitness or weight loss. In the next several sections, we will discuss some key consumer issues related to exercise and weight loss.

Common Misconceptions about Physical Fitness

There are numerous misconceptions about exercise, weight loss, and physical fitness, and a book discussing them would require hundreds of pages of text. Although debunking all exercise myths is beyond the scope of this book, we can dispel some of the most common.

Yoga Supporters of yoga offer claims that its regular practice will improve fitness, assist in weight loss, and cure a host of diseases. Unfortunately, there is little evidence to support most of these claims (6). While yoga will improve flexibility and promote relaxation, many of the yoga positions may cause joint injury, particularly if performed improperly. In short, yoga is not a panacea and should not be a major portion of one's exercise prescription.

Hand Weights The popularity of hand-held weights has increased rapidly in the past several years. Some manufacturers claim that using hand weights will greatly increase arm and shoulder strength. Although carrying hand weights will increase the energy expenditure during exercise, 1- to 3-pound hand weights do not promote significant strength gains (particularly in college-age individuals).

Further, there are some concerns about the use of hand weights. First, gripping them may increase blood pressure (7). Individuals with high blood pressure should seek a physician's advice about the use of hand weights during exercise (5, 7). Further, hand weights may aggravate existing elbow or shoulder arthritis. Finally, some aerobics instructors have banned hand weights in large classes because of the potential danger of hitting someone with an outstretched hand.

Rubber Waist Belts and Spot Reduction
Recall that spot reduction of body fat is the concept of being able to lose body fat from a specific body location. Numerous myths exist concerning the spot reduction effects of such factors as wearing nylon suits or rubber waist bands, as well as exercise focused on a specific body area (e.g., sit-ups). The bottom line is that no method of spot reduction is effective in removing fat from a specific body area (see Chapter 8). Although exercise can assist in creating a negative caloric balance and therefore promote fat loss, the loss of fat is spread throughout the body and is not localized to one particular area.

Ergogenic Aids A drug or nutritional product that improves physical fitness and exercise performance is called an **ergogenic aid.** Numerous manufacturers market products that they claim promote strength and cardiovascular fitness. The popularity of these products usually stems from their reported use by champion ath-

letes, but the key concern for the consumer is whether ergogenic aids promote fitness.

There is limited scientific evidence to support the notion that nutritional ergogenic aids promote fitness or increase athletic performance in humans (see Nutritional Links to Health and Fitness 16.1 on page 340). However, both anabolic steroids and the drug Clenbuterol have proved to increase muscle mass in animals (8, 9). Although this may seem to be good news for people who want to increase their muscle mass, the bad news is that both drugs have been shown to be harmful to health. Recent evidence has shown that prolonged use of both drugs may result in serious organ damage and, in some cases, death (10, 11). See refs. 12 and 13 for reviews on these topics.

Exercise Equipment Many types of exercise equipment are available. Every week, magazine and television ads promote a "new" exercise device designed to trim waistlines and build huge muscles overnight. In truth, there are no "miracle" exercise devices capable of promoting such changes. In fact, there is really no need to buy any exercise devices to promote fitness. A well-rounded fitness program can be designed without exercise equipment. However, if you want to purchase exercise equipment for home use, buy from a reputable and well-established company (6). Beware of mail-order products and examine the product before you buy (6). When in doubt about the usefulness of an exercise product, consult a fitness expert.

Passive Exercise Devices A **passive exercise** machine is a motor-driven device designed to move or vibrate the body without any muscular activity. Passive exercise devices come in many forms, including rolling machines, vibrating belts, pillows, and passive motion tables. Manufacturers claim that passive exercise devices improve physical fitness and assist in weight loss. Unfortunately, there is no such thing as effortless exercise. Passive exercise devices do not improve physical fitness or promote weight loss (15).

---

ergogenic aid A drug or nutritional product that improves physical fitness and exercise performance.

passive exercise Movement performed on a motor-driven device designed to move or vibrate the body without any muscular activity. Passive exercise devices come in many forms, including rolling machines, vibrating belts, pillows, and passive motion tables. Passive exercise devices do not improve physical fitness or promote weight loss.

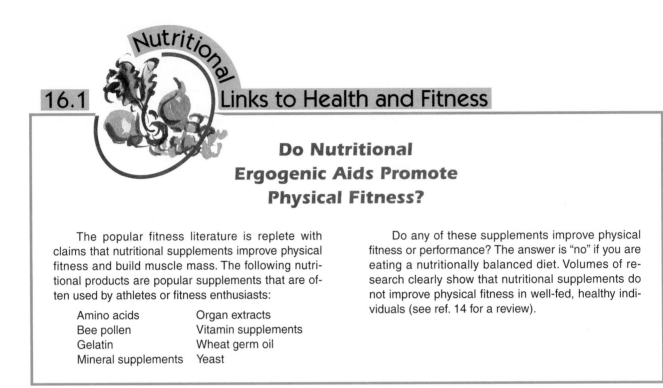

16.1 Nutritional Links to Health and Fitness

Do Nutritional Ergogenic Aids Promote Physical Fitness?

The popular fitness literature is replete with claims that nutritional supplements improve physical fitness and build muscle mass. The following nutritional products are popular supplements that are often used by athletes or fitness enthusiasts:

Amino acids	Organ extracts
Bee pollen	Vitamin supplements
Gelatin	Wheat germ oil
Mineral supplements	Yeast

Do any of these supplements improve physical fitness or performance? The answer is "no" if you are eating a nutritionally balanced diet. Volumes of research clearly show that nutritional supplements do not improve physical fitness in well-fed, healthy individuals (see ref. 14 for a review).

Hot Tubs, Saunas, and Steambaths Hot tubs, saunas, and steambaths are popular attractions at many health clubs. Although they may improve mental attitudes by promoting relaxation, none promotes fat loss or improves physical fitness. While water loss due to perspiration will reduce your body weight temporarily, it does not result in fat loss. Further, the weight will return as soon as you replace the lost fluids by eating and drinking.

There are also potential dangers in the use of saunas, steambaths, and hot tubs. One of the major problems is regulation of blood pressure. All of these forms of heat stress increase blood flow to the skin to promote cooling; this reduces blood return to the heart and may reduce brain blood flow, resulting in fainting. Therefore, when using a sauna, hot tub, or steambath, note the following precautions (6):

1. Seek a physician's advice before using hot baths if you suffer from heart disease, hypertension, diabetes, kidney disease, chronic skin problems, or if you are pregnant.

2. Don't use hot bath facilities when you are alone; if you develop a health problem, such as fainting, someone should be present to get emergency help.

3. Don't wear jewelry in hot baths (the metal will absorb heat and may burn the skin).

4. Don't drink alcohol prior to bathing because alcohol may increase your risk of fainting during heat exposure.

5. Don't exercise in a sauna, hot tub, or steam bath. The combination of exercise and a hot environment may result in overheating.

6. Do not enter a sauna, hot tub, or steambath immediately following vigorous exercise. Entering a steambath without cooling down after exercise increases your risk of fainting.

Having a championship physique does not make an individual a fitness expert.

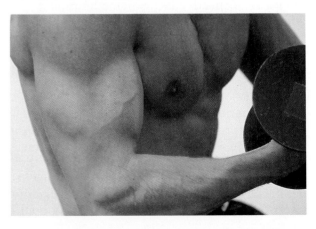

7. The duration of stay and recommended temperatures of saunas, steambaths, and hot tubs are as follows:

Sauna: Air temperature should not exceed 190°F (~88°C); stay in sauna should not exceed 15 minutes.

Steambath: Air temperature should not exceed 120°F (~38°C); stay in steambath should not exceed 10 minutes.

Hot tub (or whirlpool): Water temperature should not exceed 100°F (~38°C); stay in hot tub should not exceed 15 minutes.

Fitness Books and Magazines Book stores generally have numerous fitness-related publications on their shelves. Although many fitness books have been written by experts in the field of exercise science, others have been written by individuals with little or no formal training in exercise physiology. Dozens of fitness books and magazine articles have been written by models, movie stars, body builders, and even professional or Olympic athletes who have no academic training in exercise science. Clearly, having athletic talent or a good physique does not make an individual a fitness expert.

How do you evaluate the credibility of a fitness or weight control book? After reading and studying this book, you should be able to distinguish between fitness facts and fiction. For example, beware of texts that promise overnight results or quick, effortless weight loss. If you have doubts about the validity of a new fitness text, contact a local fitness expert for advice.

Summary

1. Exercise must be performed regularly throughout your life to achieve the benefits of physical fitness, wellness, and disease prevention.

2. Over 60% of the adults who start an exercise program quit within the first month. However, evidence exists that people who start an exercise program and continue to exercise for 6 months have an excellent chance of maintaining a regular fitness routine for years.

3. The following factors are important in maintaining a lifetime commitment to physical activity: goal setting, activity selection, regularity of exercise sessions, monitoring your progress, social support, peers as role models, and modifying your physical activity program as a result of aging.

4. Before choosing a health club, you should consider the following factors: Check the club's reputation with the local Better Business Bureau before joining; investigate programs offered throughout your community before deciding to join a particular club; before joining any facility, examine the membership contract carefully; in general, avoid clubs that advertise "overnight" fitness or weight loss success; and arrange to make several trial visits to the facility before joining. Several visits to the facility will provide you with answers regarding whether the locker room facilities are well maintained and clean, the exercise machines are in good working order, the club employees are well trained and eager to answer your fitness-related questions, and the facility is not overcrowded during the hours that you plan to use the club.

5. There is no standard definition of a *fitness expert*. However, someone can generally be considered a fitness expert if they have earned an advanced degree in exercise science, kinesiology, or exercise physiology.

6. Numerous exercise misconceptions exist. After studying this book you should be able to distinguish between fact and fiction. If you have doubts about the validity of a new fitness product or textbook, contact a local fitness expert for advice.

Study Questions

1. Outline the key factors that play a role in maintaining a regular program of exercise.

2. List five points to consider when choosing a health club.

3. Give your definition of a *fitness expert.*

4. Numerous exercise misconceptions exist. Discuss the misconceptions associated with yoga, the use of hand weights, the use of rubber weight belts to lose body fat, and nutritional ergogenic aids.

5. What factors should be considered when purchasing exercise equipment?

6. List several precautions that should be considered when using hot tubs, saunas, or steambaths.

7. Do passive exercise devices promote physical fitness and weight loss? Explain your answer.

8. What percentage of people who start an exercise program quit within the first month?

9. Discuss the importance of activity selection in maintaining physical fitness.

10. List five activities that are considered to be good or excellent modes of promoting cardiorespiratory fitness.

Suggested Reading

Howley, E., and B. D. Franks. *Health fitness: Instructors handbook.* Human Kinetics, Champaign, IL, 1997.

Margen S., et al., eds. *The wellness encyclopedia.* Houghton Mifflin, Boston, 1992.

Suggested Readings on the World Wide Web

Sympatico:
(http://www.ns.sympatico.ca/healthyway)
Articles about fitness, health, book reviews, and links to nutrition, fitness, and wellness topics.

International Association of Fitness Professionals-IDEA
(http://www.fit.org/idea/index.html)

Provides education, professional development for fitness instructors, personal trainers, and business owners on exercise training and development of healthy lifestyle programs.

American Council on Exercise (ACE)
(http://www.acefitness.org/)
A nonprofit organization that provides information on the certification of fitness professionals, plus education.

References

1. Dishman, R., ed. *Exercise adherence: Its impact on public health.* Human Kinetics, Champaign, IL, 1988.

2. Getchell, B. *Physical fitness: A way of life.* Allyn and Bacon, Needham Heights, MA, 1997.

3. Howley, E., and B. D. Franks. *Health fitness: Instructors handbook.* Human Kinetics, Champaign, IL, 1997.

4. McArdle, W., F. Katch, and V. Katch. *Exercise physiology.* Lea and Febiger, Philadelphia, 1991.

4a. McGlynn, G. *Dynamics of fitness: A practical approach.* Wm. C. Brown, Dubuque, IA, 1996.

5. Pollock, M., and J. Wilmore. *Exercise in health and disease.* W. B. Saunders, Philadelphia, 1990.

6. Corbin, C., and R. Lindsey. *Concepts of physical fitness.* Brown and Benchmark, Dubuque, IA, 1997.

7. Graves, J., M. Pollock, S. Montain, A. Jackson, and J. O'Keefe. The effect of hand-held weights on the physiological response to walking exercise. *Medicine and Science in Sports and Exercise* 19:260–265, 1987.

8. Criswell, D., S. Powers, and R. Herb. Clenbuterol-induced fiber type transition in the soleus of adult rats. 1995. (*In review*)

9. Heitzman, R. The effectiveness of anabolic agents in increasing rate of growth in farm animals; report on experiments in cattle. In: Lu F., and J. Rendell, eds. *Anabolic agents in animal production.* George Thieme, Stuttgart, Germany, 1976, pp. 89–98.

10. Palmer, R., M. Delday, D. McMillan, B. Noble, P. Bain, and C. Maltin. Effects of the cyclo-oxygenase inhibitor, fenbufen, on clenbuterol-induced hypertrophy of cardiac and skeletal muscle of rats. *British Journal of Pharmacology* 101:835–838, 1990.

11. Taylor, W., S. Snowball, C. Dickson, and M. Lesna. Alterations in liver architecture in mice treated with anabolic androgens and dimethylnitrosamine. *NATO Advanced Study Institute Series, Series A* 52:279–288, 1982.

12. Powers, S., and E. Howley. *Exercise physiology: Theory and application to fitness and performance.* Wm. C. Brown, Dubuque, IA, 1997.

13. Lamb, D., and M. Williams. *Ergogenics: Enhancement of performance in exercise and sport.* Vol. 4. Brown and Benchmark, Madison, WI, 1991.

14. Clarkson, P. Vitamins and trace minerals. In: Lamb D., and M. Williams, eds. *Ergogenics.* Brown and Benchmark, Madison, WI, 1991, pp. 123–175.

15. Martin, A. D., and G. Kauwell. Continuous assistive-passive exercise and cycle ergometer training in sedentary women. *Medicine and Science in Sports and Exercise* 22:523–527, 1990.

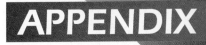

Nutritional Content of Foods, Beverages, and Fast Food Items

Part One:

Nutritional Content of Common Foods*

This food composition table has been prepared for Allyn and Bacon Publishers and is copyrighted by DINE Systems, Inc., the developer and publisher of the DINE System family of nutrition software for personal computers. The values in this food composition table were derived from the USDA Nutrient Data Base for Standard Reference Release 10 and nutrient composition information from over 300 food companies. Nutrient values used for each food were determined by collapsing similar foods into one food, using the median nutrient values. In the food composition table, foods are listed within the following eight groups. The eight groups are, in order: fruits, vegetables, beverages, alcoholic beverages, grains, dairy, fats/sweets/other, and protein foods. Further information can be obtained from:

DINE Systems, Inc.
586 N. French Road
Amherst, NY 14228
(716) 688-2492
FAX (716) 688-2502

*© 1994, DINE Systems, Inc., 586 N. French Rd., Amherst, NY 14228

Nutritional Content of Common Foods NOTE: Carbohydrate value does not include Added Sugar value.

	Amount	Weight	Calories	Protein g	Total Fat g	Sat Fat g	Carb. g	Added Sugar g	Fiber g	Chol. mg	Sodium mg	Calcium mg	Iron mg
Grains													
Bagel	1 bagel	68 g	175	7	10.22	0.22	32.5	2.25	1.5	0	325	20	1.8
Barley-cooked	1/2 cup	81 g	84	2.25	0.11	0	18.5	0	2.5	0	3	11	0.5
Biscuit	1 biscuit	30 g	100	2	3.78	1.22	13.5	0	0.5	2	262	47	0.7
Bread or roll-wheat	1 slice, 1 roll	27 g	65	2	0.89	0.22	10	2	1.4	0	106	20	0.7
Bread or roll-white	1 slice, 1 roll	28 g	70	2.75	1.11	0.33	11	2	0.5	0	132	20	0.7
Bread-mixed grain	1 slice	25 g	65	2	0.89	0.22	9.75	2.25	1.4	0	106	27	0.8
Bread-oatmeal	1 slice	37 g	90	4	1.78	0.33	10.5	4	1.5	0	140	40	1.1
Bread-pita, wheat	1 pita	57 g	145	5.5	0.89	0.22	28.5	0.5	4.1	0	360	50	1.4
Bread-pita, white	1 pita	57 g	160	6	1	0.22	30	1	1.1	0	300	80	0.7
Bread-raisin	1 slice	26 g	70	2	1	0.33	8.25	3	0.9	0	85	20	0.7
Bread-rye, pumpernickel	1 slice	30 g	80	2.75	0.89	0.11	13	1	1.1	0	185	22	1.1
Bread-wheat	1 slice	28 g	82	3	1	0.33	11.38	2	1.8	0	158.5	22.5	1
Bread-wheat, diet	1 slice	23 g	40	2.5	0.56	0.11	4.25	2	2	0	120	40	0.7
Bread-white	1 slice	27 g	67	2	1	0.22	11	1	0.7	0	135	21	0.7
Bread-white, diet	1 slice	23 g	40	3	0	0	6	1	2	0	110	40	0.7
Bread-whole wheat	1 slice	28 g	69	2.63	1.22	0.17	13	1.38	2	0	127	20	0.9
Breadsticks	1/3 large, 2 small	11 g	36	1.25	0.78	0.22	6	0.5	0.6	0	72	0	0.2
Bulgur	1/2 cup	67 g	113	4.25	0.22	0	23.5	0	3	0	3	13	3.7
Cake-nonfat	1 piece	56 g	140	3	0	0	32	15.5	1.2	0	170	0	0
Cereal-bran, fiber	1/3 cup	23 g	62	2	0.78	0.22	7.75	2.75	3.8	0	113	13	3
Cereal-granola	1/4 cup	28 g	130	3	4.89	0.89	13.5	4.5	1.7	0	55	19	0.9
Cereal-granola, fat free	1/4 cup	28 g	90	2	0	0	21	0.25	2.5	0	20	0	0.4
Cereal-oat flakes	1 cup	46 g	182	5	1.78	0.44	24.75	4.5	3.2	0	115	32	5.8
Cereal-other, cold	1 cup	29 g	110	2	0.22	0.11	19.5	3	0.6	0	226	4	1.8
Cereal-other, hot	2/3 cup	156 g	100	3	0	0	22		0.7	0	54	18	1.1
Cereal-sweetened	1 cup	29 g	120	1.25	1	0.44	13	13	0.5	0	210	0	4.5
Cereal-whole grain	3/4 cup	28 g	105	3	0.78	0.22	19	0.25	2.3	0	160	8	1.4
Cheese ravioli w/sauce	1 cup, 6 pieces	263 g	314	13	10.83	6.11	45.13	0.25	3.4	30	733	139	2
Cornbread, hushpuppies	1 square, 3 hushpuppies	51 g	166	3	5.33	1.78	25.75	0	1.6	42	421	87	0.8
Couscous	2/3 cup	108 g	120	4	0	0	26	0	4.3	0	5	0	0.7
Cracker sandwiches	2 large, 5 small	14 g	70	1.75	3.11	1.11	7.75	0.75	0.2	1	135	20	0.4
Crackers	5 crackers	14 g	60	1	2	0.44	8.75	0.75	0.4	0	120	0	0.5
Crackers-butter type	5 large, 10 small	14 g	70	1	3.56	1.11	8	0.25	0.2	1	193	4	0.4
Crackers-crispbread	1 large, 2 small	13 g	40	1	0.89	0.33	8.5	0	1.6	0	112	0	0.5
Crackers-lowfat	2 large, 5 small	14 g	60	2.25	2.33	0.33	10	0	0.6	0	100	0	0.4
Crackers-wheat	4 crackers	18 g	70	1	2.22	0.44	8	0.5	1.5	0	75	0	0.4
Croissants	1 croissant	72 g	310	7	19	11.22	27	6	2	0	240	38	1.8

© 1994, DINE Systems, Inc., 586 N. French Rd., Amherst, NY 14228

APPENDIX PART ONE (continued)

	Amount	Weight	Calories	Protein g	Total Fat g	Sat Fat g	Carb. g	Added Sugar g	Fiber g	Chol. mg	Sodium mg	Calcium mg	Iron mg
Croutons	4 tablespoons	10 g	46	1	1.78	0.44	6.25	0.25	0.3	0	124	6	0.3
English muffin	1 muffin	56 g	130	5	0.89	0.33	25	1.5	1.6	0	280	96	1.7
French toast	1 slice	59 g	151	4.25	7.33	1.89	16.25	3.5	0.5	48	277	48	1.1
Fried rice	1/2 cup	99 g	165	4	5.56	1	18.25	0.75	0.6	14	484	14	1.1
Grits	1/2 cup	124 g	73	1.5	0.11	0	16	0	0.3	0	136	0	0.8
Lasagna-meat	1 serving	308 g	350	27.5	23.11	6	31	1.5	2.6	73	1040	275	2.1
Lasagna-vegetable	1 serving	326 g	315	22	12	5.89	27	0.5	4.6	40	970	350	2.3
Macaroni	1/2 cup	66 g	95	3.25	0.33	0.11	19	0	0.9	0	4	5	0.9
Macaroni and cheese	1/2 cup	126 g	191	6	8.56	2.67	22.75	0	1.4	18	434	71	1.2
Macaroni-whole wheat	1 cup	150 g	202	8	1.11	0.22	39	0	7.4	0	10	20	4.5
Matzo or melba toast	1 matzo, 5 melba	19 g	100	3.25	0.56	0.11	22.25	0	0.9	0	6	4	0.9
Meat ravioli with sauce	1 cup, 6 pieces	227 g	324	13	8.33	2.89	46.75	0.75	3.1	20	878	54	2.1
Muffins	1 muffin	77 g	240	4.5	8.5	1.67	40	9	2	24.5	310	96.5	1.4
Muffins-fat free	1 muffin	66 g	165	3	0.17	0	38	10.63	1	0	175	60	0.7
Noodles-chow mein	1/2 cup	25 g	130	3	6.44	1.11	14.5	0	0.5	2	228	4	0.8
Noodles-egg	1/2 cup	160 g	106.5	3.75	1.17	0.22	19.88	0	0.9	26.5	69	9.5	1.3
Noodles-egg, macaroni	1 cup	145 g	190	7	0.56	0.11	37	0	1.1	0	30	14	2.1
Oatmeal-flavored	1 packet	38 g	140	4	2.22	0.44	18	8.25	2.4	0	181	100	4.5
Oatmeal-plain	2/3 cup cooked	176 g	109	4	1.78	0.33	18.25	0	3.3	0	1	15	1.9
Pancakes	1 pancake	38 g	73	2	1.22	0.44	11	1.25	0.5	7	239	50	0.6
Pasta w/parmesan cheese	1/2 cup	134 g	252	6.5	14.67	6.33	22.5	0	1.1	38	479	78	1.5
Rice cake	1 large cake	8 g	35	0.75	0	0	7.5	0	0.3	0	13	0	0
Rice-brown	1/2 cup	97 g	115	2.5	0.67	0.22	25	0	1.8	0	2	12	0.5
Rice-long grain & wild, mix	1/2 cup	88 g	137	3	2	0.56	23	2	0.9	0	579	11	1.1
Rice-seasoned	1/2 cup	107 g	150	3.5	3.78	1.67	23	1	1	5	700	13	1.2
Rice-white	1/2 cup	91 g	92	2	0	0	20.5	0	0.5	0	225	10	0.7
Roll-hamburger/hotdog, wheat	1 roll	43 g	114	4	1.11	0.22	21.25	0.75	2.5	0	242	46	1
Roll-hamburger/hotdog, white	1 roll	43 g	138	3.25	2.44	0.67	22.5	2	1.4	0	271	67	1.3
Roll-hoagie, sub	1 roll	135 g	400	11	7.11	1.78	68.5	4	1.8	0	684	100	3.8
Roll-wheat	1 roll	28 g	77	2.5	1.78	0.44	11.5	1.5	1.1	0	96	50	1
Roll-white	1 roll	34 g	105	3.25	1.67	0.44	16.25	1.75	0.6	0	148	28	1
Salad-pasta	1/2 cup	87 g	250	4	16	3.33	20.75	0	0.7	28	410	40	0.7
Spaghetti	1 cup	128 g	200	7.5	1	0.22	40.5	0	1.1	0	19	14	2
Spaghetti w/meatballs	1 cup	261 g	307	12	10.56	3.89	37	0	2.7	34	1220	53	3.3
Spaghetti-whole wheat	1 cup	144 g	200	9	1.11	0.22	39.5	0	5.8	0	10	20	2.7
Stuffing	1/2 cup	93 g	210	4.5	12.67	3	17.5	2.5	0.5	22	578	40	1.1
Taboule	1/2 cup	80 g	170	3	8.67	1.33	20	0	1.6	0	290	0	0.7

© 1994, DINE Systems, Inc., 586 N. French Rd., Amherst, NY 14228

	Amount	Weight	Calories	Protein g	Total Fat g	Sat Fat g	Carb. g	Added Sugar g	Fiber g	Chol. mg	Sodium mg	Calcium mg	Iron mg
Grains (continued)													
Taco shell	1 shell	11 g	50	0	2	1.11	8	0	0.2	0	5	0	0
Tortilla	1 tortilla	30 g	65	2	1	0.11	12	0	0.9	0	1	42	0.6
Waffles	1 waffle	39 g	110	3	4.33	0.89	13	1.75	0.8	3	279	75	1.8
Vegetables													
Artichokes	1/2 cup, 1/2 vegetable	75 g	36	2	0.11	0	7.25	0	2.6	0	42	17	0.8
Asparagus	6 spears, 1/2 cup	90 g	24	1.75	0.33	0.11	3.75	0	1.5	0	4	22	0.6
Asparagus-canned	1/2 cup	122 g	21	1.5	0.33	0.11	2.75	0	1.9	0	425	17	1.5
Bamboo shoots	1/4 cup	30 g	4	0.25	0	0	0.5	0	0.3	0	1	4	0.1
Bamboo shoots-canned	1/4 cup	33 g	6	0.5	0.11	0	1	0	0.6	0	2	1	0.1
Bean sprouts	1/2 cup	59 g	16	1.25	0	0	2.75	0	2.2	0	3	7	0.5
Bean sprouts-canned	1/2 cup	62 g	8	0.75	0	0	1.25	0	2.3	0	149	9	0.3
Beets-canned	1/2 cup	123 g	36	0.75	0	0	8	0	2.9	0	324	17	0.8
Beets-pickled	1/2 cup	119 g	82	0.75	0	0	8.5	11.25	2.8	0	250	13	0.5
Beets-raw, cooked	1/2 cup	99 g	31	0.75	0	0	6.75	0	2.5	0	49	11	0.6
Bok choy-chinese cabbage	1/2 cup	35 g	5	0.25	0	0	0.75	0	0.6	0	23	37	0.3
Broccoli-cooked	1/2 cup, 2 spear	85 g	24	1.75	0.11	0	4.25	0	2.5	0	15	68	0.8
Broccoli-raw	1/2 cup	44 g	12	0.75	0.11	0	2	0	1.5	0	12	21	0.4
Brussels sprouts	1/2 cup, 4 sprouts	78 g	32	1.5	0.33	0.11	5.75	0	2.4	0	18	24	0.8
Cabbage-raw or cooked	1/4 cup cooked, 1/2 cup raw	36 g	9	0.25	0	0	1.75	0	1	0	7	13	0.2
Carrots-canned	1/2 cup	73 g	17	0.25	0.11	0	3.75	0	2.7	0	176	19	0.5
Carrots-raw or cooked	1/2 cup, 6 sticks	69 g	26	0.5	0	0	5.75	0	2.2	0	43	21	0.4
Cauliflower-raw or cooked	1/2 cup	67 g	15	0.75	0.11	0	2.5	0	1.3	0	7	15	0.3
Celery-raw or cooked	1/2 cup, 6 sticks	68 g	10	0.25	0	0	2.25	0	1.4	0	51	25	0.2
Chef salad	1 cup	137 g	25	2.5	0.17	0	4	0	2	0	23.5	30.5	0.5
Coleslaw	1/2 cup	92 g	154	0.5	14.44	2.67	4.25	1	1.5	7	287	32	0.4
Corn	1 ear, 1/2 cup	86 g	80	1.75	0.33	0.11	17.5	0	4.6	0	4	2	0.5
Corn-canned	1/2 cup	120 g	83	1.5	0.44	0	13	5.5	4.7	0	324	5	0.4
Cucumber	1/2 cup	52 g	7	0.25	0	0	1.5	0	0.7	0	1	7	0.1
Eggplant	1/2 cup	48 g	13	0.25	0	0	3	0	1	0	2	3	0.2
French fries	1 regular, 1-1/4 cup	85.1 g	241	3	12.72	3.89	29.5	0	2.8	0	129.5	0	1
Fried vegetables/onions	1/2 cup, 6 onion rings	68 g	180	2	10.78	2.67	15.5	0	1	0	150	12	0.7

346

	Amount	Weight	Calories	Protein g	Total Fat g	Sat Fat g	Carb. g	Added Sugar g	Fiber g	Chol. mg	Sodium mg	Calcium mg	Iron mg
Green beans-canned	1/2 cup	68 g	13	0.75	0	0	2.5	0	1.5	0	170	18	0.6
Green beans-raw or cooked	1/2 cup	68 g	20	1	0	0	4	0	1.8	0	3	30	0.7
Greens-collard & mustard	1/2 cup	73 g	16	1.75	0.22	0	3.75	0	1.4	0	15	64	0.7
Greens-mustard, turnip, cooked	1/2 cup	75 g	15	1	0.11	0	2.5	0	1.4	0	16	87	0.7
Greens-mustard, turnip, raw	1/2 cup	28 g	7	0.5	0	0	1.5	0	0.9	0	9	41	0.4
Greens-turnip, canned	1/2 cup	117 g	17	1	0.22	0.11	2.5	0	2.2	0	325	138	1.8
Kale-raw or cooked	1/2 cup	55 g	20	0.75	0.11	0	3	0	1.7	0	15	47	0.6
Lettuce-endive	1/2 cup	25 g	4	0.25	0	0	0.75	0	0.7	0	6	13	0.2
Lettuce-iceberg	1 cup	55 g	7	0.5	0	0	1.25	0	0.6	0	5	11	0.3
Mixed vegetables-canned	1/2 cup	82 g	39	1.25	0.11	0	8	0	3.5	0	122	22	0.9
Mixed vegetables-frozen	1/2 cup	81 g	22	0.75	0	0	4.5	0	2	0	22	27	0.6
Mushrooms-canned	1/2 cup	78 g	19	1	0.11	0	3.25	0	1.1	0	178	1	0.6
Mushrooms-fresh, cooked	1/2 cup	96 g	25	1.75	0.11	0	4.25	0	1.5	0	1	7	1.7
Mushrooms-raw	1/2 cup	35 g	9	0.5	0	0	1.5	0	0.6	0	1	2	0.4
Okra	1/2 cup	81 g	26	1	0.11	0	5.5	0	2.1	0	5	55	0.5
Onions	1/2 cup	71 g	29	0.5	0.11	0	6.25	0	1.4	0	8	20	0.3
Parsnips	1/2 cup, 1/2 vegetable	79 g	64	0.75	0.11	0	14.75	0	3.2	0	8	30	0.5
Peas-green	1/2 cup	85 g	63	3.75	0.11	0	11.5	0	3.5	0	70	19	1.2
Peas-green, canned	1/2 cup	85 g	59	3.25	0.11	0	8	2.75	5.3	0	186	17	0.8
Peas-snowpeas	1/2 cup	79 g	35	2.25	0.11	0	5.75	0	3.4	0	4	37	1.6
Peppers-hot	2 tablespoons	19 g	8	0.25	0	0	1.5	0	0.2	0	1	3	0.2
Peppers-sweet, green	1/2 cup, 1/2 vegetable	56 g	12	0.25	0.11	0	2.25	0	0.6	0	2	3	0.6
Peppers-sweet, red	1/2 cup	50 g	12	0.25	0.11	0	2.25	0	0.8	0	2	3	0.6
Potato skins-cheese, bacon	2 halves	96 g	302	11	15.89	7.44	27.5	0	1.4	34	267	225	4.5
Potato-baked/boiled	1/2 baked, 1/2 cup	78 g	73	1.5	0.11	0	16.75	0	1.4	0	4	6	0.3
Potatoes-mashed	1/2 cup	107 g	118	1.5	4.56	1.44	17	0	1.8	4	340	40	0.3
Radishes	2 radishes	9 g	2	0	0	0	0.25	0	0.1	0	2	2	0
Romaine lettuce	1 cup	53 g	9	1	0.11	0	1.25	0	1.3	0	4	19	0.6
Rutabaga	1/2 cup	103 g	35	0.75	0.11	0	7.5	0	2.1	0	19	43	0.5
Salad-potato	1/2 cup	121 g	153	3	7.78	1.89	15	1.5	1.9	47	512	19	0.5
Salad-three bean	1/2 cup	121 g	80	2	0	0	16.25	1.75	5	0	540	20	3.6
Salsa	1/4 cup	57 g	32	0.75	0	0	4	0	0.9	0	680	0	0
Sauerkraut	1/2 cup	118 g	22	0.75	0.11	0	4.5	0	4.1	0	780	36	1.7

	Amount	Weight	Calories	Protein g	Total Fat g	Sat Fat g	Carb. g	Added Sugar g	Fiber g	Chol. mg	Sodium mg	Calcium mg	Iron mg
Vegetables (continued)													
Soup-vegetable	1 cup	251 g	81	2	1.56	0.44	11.25	2.25	0.5	2	892	16	1
Spaghetti sauce	1/2 cup	117 g	118	2	5	0.89	12.75	1.5	3.3	0	589	20	1.1
Spaghetti sauce w/ meat	1/2 cup	104 g	80	2	3.11	0.67	12.5	2	3.3	2	630	20	1.1
Spinach-canned	1/2 cup	107 g	25	1.75	0.33	0.11	3.25	0	3.9	0	29	135	2.5
Spinach-fresh, cooked	1/2 cup	93 g	24	1.75	0.11	0	3.75	0	3	0	73	131	1.7
Spinach-raw	1/2 cup	28 g	6	0.5	0	0	0.75	0	1.1	0	22	28	0.8
Squash-summer	1/2 cup	96 g	18	0.5	0.11	0	3.75	0	1.5	0	3	22	0.4
Squash-winter	1/2 cup	109 g	41	0.75	0.11	0	9.5	0	3	0	4	23	0.6
Squash-zucchini-fresh, cooked	1 cup raw, 1/2 cup cooked	112 g	18	0.75	0	0	3.5	0	1.4	0	2	19	0.5
Sweet potato	1/2 cup	154 g	98	1.25	0	0	23	0	4	0	11	30	0.5
Sweet potato-candied	1/2 cup	114 g	190	1	0	0	26.5	20	4.4	0	60	20	0.7
Tomatoes-canned or stewed	1/2 cup	121 g	34	0.75	0.11	0	6.5	0.25	2.4	0	305	33	0.7
Tomatoes-raw	1/2 cup, 4 slices	86 g	17	0.5	0.11	0	3.5	0	1.3	0	8	6	0.5
Vegetable juice	3/4 cup	182 g	35	1	0	0	8	0	1	0	650	20	0.7
Waterchestnuts-canned	1/2 cup	70 g	34	0.25	0	0	8.25	0	1.5	0	3	3	0.3
Waterchestnuts-raw	1/2 cup	62 g	66	0.75	0	0	15.75	0	1.4	0	9	7	0.4
Watercress-raw	1/2 cup	17 g	2	0.25	0	0	0.25	0	0.2	0	7	20	0
Wax beans	1/2 cup	68 g	18	1	0.11	0	4.25	0	1.5	0	6	27	0.6
Yams	1/2 cup	70 g	69	1.25	0.11	0	16.75	0	1.8	0	7	8	0.3
Fruits													
Apple cider	3/4 cup	186 g	94	0	0.11	0	17	6	0.1	0	6	7	0.4
Apples-sweetened	1/2 cup	102 g	68	0	0.11	0	12.5	3.25	2	0	4	4	0.3
Apples-unsweetened	1 fruit, 1/2 cup	133 g	77	0.25	0.44	0.11	20	0	2.1	0	0	8	0.2
Applesauce-sweetened	1/2 cup	128 g	97	0.25	0	0	12	11	1.8	0	4	4	0.4
Applesauce-unsweetened	1/2 cup	122 g	53	0.25	0	0	12.5	0	2.5	0	2	4	0.2
Apricots-sweetened	1 fruit	80 g	65	0.5	0	0	3.75	10.75	1.1	0	3	8	0.4
Apricots-unsweetened	1 fruit, 2 canned	35 g	17	0.5	0.11	0	4	0	0.8	0	0	5	0.2
Avocados	1/2 fruit, 1/2 cup	113 g	166	2	14.22	2.56	7.25	0	2.7	0	10	12	1
Banana	1 fruit, 1/2 cup	114 g	105	1	0.33	0.22	24	0	2.3	0	1	7	0.4
Blueberries-sweetened	1/2 cup	122 g	103	0.5	0.11	0	8.5	16.25	2.3	0	3	7	0.4
Blueberries-unsweetened	1/2 cup	75 g	41	0.5	0.22	0	9	0	1.7	0	2	5	0.2
Cherries-sweetened	1/2 cup	128 g	106	0.75	0	0	12.25	13	0.9	0	4	13	0.4
Cherries-unsweetened	10 fruits, 1/2 cup	93 g	44	0.75	0	0	10	0	0.9	0	2	12	0.4

© 1994, DINE Systems, Inc., 586 N. French Rd., Amherst, NY 14228

	Amount	Weight	Calories	Protein g	Total Fat g	Sat Fat g	Carb. g	Added Sugar g	Fiber g	Chol. mg	Sodium mg	Calcium mg	Iron mg
Dates	5 fruits, 1/4 cup	43 g	118	0.75	0.22	0.11	28.5	0	3.7	0	1	14	0.5
Dried fruit	1/4 cup, 8 pieces	32 g	92	1	0	0	21.75	0	2.4	0	9	11	0.7
Figs-sweetened	2 fruit	57 g	45	0.25	0	0	7	3.75	1.3	0	1	15	0.2
Figs-unsweetened	4 fruit, 1/2 cup	67 g	144	1.63	0.61	0.11	37	0	6.4	0	4	74.5	1
Fruit cocktail	1/2 cup	125 g	56	0.5	0.11	0	14.5	2.5	1.4	0	6.5	8	0.4
Fruit cocktail-sweetened	1/2 cup	127 g	83	0.5	0	0	8.75	11	1.4	0	8	8	0.3
Fruit cocktail-unsweetened	1/2 cup	123 g	50	0.5	0	0	11.5	0	1.4	0	4	6	0.3
Grapefruit-sweetened	1/2 cup	127 g	76	0.5	0	0	10	8	0.5	0	2	18	0.5
Grapefruit-unsweetened	1/2 fruit, 1/2 cup	120 g	39	0.5	0	0	9	8	0.7	0	0	14	0.2
Grapes-sweetened	1/2 cup	128 g	94	0.5	0	0	10.5	12	0.5	0	7	12	1.2
Grapes-unsweetened	20 fruits, 1/2 cup	84 g	48	0.5	0	0	11.5	0	0.5	0	2	8	0.2
Guava	1 fruit	90 g	45	0.5	0.33	0	9.5	0	5	0	2	18	0.3
Juice-unsweetened	3/4 cup	186 g	90	0.5	0	0	22.5	0	0.2	0	8	16	0.5
Kiwi fruit	1 fruit	76 g	46	0.75	0.33	0.11	10	0	2.1	0	4	20	0.3
Mango	1/2 fruit, 1/2 cup	93 g	61	0.5	0.11	0	14.25	0	1.8	0	2	9	0.2
Melon	1/2 cup	97 g	30	0.5	0	0	7	0	0.7	0	9	8	0.2
Nectarines	1 fruit	137 g	68	1	0.56	0	14.5	0	3.3	0	0	6	0.2
Olives	3 olives	12 g	15	0.25	1.56	0.22	0.25	0	0.3	0	234	8	0.2
Orange	1 fruit, 1/2 cup	134 g	63	1	0	0	14	0	3.9	0	1	53	0.2
Papaya	1/2 fruit, 1/2 cup	146 g	56	0.75	0	0	12.75	0	1.8	0	4	35	0.2
Peaches-sweetened	1/2 cup	125 g	94	0.5	0	0	5.25	17	1.2	0	8	3	0.4
Peaches-unsweetened	1 fruit, 1/2 cup	113 g	44	0.5	0	0	10.75	0	1.3	0	3	5	0.1
Pears-sweetened	2 halves	158 g	103	0.5	0	0	6	18.5	3.2	0	8	8	0.4
Pears-unsweetened	1 fruit, 1/2 cup	136 g	98	0.75	0	0	25	0	4.3	0	0	18	0.4
Pineapple-sweetened	2 slices, 1/2 cup	120 g	93	0.5	0	0	7.5	15	0.9	0	2	15	0.4
Pineapple-unsweetened	2 slice, 1/2 cup	108 g	70	0.25	0	0	17.5	0	0.9	0	2	6	0.4
Plums-sweetened	2 plums	89 g	67	0.5	0.11	0	8	7.75	0.7	0	17	9	0.7
Plums-unsweetened	1 raw, 2 canned	69 g	37	0.5	0.33	0	8.25	0	0.9	0	1	5	0.2
Prunes-cooked	1/2 cup, 7 fruits	123 g	136	1.25	0.44	0	32	0	4.9	0	3	29	1.4
Prunes-dried	1/2 cup	74 g	209	2	0.11	0	49.25	0	6.8	0	4	45	2.1
Pumpkin-canned	1/2 cup	122 g	41	0.75	0.11	0.11	8.75	0	3.5	0	6	32	1.7
Raisins	1/4 cup	38 g	109	1	0	0	26	0	2.5	0	5	19	0.8
Raspberries-sweetened	1/2 cup	132 g	117	0.75	0.11	0	12	18.25	4.2	0	0	19	0.5
Raspberries-unsweetened	1/2 cup	62 g	30	0.5	0.22	0	6.5	0	3	0	0	14	0.3
Strawberries-sweetened	1/2 cup	133 g	100	0.5	0.11	0	9	15	2	0	4	14	0.6
Strawberries-unsweetened	1/2 cup	74 g	24	0.5	0.22	0	5.5	0	1.6	0	2	11	0.5
Tangerines-sweetened	1/2 cup	126 g	76	0.5	0	0	10	8.5	0.9	0	8	9	0.4
Tangerines-unsweetened	1 fruit, 1/2 cup	102 g	43	0.5	0	0	9.75	0	0.9	0	2	14	0.1
Watermelon	1/2 cup	80 g	25	0.5	0.22	0.22	5	0	0.3	0	2	6	0.2

© 1994, DINE Systems, Inc., 586 N. French Rd., Amherst, NY 14228

	Amount	Weight	Calories	Protein g	Total Fat g	Sat Fat g	Carb. g	Added Sugar g	Fiber g	Chol. mg	Sodium mg	Calcium mg	Iron mg
Dairy													
Buttermilk	1 cup	245 g	99	8.75	2	1.33	11.25	0	0	9	257	285	0.1
Cheese spread	2 tablespoon	28 g	81	3.5	6.56	4.33	2	0	1	89	293	95	1
Cheese-American	1 ounce, 1 slice	28 g	106	6.75	8.22	5.44	0.5	0	0	27	406	174	0.1
Cheese-cheddar	1 ounce, 1 slice	28 g	113	7.5	8.67	5.89	0.5	0	0	30	177	203	0.2
Cheese-cottage	1/2 cup	109 g	113	14.5	4.78	3.11	3	0	0	17	440	65	0.2
Cheese-cottage, nonfat	1/2 cup	113 g	90	14	0	0	7	0	0	10	400	60	0
Cheese-cottage, lowfat	1/2 cup	113 g	96	15	1.22	0.78	4	0	0	5	440	74	0.2
Cheese-mozzarella	1 ounce, 1 slice	28 g	80	6	5.67	3.67	0.5	0	0	22	106	147	0.1
Cheese-mozzarella, light	1 ounce	28 g	72	7.25	4.11	2.78	0.75	0	0	16	150	183	0.1
Cheese-nonfat	1 ounce, 1 slice	28 g	40	8	0	0	1	0	0	5	290	210	0
Cheese-parmesan/romano	1 tablespoon	5 g	20	2	1.33	0.89	0.25	0	0	4	82	61	0
Cheese-provolone	1 ounce, 1 slice	28 g	100	7.75	7	4.78	0.5	0	0	20	248	214	0.2
Cheese-reduced fat	1 ounce, 1 slice	28 g	80	8	5	3	1	0	0	20	220	350	0
Cheese-ricotta	1/2 cup	124 g	216	15	14.89	10	3.75	0	0	63	104	257	0.5
Cheese-ricotta, part skim	1/2 cup	119 g	166	14.5	8.67	5.67	6.25	0	0	37	143	369	0.3
Cheese-Swiss	1 ounce	28 g	101	8	6.89	4.67	0.75	0	0	25	231	246	0.1
Hot cocoa prepared w/milk	1 cup	250 g	218	8	9	5.67	13.5	11.25	3	33	123	298	0.8
Ice cream	1/2 cup	70 g	148	2.5	7.44	4.67	4.5	11.75	0.2	30	58	88	0.3
Ice milk	1/2 cup	66 g	110	3	2.78	1.89	10	8	0.3	8	75	100	1
Lowfat chocolate milk	1 cup	258 g	175	8.5	3.78	2.33	12.25	16	1.3	12	150	294	0.7
Meal replacement drinks	1 cup	314 g	200	14	1	0.44	36	17	4	5	230	500	6.3
Milk-chocolate	1 cup	250 g	208	8.5	7.89	5.11	10.5	14.5	1.1	30	149	280	0.6
Milk-lowfat	1 cup	244 g	112	8.75	3.56	2.22	11.25	0	0	14	123	299	0.1
Milk-skim	1 cup	245 g	86	9	0.44	0.33	11.5	0	0	4	126	302	0.1
Milk-whole	1 cup	244 g	150	8.5	7.67	5	11	0	0	33	120	291	0.1
Tofutti	1/2 cup	66 g	150	2.5	6.67	1.11	9	11	1.5	0	105	1	0.6
Yogurt-frozen	1/2 cup	96 g	100	3	1.78	1.11	8	10.25	0.1	7	59	100	1
Yogurt-lowfat w/fruit	1 container	227 g	240	9	3	2	27	16	0.3	10	120	330	1
Yogurt-nonfat w/fruit	1 container	96 g	95	3.5	0	0	8	12	0	0	70	150	1
Yogurt-plain, lowfat	1 container	227 g	142	11.25	3.67	2.44	15.75	0	0	15	160	422	0.6
Yogurt-plain, nonfat	1 container	227 g	110	11	0.22	0.22	16	0	0	4	160	430	1
Yogurt-plain, whole milk	1 container	198 g	145	8.75	6.89	4.56	11.5	0	0	32	123	312	0.6
Yogurt-w/fruit, artificial sweetener	1 container	184 g	90	7	0.67	0.44	14	0	0.5	5	110	250	1

© 1994, DINE Systems, Inc., 586 N. French Rd., Amherst, NY 14228

Protein Foods

	Amount	Weight	Calories	Protein g	Total Fat g	Sat Fat g	Carb. g	Added Sugar g	Fiber g	Chol. mg	Sodium mg	Calcium mg	Iron mg
Bacon substitute	1 strip	12 g	52	3	4.11	1.56	0	0	0	13	207	1	0.2
Beans-baked	1/2 cup	121 g	140	6	1.67	0.67	15	7.5	6	8	423	60	2.1
Beans-black	1/2 cup	86 g	113	6.5	0.33	0.11	20.75	0	4.4	0	1	24	1.8
Beans-kidney, pinto	1/2 cup	86 g	115	6.5	0.33	0.11	22.25	0	4.5	0	2	33	2.4
Beans-kidney, pinto, canned"	1/2 cup	125 g	104	5.75	0.22	0	19.5	0	6.1	0	445	35	1.6
Beans-lima	1/2 cup	90 g	94	5.5	0.22	0.11	17.5	0	4.6	0	26	25	1.8
Beans-lima, canned	1/2 cup	124 g	93	4.75	0.22	0.11	17.5	0	5.8	0	309	35	2
Beans-navy, chickpeas	1/2 cup	87 g	132	6.75	1	0.22	23.75	0	4.8	0	4	52	2.4
Beans-navy, chickpeas, canned	1/2 cup	126 g	146	7	0.78	0.11	27.5	0	5	0	473	51	2
Beans-white, canned	1/2 cup	131 g	153	8.25	0.22	0.11	29.25	0	5	0	7	96	3.9
Beans-white, split peas	1/2 cup	93 g	125	7	0.22	0.11	23	0	5.3	0	2	66	2.6
Beef stew	1 cup	247 g	207	15.25	9	4.22	16.5	0.5	2.5	53	616	29	2.6
Beef-corned	3 ounces	85 g	182	18.25	12.11	5.22	0	0.25	0	65	768	11	1.5
Beef-mixed dish	1 cup	186 g	310	19.25	13.56	5.89	23.5	1.25	2.1	68	840	52	3.5
Biscuit w/egg, meat, cheese	1 biscuit	168 g	489	18.75	31.22	9.67	29	4	0.8	347	1240	151	2.9
Bologna sandwich	1 sandwich	106 g	311	11	18	6.56	22	3.75	1.7	32	845	60	2.5
Broadbeans-fava	1/2 cup	85 g	93	5.5	0.22	0	17	0	4.4	0	4	31	1.3
Broadbeans-fava, canned	1/2 cup	128 g	91	6	0.11	0	16.25	0	4.5	0	580	34	1.3
Burrito	1 burrito	230 g	213	8	7.22	3.56	29	0	3.2	33	558	53	2.3
Caviar	1 tablespoon	16 g	40	4.25	2.11	0.78	0.5	0	0	94	240	44	1.8
Cheeseburger (large) & roll	1 sandwich	280 g	711	32	43.33	16.78	33	4	1	113	1164	295	5
Cheeseburger (lowfat) & roll	1 sandwich	219 g	370	24	14	5	35	3.5	1.6	75	890	200	3.6
Cheeseburger (small) & roll	1 sandwich	172 g	461	29	27.56	13.67	25.25	3	0.8	95	906	245	3.3
Chicken breast sandwich	1 sandwich	195 g	509	26	26.89	4.78	34.75	1.75	1.7	83	1082	80	2.7
Chicken fingers/nuggets	4 fingers, 6 nuggets	98.5 g	275	15.75	14	3.11	15.25	0	0.4	49	558	7	0.8
Chicken salad	1/2 cup	84 g	179	14.75	12.22	2.89	0.75	0.75	0.3	118	329	21	0.9
Chicken wings	10 wings	257 g	617	39	46.56	13.56	15	1	0.4	198	1581	36	1.8
Chicken w/skin	3 ounces	85 g	189	22.25	9.22	2.56	0	0	0	70	60	12	1
Chicken w/out skin	3 ounces	85 g	147	24.5	3.89	1.11	0	0	0	72	63	12	0.9
Chicken-fried, no skin	4 ounces	113 g	107	19.25	4.22	1.33	0.25	0	0	50	46	9	0.8
Chicken-fried, w/skin	3 ounces	85 g	155	15.75	8.44	2.44	4.75	0	0.2	52	149	11	0.8
Chicken-mixed dish	1 cup	216 g	365	15.25	17.78	5.56	13.5	0	1	103	600	30	2.2
Chickpeas	1/2 cup	101 g	138	6.5	1.67	0.11	24.75	0	4.8	0	183	39	2

Protein Foods (continued)

	Amount	Weight	Calories	Protein g	Total Fat g	Sat Fat g	Carb. g	Added Sugar g	Fiber g	Chol. mg	Sodium mg	Calcium mg	Iron mg
Chili con carne	1 cup	247 g	286	15.75	12.44	5.78	28.5	0	6.5	43	964	86	3
Chili-vegetarian	1 cup	226 g	240	18	12	1.78	13	2	16.4	0	860	6	3.2
Chimichanga	1 chimichanga	182 g	425	18.5	17.11	8.33	41.25	0	5.2	30	933	145	4
Chop suey	1 cup	250 g	300	26	16	4.33	13	0	1.5	68	1053	60	4.8
Chow mein-beef or chicken	3/4 cup	165 g	65	6.5	1.44	0.56	5.25	0.75	1.4	26	845	80	1.3
Clams, oyster, shrimp-fried	4 pieces	43 g	103	5.25	6.11	1.11	6	0	0.1	23	183	20	0.6
Clams, oysters, shrimp	1/2 cup, 3 ounces	90 g	71	12.25	1.22	0.33	2.5	0	0	62	108	41	6
Coconut-shredded	2 tablespoon	10 g	44	0.25	3	2.67	2.25	2.25	0.4	0	24	1	0.2
Crabmeat	3 ounces	85 g	86	12.5	1	0.22	4.5	0	0	26	713	25	0.4
Egg salad	1/2 cup	103 g	267	11	22.89	5.78	1	3	0.3	418	513	43	1.8
Egg-boiled, poached	1 egg	50 g	79	6.5	5.56	2.11	0.5	0	0	274	69	28	1
Egg-fried, scrambled	1 egg	55 g	89	6.25	6.78	3	1	0	0	281	150	37	0.9
Egg-omelet	1 omelet (3 eggs)	228 g	382.5	24.13	25.17	7.33	6	0	0.4	675	625	171.5	2.6
Egg-substitute	1/4 cup	56 g	43	5.5	1.56	0.22	1.5	0	0	0	115	30	0.8
Eggroll	1 eggroll	85 g	173	6.75	4.56	0.89	25	3	0.8	7	471	20	1.1
Enchilada	1 enchilada	178 g	322	10.5	16.89	9.67	30	0	5.8	42	1052	276	2.2
Fish casserole	1 cup	259 g	407	18.5	23.78	7.56	26.25	0.75	1.8	70	1314	182	2.3
Fish sandwich	1 sandwich	177 g	488	19	26.56	5.89	39.25	3.75	1.5	70	928	46	2
Fish sticks	3 pieces	57 g	150	6.75	8.22	2.22	12	0.75	0.7	15	280	0	0.5
Fish-fried	3 ounces	85 g	209	8.75	11.56	2.67	16.25	1.25	0.7	39	350	0	0.5
Fish-not fried	3 ounces	85 g	81	17	1	0.33	0	0	0	45	57	13	0.4
Fish-smoked, pickled	1 ounce	28 g	56	6.25	2.33	0.67	0	0	0	14	235	5	0.3
Grilled cheese sandwich	1 sandwich	120 g	442	17	30.67	13.78	23	2.25	1.7	53	1200	402	1.8
Ground beef-lean	3 ounces, 3/4 cup	85 g	228	22.5	13.94	5.44	0	0	0	76.5	62.5	8	2.1
Ground beef-regular	3 ounces, 3/4 cup	85 g	246	20.75	17.56	6.89	0	0	0	80	71	9	2.1
Ham	3 ounces	85 g	124	15.75	6.56	2.33	0	0	0	41	1064	6	0.8
Ham sandwich	1 sandwich	140 g	343	23.5	15.89	7.67	23	2	1.7	60	1577	229	2.5
Hamburger (large) & roll	1 sandwich	228 g	594	27.5	33	12.67	33.25	2	0.9	101	688	87	4.8
Hamburger (lowfat) & roll	1 sandwich	206 g	320	22	10	4	35	3.5	1.6	60	670	150	3.6
Hamburger (small) & roll	1 sandwich	137 g	355	22	19.33	8.22	22.25	3	1.7	95	556	71	3.2
Hot dog	1 hot dog	50 g	144	5.75	12.89	5.22	0.25	1.25	0.7	30	547	20	0.7
Hot dog and roll	1 sandwich	105 g	298	9.25	17.56	6.67	20	2.5	0.7	29	880	60	2.2
Julienne salad	2 cup	483 g	489	47.5	29	13.89	7.5	0	3.5	281	1340	360	3.4
Lamb	3 ounces	85 g	169	19.75	11.11	5.33	0	0	0	68	49	8	1.5
Lentils	1/2 cup	99 g	115	7.75	0.22	0	20.25	0	2.8	0	2	19	3.3
Liver	3 ounces	85 g	127	17.75	4.56	2	2.5	0	0	258	52	8	5.8

© 1994, DINE Systems, Inc., 586 N. French Rd., Amherst, NY 14228

APPENDIX PART ONE (continued)

	Amount	Weight	Calories	Protein g	Total Fat g	Sat Fat g	Carb. g	Added Sugar g	Fiber g	Chol. mg	Sodium mg	Calcium mg	Iron mg
Luncheon meat-beef, pork	2 slice	56 g	152	8.5	12.22	5.11	0	1	0	36	696	6	0.8
Luncheon meat-chicken, turkey	2 slice	56 g	64	11.5	1.33	0.44	0	0	0	24	716	6	0.6
Luncheon meat-lean	2 slice	56 g	90	8	4	3.11	3	1.5	0	30	586	0	0.8
Meatloaf	3 ounces	85 g	204	16	12	4.44	7	0.25	0.7	104	303	18	2
Miso	1/2 cup	138 g	284	14.25	7.33	1.11	39.25	0	7.4	0	5032	92	3.8
Nuts-mixed	3 tablespoons, 26 nuts	28 g	170	4.25	13.56	2.22	6.25	0	1.6	0	170	20	1.1
Pate	1 tablespoon	13 g	41	2	3.67	1.44	0	0	0	51	91	9	0.7
Peanut butter	2 tablespoon	32 g	190	9	14.56	2.78	4.5	2	2.4	0	150	11	0.6
Peanut butter & jelly sandwich	1 sandwich	101 g	371	12.25	17.89	3.56	26.5	17.75	3.8	0	426	66	2.2
Peanuts	3 tablespoons, 32 nuts	28 g	164	6.25	12.33	1.78	5.25	0	2.5	0	110	7	0.5
Peas-black eyed	1/2 cup	86 g	100	5.75	0.33	0.11	18.25	0	8.3	0	3	21	2.2
Peas-black eyed, canned	1/2 cup	120 g	92	5	0.33	0.11	16.5	0	8.2	0	359	24	1.2
Pepperoni	3 ounces	85 g	440	16.5	41.56	14.56	2.25	2	0	72	1589	5	0.6
Pizza-cheese & vegetable	1 slice	130 g	249	12.5	9.22	5.11	30	0.5	4	15	518	195	2.3
Pizza-cheese topping	1 slice	65 g	199	11.5	8.44	4.44	28.25	0.5	2	17	456	250	1.2
Pizza-cheese, meat & vegetable	1 slice	120 g	270	16	12.44	6	26.5	0.5	3.5	27	682	230	2.5
Pizza-French bread	1 slice	164 g	410	17.5	19.22	8	39	2	2	35	1030	200	2.7
Pizza-meat topping	1 slice	106 g	271	11.5	13	5.33	27	0.5	1.2	20	733	132	1.8
Pork and beans	1/2 cup	126 g	134	6.5	1.89	0.67	17	8	6.6	9	521	71	2.1
Pork chop	3 ounces	85 g	217	23.5	12.89	4.89	0	0	0	70	48	21	0.8
Pork chop-lean cut	3 ounces	85 g	177	0	8	0	0	0	0	0	0	0	0
Pork feet	8 ounces	227 g	138	14.5	8.78	3.22	0	0	0	71	597	32	1.1
Pork rinds	3 ounces	113 g	458	51.75	26	10	0	0	0	80	2275	19	0.5
Pork roast	3 ounces	85 g	232	23	15	5.56	0	0	0	78	53	16	1
Pork roast-lean cut	3 ounces	85 g	180	24	8.33	3.11	0	0	0	78	55	14	1.2
Pork spareribs	3 ounces	113 g	132	10.25	9.89	3.89	0	0	0	41	31	16	0.6
Pork-fresh, fried	3 ounces	114 g	144	11	11.22	4.22	0	0	0	41	25	4	0.4
Pork-fresh, roasted	4 ounces	114 g	164	15.75	10.22	3.89	0	0	0	54	37	4	0.6
Refried beans	1/2 cup	113 g	135	6	1.33	0.56	18	0	6	0	400	40	2.2
Roast beef sandwich	1 sandwich	164 g	353	27.25	14.89	7.33	30.25	2.25	1.7	49	766	87	4.1
Roast beef-lean cut	3 ounces	85 g	156	24.75	5.67	1.89	0	0	0	69	54	4	2.7
Roast beef-regular	3 ounces	85 g	222.5	22.75	13.5	5.11	0	0	0	69.5	53	5	2.4
Sausage	3 ounces	85 g	264	12	22.33	8.67	0	1.5	0	42	774	12	1.2

	Amount	Weight	Calories	Protein g	Total Fat g	Sat Fat g	Carb. g	Added Sugar g	Fiber g	Chol. mg	Sodium mg	Calcium mg	Iron mg
Protein Foods (continued)													
Seafood or fish salad	1/2 cup	104 g	160	13.5	9.78	2.33	1.75	0.25	0.4	142	250	31	0.9
Sloppy Joe sandwich	1 sandwich	146 g	302	18.5	13.78	6	23.75	2.5	1.4	63	509	71	3.5
Soybeans-roasted	1/4 cup	44 g	205	14.25	10.22	1.56	13.5	0	1.9	0	1	89	2
Steak	3 ounces	85 g	191	24	9.33	3.44	0	0	0	71	54	7	2.7
Steak-lean cut	3 ounces	85 g	176	24.5	7.89	3	0	0	0	69	56	5	2.4
Submarine/hoagy	1 submarine	401 g	934	34.5	51.22	12.67	73.25	3.75	3.1	87	1538	294	5.7
Sweet & sour chicken, pork	1 cup	258 g	426	17.5	13.89	3.33	23.5	31.75	1.3	83	1209	27	1.9
Taco	1 taco	171 g	370	21	18.44	11.11	26.5	0	3.4	57	802	221	2.4
Taco salad	1-1/2 cup	198 g	279	13.5	13.33	6.67	24	0	4.3	44	763	192	2.3
Tahini	1 tablespoon	16 g	92	2.5	7.33	1.11	3.75	0	1.5	0	10	109	2.2
Tofu	3 ounces	85 g	65	6.75	2.33	0.33	2.25	0	1	0	8	68	1.1
Tostada	1 tostada	198 g	325	13.75	13.89	9.67	28	0	7.5	40	834	214	2.2
Tripe	4 ounces	114 g	61	12.5	1.11	0.67	0	0	0	58	44	77	0.3
Tuna casserole	1 cup, 18 chips	231 g	248	16	10.44	3.33	26.75	0	0.7	36	1072	120	1.4
Tuna in oil	1/2 cup	74 g	142	22	5.44	1.11	0	0	0	18	275	7	0.8
Tuna in water	1/2 cup	74 g	90	19.25	1.44	0.44	0	0	0	28	400	0	0.7
Tuna salad	1/2 cup	102 g	183	14	9.44	1.89	2.25	0	0.4	13	412	23	0.8
Tuna sandwich	1 sandwich	120 g	364.5	16.25	23	4.11	24.13	2.25	1.7	25	599	53	2
Turkey hot dog	1 hot dog	45.4 g	102	6.5	8	3.11	0.25	1.5		51	641	51	0.9
Turkey sandwich	1 sandwich	194 g	355	30.25	14.67	2.67	23.5	2.25	1.7	76	385	75	3.3
Turkey w/skin	3 ounces	85 g	168	24	7.89	2.11	0	0	0	70	57	20	1.5
Turkey w/out skin	3 ounces	85 g	137	25.5	3.22	1	0	0	0	72	64	19	1.5
Veal	3 ounces	85 g	195	25.63	10.17	4	0	0	0	95.5	69.5	16.5	1
Veal-lean cut	3 ounces	85 g	167	27	5.33	1.67	0	0	0	98	76	20	1
Veal-mixed dish	1 serving	168 g	327	28.25	17.78	9.78	9.5	0.75	1.7	137	634	138	3.7
Venison	3 ounces	85 g	147	25.75	3.11	1.22	0	0	0	95	280	6	3.8
Beverages													
Beer-nonalcoholic	12 fluid ounces, 1-1/2 cup	359 g	55	0.75	0	0	11	0	0	0	19	25	0.1
Coffee	1 cup	237 g	5	0.25	0	0	1	0	0	0	7	6	0.6
Coffee-decaffeinated	1 cup	239 g	3	0.25	0	0	0.75	0	0	0	8	8	0.1
Cola	12 fluid ounces	366 g	150	0	0	0	0	37	0	0	70	0	0
Cola-diet	12 fluid ounces	360 g	2	0.25	0	0	0.25	0	0	0	70	0	0
Cola-diet, no caffeine	12 fluid ounces	358 g	2	0	0	0	0	0	0	0	70	0	0
Cola-no caffeine	12 fluid ounces	363 g	155	0	0	0	0	38.75	0	0	73	0	0
Juice drink	3/4 cup, 1 juice box	190 g	106	0	0	0	6.5	19.5	0	0	7	1	1

Food	Amount	Weight	Calories	Protein g	Total Fat g	Sat Fat g	Carb. g	Added Sugar g	Fiber g	Chol. mg	Sodium mg	Calcium mg	Iron mg
Mellow Yellow, Mountain Dew	12 fluid ounces	371 g	177	0	0	0	0	44	0	0	30	0	0
Noncola-diet, no caffeine	12 fluid ounces	342 g	4	0	0	0	0.5		0	0	42	0	0
Noncola-no caffeine	12 fluid ounces	364 g	157	0	0	0	0	37.75	0	0	46	2	0.1
Postum	1 teaspoon	3 g	12	0	0	0	3	0	1.3	0	0	0	0
Tea-herbal, no caffeine	1 cup	240 g	4	0	0	0	0.75	0	0	0	3	5	0.2
Tea-plain	1 cup	239 g	3	0	0	0	0.5	0	0	0	0	0	0
Wine-nonalcoholic	5 fluid ounces	136 g	42	0.5	0	0	9.75	0	0	0	7	12	0.6
Beverages-Alcoholic													
Beer	12 fluid ounces, 1-1/2 cup	360 g	145	1	0	0	13.25	0	0	0	8	12	0
Beer-light	12 fluid ounces, 1-1/2 cup	355 g	110	1	0	0	7	0	0	0	8	15	0
Chianti	5 fluid ounces	148 g	106	0.25	0	0	2.5	0	0	0	8	12	0.6
Cocktail-mixed drink	1 cocktail	134 g	139	0	0	0	1	1.5	0	0	6	4	0.1
Liqueur	1 glass, 1-1/2 ounce	50 g	167	0	0.11	0	8.5	9.5	0	0	4	1	0
Liquor	1 jigger, 1-1/2 fluid ounces	42 g	110	0	0	0	0	0	0	0	0	0	0
Vermouth	5 fluid ounces	148 g	100	0.25	0	0	1	0	0	0	8	12	0.4
Wine	5 fluid ounces	148 g	104	0.25	0	0	2.5	0	0	0	12	12	0.4
Wine cooler	12 fluid ounces, 1-1/2 cup	360 g	173	0.75	0	0	7.75	9.75	0	0	25	32	1.4
Wine-light	5 fluid ounces	148 g	73	0.5	0	0	1		0	0	10	13	0.6
Fats/Sweets/Other													
Bacon	1 slice, 1-1/2 tablespoon	9.25 g	37	2.35	3.11	1.16	0.09	0.05	0	8	160.5	0.88	0.2
Bacon bits	1 tablespoon	7 g	21	2.5	1.11	0.33	0	0	0	6	181	1	0.1
Breakfast milk powder	1 packet	36 g	130	6	0	0	0	26.25	0.4	0	185	80	4.5
Brownie	1 square	38 g	150	2	6.22	1.67	6.5	15	0.9	10	105	1	0.7
Butter	1 teaspoon, 1 pat	5 g	34.7	0	3.81	2.41	0	0	0	10.7	39.7	0.7	0.3
Cake	1 piece	98 g	280	4	11.33	3	15.25	22.25	0.5	56	285	57	1
Candy-chewy	1 ounce	28 g	109	0	1	0.56	1.5	20.5	0	0	32	1	0

© 1994, DINE Systems, Inc., 586 N. French Rd., Amherst, NY 14228

Fats/Sweets/Other (continued)

	Amount	Weight	Calories	Protein g	Total Fat g	Sat Fat g	Carb. g	Added Sugar g	Fiber g	Chol. mg	Sodium mg	Calcium mg	Iron mg
Candy-chocolate & peanut butter	1 package, 1-1/2 ounces	47 g	237	6	13.78	5.89	4	22	2.5	3	90	34	0.7
Candy-chocolate	1 ounce	28 g	150	2	8.22	4.78	2.25	15	0.8	6	24	50	0.3
Candy-chocolate covered	1 ounce	28 g	132	1.25	5.56	2.11	3	13.25	1.5	3	43	33	0.4
Candy-fudge	1 cube	28.4 g	119	1	4.06	1.06	1.7	17.93	0.4	2.7	54.1	27	0.3
Candy-hard	5 pieces	28 g	110	0	0	0	0	27.5	0	0	7	1	0.1
Catsup	1 tablespoon	15 g	17	0	0	0	2.75	1.5	0.2	0	168	3	0.1
Cheese puffs	1 cup	28 g	160	2	9.78	1.78	16	0	0.3	0	330	3	0.4
Cheese sauce	1/4 cup	70 g	71	3.5	3.56	1.89	6.5	0	0.3	10	412	139	0.1
Chili sauce	1 tablespoon	15 g	17	0.25	0	0	2.75	1.25	0.9	0	196	2	0.1
Chip dip	1/4 cup	60 g	120	2	10	6	4	0.5	0	40	360	80	1
Coffee whitener	1 tablespoon	11 g	22	0	2.11	1.33	0	1	0	1	12	1	1
Cookies-fig bars	2 bar	28 g	100	1	1.78	0.44	10.5	10.5	1.2	1	90	20	0.7
Cookies-nonfat	2 cookies	23 g	75	1	0	0	17.5	6.5	0.6	0	115	0	0.2
Cookies-oatmeal raisin	3 cookies	40 g	195	2.25	8.11	1.89	13.5	13.5	1.4	1	150	0	0.8
Cookies-other	3 cookies	42 g	180	1.5	8.11	2.89	10	15	0.3	3	131	1	0.7
Corn chips	1 cup	28 g	152	2	9.44	1.33	16	0	1.3	0	205	36	0.2
Cream cheese	2 tablespoon	30 g	106	2.5	10.22	6.67	1	0	0	34	90	24	0.4
Cream cheese-light	2 tablespoon	28 g	80	3	7	4	1	0	0	25	115	20	1
Cream-coffee, half & half	1 tablespoon	15 g	25	0.5	2.22	1.44	0.5	0	0	8	6	15	0
Cream-whipped	1 tablespoon	5 g	15	0.25	1.33	1.11	0.25	0.25	0	2	4	3	1
Cupcakes	1 cupcake	39 g	140	1.25	4.56	1.89	8.5	15	0.7	12	121	24	0.6
Danish	1 danish	71 g	252	4.5	11.67	3.67	10.25	19	0.7	14	249	36	1.1
Danish-nonfat	1 danish	33 g	90	2	0	0	20	9.75	0.2	0	85	20	0
Dessert topping-no sugar	1 tablespoon	5 g	5	0	0.56	0.44	0.56	0	1	4	5	2	1
Diet bar	1 bar	31 g	120	2	4	1.44	19	9.5	3	1	30	150	2.7
Doughnut or sweet roll	1 doughnut, 1 sweetroll	60 g	220	3.75	9.89	3.33	29.5	18	1	5	230	22	1.1
Frozen desserts-nonfat	1/2 cup	68 g	100	2	0.22	0.11	23.5	9.5	0.4	1	48	100	0
Frozen yogurt cone-lowfat	1 serving	85 g	105	4	1	0.56	22	13	0.1	3	80	112	0.2
Frozen yogurt sundae-lowfat	1 sundae	171 g	240	6	3	2.33	50.5	43	0.8	6	170	190	0.1
Gelatin	1/2 cup	127 g	105	2	1	1	23	22	0	0	57	0	0
Gelatin-sugar free	1/2 cup	121 g	8	1.5	0	0	0	0	0	0	31	0	0
Granola bars	1 bar	28 g	133	2	6	2	18.25	13	0.6	0	70	20	0.5
Gravy	1/4 cup	60 g	30	1	1.44	0.56	2.25	0.5	0.1	1	260	3	0.4
Hollandaise sauce	1/4 cup	64 g	230	2.25	23.22	8.44	2.5	0	0	140	316	50	1

© 1994, DINE Systems, Inc., 586 N. French Rd., Amherst, NY 14228

	Amount	Weight	Calories	Protein g	Total Fat g	Sat Fat g	Carb. g	Added Sugar g	Fiber g	Chol. mg	Sodium mg	Calcium mg	Iron mg
Honey	2 teaspoon	14 g	42	0	0	0	0	10.5	0	0	1	1	0.1
Hot cocoa mix	1 envelope	26 g	110	1.5	2.78	1.56	3.5	16	1.1	2	165	40	0.7
Ice cream bar	1 bar	57g	172	2	11.78	7.11	6	11.5	0.3	17	50	80	0
Jam or jelly	2 teaspoon	13 g	35	0	0	0	1	7.5	0.1	0	1	1	0
Lard	1 tablespoon	13 g	115	0	12.22	5	0	0	0	12	0	1	1
Margarine-stick	1 teaspoon, 1 pat	5 g	33.7	0	3.52	0.67	0	0	0	0	44.3	1.3	0
Margarine-stick, light	1 teaspoon, 1 pat	5 g	20	0	2.22	0.33	0	0	0	0	36.7	0.33	0
Margarine-tub	1 tablespoon	14 g	101	0	8.89	2	0	0	0	0	152	4	0.3
Margarine-tub, light	1 tablespoon	14 g	50	0	5.89	1	0	0	0	0	110	1	1
Marshmallows	2 piece	14g	47	0.25	0	0	0	11.75	0	0	7	2	0.1
Mayonnaise	1 tablespoon	14 g	100	0.25	11	1.89	0.25	0.25	0	8	74	1	1
Mayonnaise-light	1 tablespoon	14 g	48	0.25	4.56	1	0.75	1	0	5	95	1	1
Mayonnaise-nonfat	1 tablespoon	16 g	12	0	0	0	3	3	0	0	190	0	0
Meal replacement bar	1 serving	48 g	270	11	14	5	24	22.5	0	0	330	250	4.5
Milkshake	10 fluid ounces, 1-1/4 cup	290 g	368	10	12.78	8.22	26.5	19.25	0.5	54	243	375	0.5
Milkshake-lowfat	1 serving	293 g	320	10.75	1.33	0.56	66	44.75	0	10	170	327	0.1
Miracle Whip	1 tablespoon	14 g	64	0	5.89	0.89	2.5	0.5	0	5	95	2	1
Miracle Whip-nonfat	1 tablespoon	16 g	20	0	0	0	5	5	0	0	210	0	0
Molasses	1 tablespoon	20 g	55	0	0	0	0	14.5	0	0	11	75	1.8
Mustard	1 teaspoon	5 g	6	0.25	0.33	0	0.25	0	0	0	60	0	0
Noncola-diet	12 fluid ounces, 1-1/2 cup	369 g	2	0	0	0	0.5	0.25	0	0	8	0	0
Nutrasweet-Equal	1 packet	1 g	4	0.5	0	0	0	0	0	0	0	0	0
Oil	1 tablespoon	14 g	120	0	12.78	1.89	0	0	0	0	0	0	0.1
Pickles-dill	2 spear	61 g	7	0	0.11	0	1	0.75	0.9	0	584	9	0.4
Pickles-sweet	1 pickle, 3 slices	18 g	18	0	0.5	0	0.5	4	0.3	0	107	2	0.2
Pie-custard or cream	1 slice	152 g	346	6.75	13.11	6.22	20.75	25.75	1	125	375	122	0.8
Pie-fruit	1 slice	158 g	405	4	16.22	5.33	34.75	25.25	4	6	423	17	1.6
Pie-pecan	1/6 of 9" pie	138 g	575	7	29.67	5.67	33	37.25	2.2	100	305	65	4.6
Popcorn	1 cup	11 g	32	0.75	1.44	0.44	5.5	0	0.8	0	68	0	0.2
Popsicle	1 popsicle	69 g	50	0	0	0	0	13	0	0	10	0	0
Potato chips	1 cup, 20 chips	28 g	150	2	9.67	2	15	0	1.4	0	190	0	0.4
Pretzels	2/3 cup	28 g	110	2.75	0.89	0.22	21.75	1	0.9	0	610	9	1.4
Pudding	1/2 cup	147 g	150	4.5	2.22	1.44	10	18	0	9	443	152	0.1
Pudding-diet	1/2 cup	132 g	90	4	2.44	1.56	13	0	0.4	9	423	152	0.2
Relish	2 tablespoon	28 g	35	0	0	0	1.25	7.5	0.2	0	243	6	0.1
Saccharin	1 packet	1 g	2	0	0	0	0.25	0	0	0	2	0	0
Salad dressing	1 tablespoon	16 g	80	0	8.22	1.33	0.25	0.25	1	0	146	2	1

© 1994, DINE Systems, Inc., 586 N. French Rd., Amherst, NY 14228

Food	Amount	Weight	Calories	Protein g	Total Fat g	Sat Fat g	Carb. g	Added Sugar g	Fiber g	Chol. mg	Sodium mg	Calcium mg	Iron mg
Fats/Sweets/Other (continued)													
Salad dressing-light	1 tablespoon	15 g	16	0.25	0.33	0.11	0.75	0.5	0.3	0	137	1	1
Salad dressing-no oil	1 tablespoon	17 g	12	0	0	0	2.5	0	0.7	0	0	1	1
Salad dressing-nonfat	1 tablespoon	15 g	16	0	0	0	3	3	0	0	143	0	0
Salt	4 shakes	0 g	0	0	0	0	0	0	0	0	64	0	0
Sherbet	1/2 cup	97 g	136	1	1.89	1.22	6	23.5	0	7	44	52	0.2
Soft drinks	12 fluid ounces, 1-1/2 cup	369 g	156	0	0	0	0	39.5	0	0	22	0	0
Soup-beef or chicken	1 cup	266 g	74	4.25	2.22	0.67	8.5	0	1	7	910	17	0.9
Soup-bouillon, broth	1 cube, packet(s),	5 g	9	0.75	0.22	0.11	0.25	1	0	0	965	1	0.1
Soup-broth based, no salt	1 cup	241 g	135	5.75	3.89	0.78	16.5	0	2.8	1	115	47	1.8
Soup-cream, chowder	1 cup	246 g	140	5.5	6.11	2.89	14	0	0.9	22	1010	150	0.6
Soup-low salt	1 cup	246 g	110	4	3	1	12	0	0.5	2	100	17	1.3
Soup-miso	1 cup	199 g	152	4.5	6.44	0.89	19	0	3	0	490	20	1.3
Sour cream	2 tablespoon	24 g	52	0.5	5.11	3.11	1	0	0	10	34	28	0
Sour cream-imitation	2 tablespoon	26 g	50	1.5	4.67	4	1.5	0	0	2	20	14	0
Sour cream-nonfat	2 tablespoon	28 g	16	2	0	0	2	0	0	0	20	40	0
Soy sauce	1 tablespoon	18 g	10	1.25	0	0	1.25	0	0	0	1015	3	0.4
Steak/Worcestershire sauce	1 tablespoon	15 g	11	0	0	0	1	1.75	0	0	143	0	0
Sugar	1 teaspoon	4 g	15	0	0	0	0	3.75	0	0	0	0	0
Sunflower seeds	2 tablespoon	19 g	116	3.75	10.78	1.11	4	0	1.7	0	1	11	1.3
Syrup-pancake, table	2 tablespoon	40 g	110	0	0	0	0	27.5	0	0	21	1	1
Tortilla chips	1 cup, 10 chips	19 g	95	1.25	4.67	1.33	12	0	0.9	0	123	23	0.3
White sauce	1/4 cup	63 g	99	2.5	5.67	2.22	6	0	0.1	8	222	73	0.2

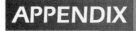

Nutritional Content of Foods, Beverages, and Fast Food Items

(continued)

Part Two:

Nutritional Content of Fast Foods

- **Burger King**
- **Domino's Pizza**
- **Kentucky Fried Chicken**
- **McDonald's**
- **Taco Bell**
- **Wendy's**

Nutritional Content of Fast Foods (continued)

Burger King	Serving Size (g)	Calories	Calories from Fat	Total Fat (g)	Saturated Fat (g)	Cholesterol (mg)	Sodium (mg)	Total Carbohydrate (g)	Dietary Fiber (g)	Sugars (g)	Protein (g)	% Daily Value‡ Vitamin A	Vitamin C	Calcium	Iron
Burgers															
Whopper® Sandwich	270	640	350	39	11	90	870	45	3	8	27	10	15	8	25
Whopper® with Cheese Sandwich	294	730	410	46	16	115	1300	46	3	8	33	15	15	25	25
Double Whopper® Sandwich	351	870	500	56	19	170	940	45	3	8	46	10	15	8	40
Double Whopper® with Cheese Sandwich	375	960	570	63	24	195	1360	46	3	8	52	15	15	25	40
Whopper JR.® Sandwich	168	420	220	24	8	60	570	29	2	5	21	4	8	6	20
Whopper JR.® with Cheese Sandwich	180	460	250	28	10	75	780	29	2	5	23	8	8	15	20
Hamburger	129	330	140	15	6	55	570	28	1	4	20	2	0	4	15
Cheeseburger	142	380	170	19	9	65	780	28	1	5	23	6	0	15	15
Double Cheeseburger	213	600	320	36	17	135	1040	29	1	5	41	8	0	20	25
Double Cheeseburger with Bacon	221	640	350	39	18	145	1220	29	1	5	44	8	0	20	25
Sandwiches/Side Orders															
BK Big Fish Sandwich	255	720	390	43	8	60	1090	59	2	4	25	2	2	6	20
BK Broiler® Chicken Sandwich	248	540	260	29	6	80	480	41	2	3	30	4	10	4	30
Chicken Sandwich	229	700	380	43	9	60	1400	54	2	4	26	*	*	10	20
Chicken Tenders® (6 piece)	88	250	110	12	3	35	530	14	2	0	16	*	*	*	4
Broiled Chicken Salad†	302	200	90	10	5	60	110	7	3	4	21	100	25	15	20
Garden Salad†	215	90	45	5	3	15	110	7	3	0	6	110	50	15	6
Side Salad†	133	50	25	3	2	5	55	4	2	0	3	50	20	6	2
French Fries (medium, salted)	116	400	180	20	5	0	240	43	3	0	5	*	4	*	6
Onion Rings	124	310	130	14	2	0	810	41	5	6	4	*	*	*	*
Dutch Apple Pie	113	310	140	15	3	0	230	39	2	22	3	*	10	*	8

Nutritional Content of Fast Foods (continued)

Burger King (continued)	Serving Size (g)	Calories	Calories from Fat	Total Fat (g)	Saturated Fat (g)	Cholesterol (mg)	Sodium (mg)	Total Carbohydrate (g)	Dietary Fiber (g)	Sugars (g)	Protein (g)	% Daily Value‡ Vitamin A	Vitamin C	Calcium	Iron
Drinks															
Vanilla Shake (medium)	284	310	60	7	4	20	230	53	1	47	9	6	6	30	*
Chocolate Shake (medium)	284	310	60	7	4	20	230	54	3	48	9	6	*	20	10
Chocolate Shake (medium, syrup added)	341	460	70	7	4	20	300	87	1	22	11	6	6	30	*
Strawberry Shake (medium, syrup added)	341	430	60	7	4	20	260	83	1	47	9	6	6	30	*
Coca-Cola® Classic (medium)	22 (fl oz)	260	0	0	0	0	@	70	0	70	0	*	*	*	*
Diet Coke® (medium)	22 (fl oz)	1	0	0	0	0	@	<1	0	<1	0	*	*	*	*
Sprite® (medium)	22 (fl oz)	260	0	0	0	0	@	66	0	66	0	*	*	*	*
Tropicana® Orange Juice	311	140	0	0	0	0	0	33	0	28	2	0	100	0	0
Coffee	355	5	0	0	0	0	5	1	0	0	0	*	*	*	*
Milk, 2% Low fat	244	120	40	5	3	20	120	12	0	0	8	10	4	30	*
Breakfast															
Croissan'wich® with Bacon, Egg and Cheese	118	350	220	24	8	225	790	18	<1	2	15	8	*	15	10
Croissan'wich® with Sausage, Egg and Cheese	159	530	370	41	14	255	1000	21	<1	2	20	8	*	15	15
Croissan'wich® with Ham, Egg and Cheese	144	350	200	22	7	230	1390	19	<1	2	18	8	*	15	10
French Toast Sticks	141	500	240	27	7	0	490	60	1	11	4	•	•	6	15
Hash Browns	71	220	110	12	3	0	320	25	2	0	2	10	8	*	2
A.M. Express® Grape Jam	12	30	0	0	0	0	0	7	0	6	0	0	0	0	0
A.M. Express® Strawberry Jam	12	30	0	0	0	0	5	8	0	5	0	0	0	0	0

‡Percent Daily Values are based on a 2,000 calorie diet.
* Contains less than 2% of the daily value of this nutrient.

†Without dressing
@Depends on the water supply.
#Regular Italian Dressing: 150 calories, 16 grams (g) fat.

Source: © Burger King Corporation. The nutritional information on this brochure was updated in December, 1994. For the latest nutritional information, please check your local Burger King® restaurant. "Nutritional Information Chart" reprinted by permission.

Nutritional Content of Fast Foods (continued)

Domino's Pizza

	Serving Size (g)	Calories (kcal)	Calories from Fat (kcal)	Protein (g)	Carbohydrates (g)	Sugars (g)	Dietary Fiber (g)	Fat-total (g)	Saturated Fat (g)	Cholesterol (mg)	Ash (g)	Water (g)	Vitamin A (IU)	Vitamin C (mg)	Calcium (mg)	Iron (mg)	Sodium (mg)
12" Hand-Tossed																	
Cheese	Per 2 of 8 slices (147.4 g)	344.2	90	14.8	50.0	1.0	2.4	9.5	4.4	19.1	3.4	68.7	456.2	2.6	277.8	4.0	980.5
Pepperoni	Per 2 of 8 slices (159.4 g)	406.2	140	17.5	50.2	1.0	2.5	15.1	6.6	32.1	4.1	71.5	467.6	2.7	282.3	4.3	1179.0
X-Tra Cheese & Pepperoni	Per 2 of 8 slices (175.3 g)	455.0	170	20.9	50.5	1.0	2.5	18.8	8.6	41.7	4.6	79.2	578.7	2.7	411.8	4.5	1304.0
Ham	Per 2 of 8 slices (160.7 g)	361.6	90	17.2	50.3	1.2	2.4	10.2	4.6	26.1	4.0	78.1	456.5	2.7	279.3	4.2	1143.0
Italian Sausage & Mushroom	Per 2 of 8 slices (176 g)	402.4	120	17.5	52.2	1.3	2.9	13.9	6.1	30.5	4.2	87.2	483.0	3.2	286.5	4.5	1151.0
Veggie*	Per 2 of 8 slices (176 g)	360.0	90	15.2	51.7	1.2	3.0	10.4	4.5	19.1	3.6	93.9	493.5	12.7	285.9	4.4	1028.8
12" Thin Crust																	
Cheese	1/3 pizza (140.9 g)	364.3	140	16.1	40.1	2.2	1.9	15.5	6.3	25.5	3.7	64.2	567.4	3.5	422.3	1.5	1012.0
Pepperoni	1/3 pizza (156.7 g)	447.1	210	19.7	40.4	2.3	2.0	23.0	9.2	42.8	4.7	67.8	582.6	3.5	428.4	1.8	1277.0
X-Tra Cheese & Pepperoni	1/3 pizza (177.7 g)	512.3	250	24.2	40.8	2.3	2.0	28.0	12.0	55.6	5.3	77.8	731.0	3.5	601.1	2.1	1443.0
Ham	1/3 pizza (158.5 g)	387.7	150	19.3	40.5	2.5	1.9	16.5	6.6	34.8	4.4	76.5	567.9	3.6	424.3	1.7	1229.0
Italian Sausage & Mushroom	1/3 pizza (178.7 g)	442.3	190	19.8	43.1	2.6	2.5	21.4	8.6	40.7	4.8	88.5	603.5	4.2	434.0	2.1	1240.0
Veggie*	1/3 pizza (178.7 g)	385.7	150	16.7	42.5	2.5	2.6	16.7	6.5	25.5	3.9	97.5	617.5	16.9	433.3	2.0	1076.0

Nutritional Content of Fast Foods (continued)

Domino's Pizza (continued)

	Serving Size (g)	Calories (kcal)	Calories from Fat (kcal)	Protein (g)	Carbohydrates (g)	Sugars (g)	Dietary Fiber (g)	Fat-total (g)	Saturated Fat (g)	Cholesterol (mg)	Ash (g)	Water (g)	Vitamin A (IU)	Vitamin C (mg)	Calcium (mg)	Iron (mg)	Sodium (mg)
12" Deep Dish																	
Cheese	Per 2 of 8 slices (205.3 g)	559.7	210	23.5	63.2	4.3	3.2	23.8	9.0	31.5	4.4	92.2	763.9	3.0	451.4	4.8	1184.0
Pepperoni	Per 2 of 8 slices (218 g)	621.8	260	26.2	63.4	4.4	3.2	29.4	11.2	44.5	5.1	95.7	775.3	3.0	455.9	5.0	1383.0
X-Tra Cheese & Pepperoni	Per 2 of 8 slices (234.9 g)	670.7	300	29.6	63.7	4.4	3.2	33.1	13.3	54.0	5.5	104.3	886.6	3.0	585.5	5.2	1508.0
Ham	Per 2 of 8 slices (219.4 g)	577.2	220	25.9	63.5	4.5	3.2	24.5	9.3	38.4	4.9	102.3	764.3	3.1	452.9	4.9	1347.0
Italian Sausage & Mushroom	Per 2 of 8 slices (235.7 g)	618.2	250	26.2	65.5	4.6	3.7	28.2	10.8	42.9	5.1	112.4	791.0	3.5	460.2	5.2	1356.0
Veggie*	Per 2 of 8 slices (235.7 g)	575.8	220	24.0	65.0	4.5	3.7	24.7	9.2	31.5	4.5	119.1	801.5	13.0	459.6	5.1	1233.0

*Veggie includes fresh mushrooms, onions, green peppers, & ripe olives.
Data is based on minimal portioning requirements. Nutrient values may vary slightly by location and supplier base.

Source: ©1994 Domino's Pizza, Inc. Reprinted by permission of Domino's Pizza, Inc.

Nutritional Content of Fast Foods (continued)

Kentucky Fried Chicken	Serving Size (g)	Calories	Calories from Fat	Total Fat (g)	% Daily Value	Saturated Fat (g)	% Daily Value	Cholesterol (mg)	% Daily Value	Sodium (mg)	% Daily Value	Carbohydrates (g)	% Daily Value	Dietary Fiber (g)	% Daily Value	Sugars (g)	Protein (g)	Vitamin A	Vitamin C	Calcium	Iron
																	% Daily Value			
Colonel's Rotisserie Gold® Chicken Quarter—Breast and Wing	6.2 oz	335	168	18.7	29	5.4	27	157	52	1104	46	1	—	—	—	—	40	<2	<2	<2	<2
Colonel's Rotisserie Gold® Chicken Quarter—Breast and Wing with skin and wing removed by customer	4.1 oz	199	53	5.9	9	1.7	9	97	32	667	28	0	—	—	—	—	37	<2	<2	<2	<2
Original Recipe® Chicken Breast	4.8 oz	360	180	20	31	5	27	115	38	870	36	12	4	1	4	0	33	—	—	4	6
Extra Tasty Crispy™ Chicken Breast	5.9 oz	470	250	28	42	7	35	80	27	930	39	25	8	1	4	0	31	—	—	4	6
Hot & Spicy Chicken Breast	6.5 oz	530	310	35	54	8	42	110	36	1110	46	23	8	2	9	0	32	—	—	4	6
Mashed Potatoes with Gravy	4.2 oz	109	45	5	8	<1	<5	<1	<1	386	16	16	5	2	8	<1	1	—	—	—	—
Cornbread	2.0 oz	228	117	13	20	2	11	42	14	194	8	25	8	1	4	10	3	1	0	6	4
Corn on the Cob	5.3 oz	222	104	12	18	2	9	0	0	76	3	27	9	8	31	4	4	4	3	0	2

Source: Courtesy of Kentucky Fried Chicken (KFC) Corp.

APPENDIX PART TWO

Nutritional Content of Fast Foods (continued)

McDonald's	Serving Size (g)	Calories	Calories from Fat	Total Fat (g)	% Daily Value	Saturated Fat (g)	% Daily Value	Cholesterol (mg)	% Daily Value	Sodium (mg)	% Daily Value	Carbohydrates (g)	% Daily Value	Dietary Fiber (g)	% Daily Value	Sugars (g)	Protein (g)	Vitamin A	Vitamin C	Calcium	Iron
Sandwiches																					
Hamburger	106 g	250	80	9	14	3.5	15	40	12	490	20	32	11	2	7	1	12	4	4	10	15
Cheeseburger	119 g	300	120	13	20	5	25	50	17	730	30	33	11	2	7	1	15	8	4	20	15
Quarter Pounder	166 g	400	180	20	31	8	40	85	28	640	27	35	12	2	8	2	23	4	6	15	20
Quarter Pounder with Cheese	191 g	490	250	27	43	10	55	115	38	1090	46	36	12	2	8	3	28	15	6	30	20
McLean Delux™	206 g	320	90	10	15	4	20	60	20	670	28	35	12	3	10	3	22	10	10	15	20
McLean Delux™ with Cheese	219 g	370	130	14	22	5	25	75	25	890	37	35	12	3	10	3	24	15	10	20	20
Big Mac®	215 g	490	240	27	40	9	45	90	33	890	37	49	13	2	9	1	24	6	2	25	20
Filet-O-Fish®	141 g	370	160	18	28	4	20	50	17	730	30	38	13	2	7	0	14	2	*	15	20
McGrilled Chicken Sandwich	240 g	400	110	12	18	4	20	80	27	680	28	42	14	1	4	2	31	8	15	15	8
McChicken® Sandwich	182 g	490	270	30	45	6	28	45	15	760	32	43	14	3	11	1	16	4	2	15	15
Chicken Fajita	82 g	190	70	8	12	2	10	35	12	310	13	20	7	1	5	1	11	2	10	8	4
French Fries																					
Small French Fries	68 g	220	110	12	18	2.5	13	0	0	110	5	26	9	2	9	0	3	*	15	*	2
Large French Fries	122 g	400	200	22	34	5	25	0	0	200	8	46	16	4	16	1	6	*	25	*	6
Salads																					
Chef Salad	265 g	170	80	9	14	4	20	110	37	400	17	8	3	2	9	4	17	100	35	15	8
Chunky Chicken Salad	255 g	150	35	4	6	1	5	80	27	230	10	7	2	2	9	3	25	170	45	4	6
Garden Salad	189 g	50	20	2	3	0.5	3	65	22	70	3	6	2	2	10	4	4	90	35	4	8
Breakfast																					
Egg McMuffin®	135 g	280	100	11	17	4	20	235	78	710	30	28	9	1	6	2	18	10	*	25	15
Sausage McMuffin®	135 g	350	180	20	31	7	35	60	20	770	32	27	9	1	6	2	15	4	*	20	15
Sausage McMuffin® with Egg	159 g	430	230	25	38	8	40	270	90	920	38	27	9	1	6	2	21	10	*	25	20
English Muffin	58 g	170	35	4	6	1	5	0	0	290	12	26	9	2	6	2	5	2	*	15	8
Sausage Biscuit	118 g	420	250	28	43	8	40	45	15	1040	43	32	11	0	0	0	12	*	*	8	10

% Daily Value

Nutritional Content of Fast Foods (continued)

McDonald's (continued)

	Serving Size (g)	Calories	Calories from Fat	Total Fat (g)	% Daily Value	Saturated Fat (g)	% Daily Value	Cholesterol (mg)	% Daily Value	Sodium (mg)	% Daily Value	Carbohydrates (g)	% Daily Value	Dietary Fiber (g)	% Daily Value	Sugars (g)	Protein (g)	Vitamin A	Vitamin C	Calcium	Iron
Breakfast																					
Sausage Biscuit with Egg	175 g	520	310	34	51	11	50	270	87	1240	50	33	11	0	0	3	19	6	*	10	20
Bacon, Egg & Cheese Biscuit	153 g	440	240	26	40	8	40	240	80	1220	51	33	11	0	0	1	15	10	*	20	15
Biscuit	75 g	260	120	13	20	3	15	1	0	730	30	32	11	1	5	3	5	*	*	8	8
Sausage	43 g	160	140	15	23	5	25	45	15	310	13	0	0	0	0	0	7	*	*	*	4
Scrambled Eggs (2)	100 g	140	90	10	15	3	15	425	142	290	12	1	0	0	0	0	12	10	2	6	10
Hash Browns	53 g	130	70	7	11	1	5	0	0	330	14	15	5	1	4	0	1	*	*	*	*
Hotcakes (plain)	126 g	250	35	4	8	1	5	10	3	570	2	43	14	0	0	10	8	*	*	10	11
Hotcakes with Syrup & Margarine (2 pats)	174 g	410	80	9	18	1.5	10	10	3	670	28	75	25	0	0	30	8	4	*	10	10
Desserts/Shakes																					
Vanilla Lowfat Frozen Yogurt Cone	84 g	110	10	1	2	0.5	3	5	2	80	3	22	8	0	0	19	4	2	*	10	*
Strawberry Lowfat Frozen Yogurt Sundae	172 g	210	10	1	2	0.5	3	5	2	100	4	49	16	0	0	48	6	4	2	20	*
Hot Fudge Lowfat Frozen Yogurt Sundae	168 g	240	25	3	5	2	10	5	2	170	7	50	16	0	0	44	7	4	*	25	2
Baked Apple Pie	84 g	280	140	15	23	2	10	0	0	90	4	35	11	1	6	15	3	*	*	2	6
McDonaldland Cookies®	1 pkg.	290	80	9	14	1	5	0	0	300	13	47	16	1	5	21	4	*	*	*	10
Chocolaty Chip Cookies	1 pkg.	330	140	15	23	4	20	5	2	280	12	42	14	2	7	15	4	*	*	2	10
Vanilla Shake, small (16 fl oz)	480 ml	310	45	5	8	3	15	25	8	170	7	55	17	0	0	51	12	4	*	35	2
Chocolate Shake, small (16 fl oz)	480 ml	350	60	6	9	4	20	25	8	240	10	62	19	0	0	58	13	4	4	35	6
Strawberry Shake, small (16 fl oz)	480 ml	340	45	5	8	3	15	25	8	170	7	63	20	0	0	59	12	4	4	35	2

Source: ©1994 McDonald's Corporation. Rev. 3/94, McD 2–1023, –030.

Nutritional Content of Fast Foods (continued)

Taco Bell

	Serving Size (g)	Calories	% Calorie Reduction	Calories from Fat	Total Fat (g)	% Fat Reduction	Cholesterol (mg)	Protein (g)	Carbohydrates (g)
Taco	78	180	—	100	11	—	30	10	11
LIGHT Taco	78	140	22	50	5	55	20	11	11
Soft Taco	99	220	—	100	11	—	30	12	19
LIGHT Soft Taco	99	180	18	50	5	55	25	13	19
Taco Supreme™	106	230	—	140	15	—	45	11	12
LIGHT Taco Supreme™	106	160	30	50	5	67	20	13	14
Soft Taco Supreme®	128	270	—	140	15	—	45	13	21
LIGHT Soft Taco Supreme®	128	200	26	50	5	67	25	14	23
Bean Burrito	198	390	—	110	12	—	5	13	58
LIGHT Bean Burrito	198	330	15	60	6	50	5	14	55
7-Layer Burrito (no longer offered)	276	540	—	210	23	—	20	17	65
LIGHT 7-Layer Burrito	276	440	19	80	9	61	5	19	67
Burrito Supreme	248	440	—	170	19	—	45	18	50
LIGHT Burrito Supreme	248	350	20	70	8	58	25	20	50
Taco Salad	535	860	—	500	55	—	80	32	64
LIGHT Taco Salad (with chips)	535	680	21	230	25	55	50	35	81
(without chips)	464	330	—	80	9	—	50	30	35

LIGHT = 50% less fat per serving.

Source: Nutritional Brochure ©1995 TACO BELL CORP. ITEM#2582.

Nutritional Content of Fast Foods (continued)

Wendy's

	Serving Size	Weight (g)	Calories	Calories from Fat	Total Fat (g)	Saturated (g)	Cholesterol (mg)	Sodium (mg)	Total Carbohydrates (g)	Dietary Fiber (g)	Sugars (g)	Protein (g)	Vitamin A	Vitamin C	Calcium	Iron
Sandwiches																
Plain Single	1 ea.	133	300	140	16	6	65	460	31	2	5	25	0	0	10	20
Single with everything	1 ea.	219	420	180	20	7	70	810	32	3	9	26	6	10	10	30
Big Bacon Classic	1 ea.	287	610	290	33	13	105	1510	45	3	11	36	15	25	25	35
Jr. Hamburger	1 ea.	117	270	90	10	3	30	560	34	2	7	15	2	2	10	20
Jr. Cheeseburger	1 ea.	129	320	120	13	6	45	770	34	2	7	17	6	2	15	20
Jr. Bacon Cheeseburger	1 ea.	170	410	190	21	8	60	910	34	2	7	22	8	15	15	25
Jr. Cheeseburger Deluxe	1 ea.	179	360	150	16	6	45	840	36	3	8	18	10	10	15	20
Hamburger, Kids' Meal	1 ea.	111	270	90	10	3	30	560	33	2	7	15	2	0	10	20
Cheeseburger, Kids' Meal	1 ea.	123	320	120	13	6	45	770	33	2	7	17	6	0	15	20
Grilled Chicken Sandwich	1 ea.	177	290	60	7	1.5	55	720	35	2	8	24	4	10	10	15
Breaded Chicken Sandwich	1 ea.	208	440	160	18	3	60	840	44	2	6	26	4	10	10	80
Chicken Club Sandwich	1 ea.	220	500	200	23	5	70	1090	44	2	7	30	4	15	10	80
French Fries																
Small	3.2 oz	91	260	120	13	2.5	0	85	33	3	0	3	0	8	2	4
Medium	4.6 oz	130	380	170	19	4	0	120	47	5	0	5	0	10	2	6
Biggie	5.6 oz	159	460	200	23	5	0	150	58	6	0	6	0	15	2	8
Baked Potato																
Plain	10 oz	284	310	0	0	0	0	25	71	7	5	7	0	60	2	20
Bacon & Cheese	1 ea.	380	540	160	18	4	20	1430	78	7	5	17	10	60	20	25
Broccoli & Cheese	1 ea.	411	470	120	14	3	5	470	80	9	6	9	35	120	20	25
Cheese	1 ea.	383	570	210	23	9	30	640	78	7	5	14	15	60	40	20
Chili & Cheese	1 ea.	439	620	220	24	9	40	780	83	9	7	20	20	60	35	35
Sour Cream & Chives	1 ea.	314	380	60	6	4	15	40	74	8	6	8	30	80	8	25
Sour Cream	1 pkt.	28	60	50	6	4	10	15	1	0	1	1	4	0	4	0
Whipped Margarine	1 pkt.	14	60	60	7	1	0	110	0	0	0	0	10	0	0	0

% Daily Value columns: Vitamin A, Vitamin C, Calcium, Iron

Nutritional Content of Fast Foods (continued)

Wendy's (continued)

	Serving Size	Weight (g)	Calories	Calories from Fat	Total Fat (g)	Saturated (g)	Cholesterol (mg)	Sodium (mg)	Total Carbohydrates (g)	Dietary Fiber (g)	Sugars (g)	Protein (g)	% Daily Value Vitamin A	% Daily Value Vitamin C	% Daily Value Calcium	% Daily Value Iron
Chili																
Small	8 oz	227	210	60	7	2.5	40	800	21	5	5	15	8	6	8	15
Large	12 oz	340	310	90	10	4	45	1190	32	7	8	23	10	10	10	25
Cheddar Cheese, shredded	2 T.	17	70	50	6	3	15	110	1	0	0	4	4	0	10	0
Saltine Crackers	2 ea.	6	25	5	0.5	0	0	80	4	0	0	0	0	0	0	2
Chicken Nuggets																
6 piece	6	94	280	180	20	5	50	600	12	0	N/A	14	0	0	2	4
Barbeque Sauce	1 pkt.	28	50	0	0	0	0	100	11	N/A	N/A	1	6	0	0	4
Honey	1 pkt.	14	45	0	0	0	0	0	12	0	12	0	0	0	0	0
Sweet & Sour Sauce	1 pkt.	28	45	0	0	0	0	55	11	N/A	N/A	0	0	0	0	2
Sweet Mustard Sauce	1 pkt.	28	50	10	1	0	0	140	9	N/A	N/A	1	0	0	0	0

Source: ©1994 Wendy's International, Inc. Reprinted by permission.

GLOSSARY

acclimatize Refers to the physiological adaptations that occur to assist the body in adjusting to environmental extremes. Exercise in a hot or even moderately hot environment will cause the body to adapt to these conditions.

acute muscle soreness This condition may develop during or immediately following an exercise bout that has been too long or too intense. Acute muscle soreness is likely caused by alterations in the chemical balance within muscle, increased fluid accumulation in muscle, or injury to muscle tissue.

adenosine triphosphate (ATP) A high-energy compound that is synthesized and stored in small quantities in muscle and other cells. The breakdown of ATP results in a release of energy that can be used to fuel muscular contraction. ATP is the only compound in the body that can provide this immediate source of energy.

aerobic Means "with oxygen"; as pertains to energy-producing biochemical pathways in cells that use oxygen to produce energy.

aerobics A common term to describe all forms of low-intensity exercise designed to improve cardiorespiratory fitness (e.g., jogging, walking, cycling, and swimming). Because aerobic exercise has proved effective in promoting weight loss and reducing the risk of cardiovascular disease, many exercise scientists consider cardiorespiratory fitness to be one of the most important components of health-related physical fitness.

AIDS A fatal disease that develops from infection by the human immunodeficiency virus, or HIV.

amino acids The basic structural unit of proteins. Twenty different amino acids exist and can be linked end to end in various combinations to create different proteins with unique functions.

anabolic steroids Hormones produced by the body which enhance muscle growth. Usually refers to the synthetic form of the hormone testosterone.

anaerobic threshold The work intensity during graded, incremental exercise at which there is a rapid accumulation of blood lactic acid. This usually occurs at 50% to 60% of VO_2 and contributes to muscle fatigue.

anaerobic Means "without oxygen"; as pertains to energy-producing biochemical pathways in cells that do not require oxygen to produce energy.

anorexia nervosa A common eating disorder that is unrelated to any specific physical disease. The end result of extreme anorexia nervosa is a state of starvation in which the individual becomes emaciated due to a refusal to eat.

antagonist The muscle on the opposite side of the joint.

antioxidants Chemicals that prevent a damaging form of oxygen (called *oxygen free radicals*) from causing destruction to the cells. Although free radicals are constantly produced by the body, excess production of these compounds has been implicated in cancer, lung disease, heart disease, and even the aging process.

arteries The blood vessels that transport blood away from the heart.

arteriosclerosis A group of diseases characterized by a narrowing or "hardening" of the arteries. The end result of any form of arteriosclerosis is that blood flow to vital organs may be impaired due to a progressive blockage of the artery.

arthroscopic surgery A common type of surgery that can repair joint injuries without causing undue trauma to the joint.

asthma A disease that reduces the size of airways leading to the lungs and can result in a sudden difficulty in breathing. It is promoted by a number of factors, such as air pollution, pollen, and exercise.

atherosclerosis A special type of arteriosclerosis that results in arterial blockage due to collection of a fatty deposit (called *atherosclerotic plaque*) inside the blood vessel.

behavior modification A technique used in psychological therapy to promote desirable changes in behavior.

body composition The relative amounts of fat and lean body tissue (muscle, organs, bone) found in the body.

body mass index A useful technique for categorizing people with respect to their degree of body fat. The body mass index (BMI) is simply the ratio of the body weight (kilograms; kg) divided by the height squared (meters^2).

breathing exercises A simple means of achieving relaxation.

bulimia An eating disorder that involves overeating (called *binge eating*) followed by vomiting (called *purging*).

calorie The unit of measure used to quantify food energy or the energy expended by the body. Technically, a calorie is the amount of energy necessary to raise the temperature of 1 gram of water 1°C.

cancer A class of over 100 different diseases that can influence almost every body tissue. Cancer is caused by the uncontrolled growth and spread of abnormal cells.

capillaries Thin-walled vessels that permit the exchange of gases (oxygen and carbon dioxide) and nutrients to occur between the blood and tissues.

carbohydrates One of the macronutrients that is especially important during many types of physical activity because they are a key energy source for muscular contraction. Dietary sources of carbohydrates are breads, cereals, fruits, and vegetables.

carbon monoxide A gas produced during the burning of fossil fuels such as gasoline and coal; also contained in cigarette smoke. This pollutant binds to hemoglobin in the blood and reduces the blood's oxygen carrying capacity.

carcinogens Cancer-causing agents which include radiation, chemicals, drugs, and other toxic substances.

cardiac output The amount of blood the heart pumps per minute.

cardiovascular disease Any disease that affects the heart or blood vessels.

cartilage A tough, connective tissue that forms a pad on the end of bones in certain joints, such as the elbow, knee, and ankle. Cartilage act as a shock absorber to cushion the weight of one bone on another and to provide protection from the friction due to joint movement.

cellulite The "lumpy" hard fat that often gives skin a dimpled look. Cellulite is just plain fat and not a special category of fat.

chemical dependency A term for drug addiction.

chlamydia The most common sexually transmitted disease among heterosexuals in the United States. The disease is caused by a bacterial infection within the reproductive organs and is spread through vaginal, anal, and oral sex.

cholesterol A type of derived fat in the body which is necessary for cell and hormone synthesis. Can be acquired through the diet or can be made by the body.

chondromalacia Sometimes called "runner's knee"; it is a common exercise-induced injury which is manifest as pain behind the knee cap. In sports injury clinics, chondromalacia may account for almost 10% of all visits, or 20% to 40% of all knee problems.

cocaine Cocaine is a powerful stimulant derived from the leaves of the South American coca shrub, which grows primarily in the Andes mountains. Cocaine is extracted from the coca leaves using a multistep process to produce a white powder.

complete proteins Contain all the essential amino acids and are found only in foods of animal origin (meats and dairy products).

complex carbohydrates A term that refers to carbohydrates that provide both micronutrients and the glucose necessary for producing energy. They are contained in starches and fiber.

concentric contractions Isotonic muscle contractions that result in muscle shortening.

contributory risk factors; also called *secondary risk factors* Factors that increase the risk of CHD, but their direct contribution to the disease process has not been precisely determined.

convection Heat loss by the movement of air (or water) around the body.

cool-down The cool-down (sometimes called a *warm-down*) is a 5 to 15 minute period of low-intensity exercise that immediately follows the primary conditioning period.

coronary artery disease See *coronary heart disease.*

coronary heart disease (CHD); also called *coronary artery disease* CHD is the result of atherosclerotic plaque forming a blockage of one or more coronary arteries (the blood vessels supplying the heart).

creeping obesity A slow increase in body fat collected over a period of several years.

cross training The use of a variety of activity modes for training the cardiorespiratory system.

cryokinetics A relatively new rehabilitation technique which is implemented after the acute injury and healing period have been completed. It incorporates varying periods of treatment using ice, rest, and exercise.

cycle ergometer fitness test A submaximal exercise test designed to evaluate cardiorespiratory fitness.

delayed-onset muscle soreness (DOMS) This condition develops within 24 to 48 hours after a bout of exercise that is excessive in duration or intensity. It is common following new or unique physical activities that use muscle groups unaccustomed to exercise.

derived fats A class of fats which does not contain fatty acids but are classified as fat because they are not soluble in water.

diabetes A metabolic disorder characterized by high blood glucose levels. Chronic elevation of blood glucose is associated with increased incidence of heart disease, kidney disease, nerve dysfunction, and eye damage.

diastolic blood pressure The pressure of the blood in the arteries at the level of the heart during the resting phase of the heart (diastole).

duration of exercise The amount of time invested in performing the primary workout.

dynamic Means "movement"; in reference to muscle contractions, dynamic is synonymous with isotonic contraction.

eccentric contractions Isotonic contractions in which the muscle exerts force while the muscle lengthens (also called *negative contractions*).

ergogenic aid A drug or nutritional product that improves physical fitness and exercise performance.

essential amino acids Amino acids which cannot be manufactured by the body and, therefore, must be consumed in the diet.

eustress A stress level that results in improved performance.

evaporation The conversion of water (or sweat) to a gas (water vapor). The most important means of removing heat from the body during exercise.

exercise metabolic rate (EMR) The energy expenditure during any form of exercise.

exercise prescription The correct dosage of exercise to effectively promote physical fitness. Exercise prescriptions should be tailored to meet the needs of the individual and include fitness goals, mode of exercise, a warm-up, a primary conditioning period, and a cool-down.

exercise stress test A diagnostic test designed to determine if the patient's cardiovascular system has a normal response to exercise. The test is generally performed on a treadmill while a physician monitors heart rate, blood pressure, and EKG.

fartlek training *Fartlek* is a Swedish word meaning "speed play," and it refers to a popular form of training for long-distance runners. It is much like interval training, but it is not as rigid in its work-to-rest interval ratios. It consists of "free-form" running done out on trails, roads, golf courses, and so on.

fast-twitch fibers Muscle fibers that contract rapidly but fatigue quickly. These fibers are white and have a low aerobic capacity, but they are well equipped to produce ATP anaerobically.

fat An efficient storage form for energy, because each gram of fat holds over twice the energy content of either carbohydrate or protein. Excess fat in the diet is stored in fat cells (called *adipose tissue*) located under the skin and around internal organs.

fatty acids The basic structural unit of triglycerides that are important nutritionally, not only because of their energy content, but also because they play a role in cardiovascular disease.

fiber A stringy, nondigestible carbohydrate found in whole grains, vegetables, and fruits in its primary form, cellulose.

flexibility The ability to move joints freely through their full range of motion.

frequency of exercise The number of times per week that one intends to exercise.

fructose Also called *fruit sugar*; a naturally occurring sugar found in fruits and in honey.

galactose A simple sugar found in the breast milk of humans and other mammals.

glucose The most noteworthy of the simple sugars because it is the only sugar molecule that can be used by the body in its natural form. All other carbohydrates must first be converted to glucose to be used for fuel.

glycogen The storage form of glucose in the liver and skeletal muscles.

gonorrhea A common sexually transmitted disease. The infection can be transmitted through vaginal, anal, and oral sex. Gonorrhea is caused by a bacterial infection and is curable by antibiotics.

heart attack; also called *myocardial infarction* Stoppage of blood flow to the heart, resulting in the death of heart cells.

heart rate Number of heart beats per minute.

heat injuries; also called *heat illness* Bodily injury that can occur when the exercise heat load exceeds the body's ability to regulate body temperature. They are serious and can result in damage to the nervous system and, in extreme cases, death.

herpes A general term for a family of diseases that are also caused by viral infections. Herpes is highly contagious and can be transmitted through any form of sexual contact (e.g., hand-to-genital contact, oral sex, or intercourse).

high-density lipoproteins (HDL) A combination of protein, triglycerides, and cholesterol in the blood, composed of relatively large amounts of protein. Protects against the fatty plaque accumulation in the coronary arteries of the heart that leads to heart disease. Research has shown that individuals with high blood HDL-cholesterol levels have a decreased risk of CHD. Therefore, HDL-cholesterol is often called "good cholesterol".

homeotherms Animals that regulate their body temperature around a constant level; that is, body temperature is regulated around a set point. Humans regulate their body temperature around the set point of 98.6°F or 37°C.

humidity The amount of water vapor in the air. If the relative humidity is high, meaning the air is relatively saturated with water, and the air temperature is high, evaporation is retarded and body heat loss is drastically decreased.

hydrostatic weighing A method of determining body composition that involves weighing the individual both on land and in a tank of water.

hyperplasia An increase in the number of muscle fibers.

hypertension (high blood pressure) Usually considered to be a blood pressure of greater than 140 for systolic or 100 for diastolic.

hypertrophy An increase in muscle fiber size.

incomplete proteins Proteins that are missing one or more of the essential amino acids; can be found in numerous vegetable sources.

intensity of exercise The amount of physiological stress or overload placed on the body during exercise.

intermediate fibers Muscle fibers that possess a combination of the characteristics of fast- and slow-twitch fibers. They contract rapidly and are fatigue resistant due to a well-developed aerobic capacity.

interval training Repeated bouts or intervals of relatively intense exercise. The duration of the intervals can be varied, but a 1- to 5-minute duration is common. Each interval is followed by a rest period, which should be equal to or slightly greater than the interval duration.

isocaloric balance Food energy intake that equals energy expenditure.

isokinetic A muscle contraction that is a subtype of isotonic contraction; isokinetic contractions are concentric or eccentric isotonic contractions performed at a constant speed.

isometric Refers to muscle contractions in which muscular tension is developed but no movement of body parts takes place.

isotonic Refers to muscle contractions in which there is movement of a body part. Most exercise or sports skills use isotonic contractions.

lactic acid A by-product of glucose metabolism. Produced primarily during intense exercise (i.e., greater than 50%–60% of maximal aerobic capacity). Results in inhibition of muscle contraction and, therefore, fatigue.

lactose A simple sugar found in milk products; it is composed of galactose and glucose.

ligaments Connective tissue within the joint capsule which holds bones together.

lipoproteins Combinations of protein, triglycerides, and cholesterol in the blood that are important because of their role in promoting heart disease.

long, slow distance training The term utilized to indicate continuous exercise which requires a steady, submaximal exercise intensity (i.e., the intensity is generally around 70% HRmax).

low-density lipoproteins (LDL) A combination of protein, triglycerides, and cholesterol in the blood, composed of relatively large amounts of cholesterol. Promotes the fatty plaque accumulation in the coronary arteries of the heart that leads to heart disease. The association between elevated total blood cholesterol and the increased risk of CHD is due primarily to LDL cholesterol. Research has shown that individuals with high blood LDL cholesterol levels have an increased risk of CHD. Because of this relationship, LDL cholesterol has been labeled "bad cholesterol."

macronutrients Carbohydrates, fats, and proteins, which are necessary for building and maintaining body tissues and providing energy for daily activities.

major risk factors; also called *primary risk factors* Factors considered to be directly related to the development of CHD and stroke.

maltose A simple sugar found in grain products; it is composed of two glucose molecules linked together.

marijuana A plant mixture (stems, leaves, or seeds) from either the *Cannabis sativa* or *Cannabis indica* (hemp) plants. The active chemical in marijuana that produces physical effects is tetrahydrocannabinol (THC); the higher the THC concentration in marijuana, the greater the effect.

meditation A method of relaxation that has been practiced for ages in an effort to produce relaxation and achieve inner peace. There are many types of meditation, and there is no scientific evidence that one form is superior to another.

micronutrients Nutrients in food, such as vitamins and minerals, that regulate the functions of the cells.

minerals Chemical elements (e.g., sodium and calcium) that are required by the body for normal functioning.

mode of exercise The specific type of exercise to be performed. For example, to improve cardiorespiratory fitness, one could select from a wide variety of exercise modes, including running, swimming, or cycling.

motor unit A motor nerve and each of the muscle fibers that it innervates.

muscular endurance The ability of a muscle to generate force over and over again.

muscular strength The maximal ability of a muscle to generate force.

myocardial infarction (MI) Damage to the heart due to a reduction in blood flow, resulting in the death of heart muscle cells.

negative caloric balance Expending more calories than are consumed.

nonessential amino acids Eleven amino acids that the body can make and are therefore not necessary in the diet.

nutrients Substances contained in food which are necessary for good health.

obesity A term applied to individuals with a high percentage of body fat, generally over 25% for men and over 30% for women.

omega-3 fatty acid A type of unsaturated fatty acid that lowers both blood cholesterol and triglycerides and is found primarily in fresh or frozen mackerel, herring, tuna, and salmon.

1-mile walking test See *Walk (1 mile) test.*

1.5-mile run test A fitness test designed to evaluate cardiorespiratory fitness. The objective of the test is to complete a 1.5-mile distance (preferably on a track) in the shortest possible time.

one-repetition maximum (1 RM) test Measurement of the maximum amount of weight that can be lifted one time.

organic Refers to foods that are grown without pesticides.

osteoporosis The loss of bone mass and strength, which increases the risk of bone fractures.

overload principle A basic principle of physical conditioning. The overload principle states that in order to improve physical fitness, the body or specific muscles must be stressed. For example, for a skeletal muscle to increase in strength, the muscle must work against a heavier load than normal.

overtraining Failure to get enough rest between exercise training sessions. Overtraining may lead to chronic fatigue and/or injuries.

overtraining syndrome A phenomenon resulting from improper training techniques which results in exercise-related injuries. Overtraining results from too much exercise and not enough recovery time between workouts. The symptoms may include increased resting heart rate, reduced appetite, weight loss, irritability, disturbed sleep, elevated blood pressure, frequent injuries, increased incidence of infections, and chronic fatigue.

ozone A gas produced by a chemical reaction between sunlight and the hydrocarbons emitted from car exhausts. This form of pollution is extremely irritating to the lung and airways. It causes tightness in the chest, coughing, headaches, nausea, throat and eye irritation, and, worst of all, bronchoconstriction.

palpation Touching the skin in order to feel the pulse.

passive exercise Movement performed on a motor-driven device designed to move or vibrate the body without any muscular activity. Passive exercise devices come in many forms, including rolling machines, vibrating belts, pillows, and passive motion tables. Passive exercise devices do not improve physical fitness or promote weight loss.

patella-femoral pain syndrome (PFPS) A common exercise-induced injury that is manifest as pain behind the knee cap (patella).

pelvic inflammatory disease An inflammatory infection of the lining of the abdominal and pelvic cavities. Common symptoms of pelvic inflammatory disease include pain in the lower abdominal cavity, fever, and menstrual irregularities.

positive caloric balance Consuming more calories than are expended.

principle of progression A principle of training which dictates that overload should be increased gradually during the course of a physical fitness program.

principle of recuperation The principle of recuperation that the body requires recovery periods between exercise training sessions in order to adapt to the exercise stress. Therefore, a period of rest is essential to achieve maximal benefit from exercise.

principle of reversibility The loss of fitness due to inactivity.

principle of specificity The principle that the exercise training effect is specific to those muscles involved in the activity.

progressive resistance exercise (PRE) The application of the overload principle applied to strength and endurance exercise programs. Even though the overload principle and PRE can be used interchangeably, PRE is preferred when discussing weight training.

proprioceptive neuromuscular facilitation (PNF) Combines stretching with alternating contracting and relaxing of muscles to improve flexibility. There are two common types of PNF stretching. One is called contract-relax (C-R) stretching, while the second is called contract-relax/antagonist contract (CRAC) stretching.

pulmonary circuit The blood vascular system which circulates blood from the right side of the heart, through the lungs, and back to the left side of the heart.

push-up test A fitness test designed to evaluate muscular endurance of shoulder and arm muscles.

R.I.C.E. An acronym representing a treatment protocol for exercise-related injuries. It stands for a combination of rest-*R*, ice-*I*, compression-*C*, and elevation-*E*.

recovery index Measurement of heart rate during three 30-second recovery periods following a submaximal step test.

recruitment The process of involving more muscle fibers to produce increased muscular force.

repetition maximum (RM) The measure of the intensity of exercise in both isotonic and isokinetic weight training programs. The RM is the maximal load that a muscle group can lift a specified number of times before tiring. For example, 6 RM is the maximal load that can be lifted six times.

resting metabolic rate (RMR) The amount of energy expended during all sedentary activities.

saturated A type of fatty acid that comes primarily from animal sources (meat and dairy products) and is solid at room temperature.

set The number of repetitions performed consecutively without resting.

set point theory A theory of weight regulation that centers around the concept that body weight is controlled at a set point by a weight-regulating control center within the brain.

sexually transmitted diseases (STDs) A group of more than 20 diseases that are generally spread through sexual contact.

sit and reach test A fitness test that measures the ability to flex the trunk (i.e., stretching the lower back muscles and the muscles in the back of the thigh).

sit-up test A field test to evaluate abdominal muscle endurance.

skinfold test A field test to estimate body composition. The test works on the principle that over 50% of the body fat lies just beneath the skin. Therefore, measurement of representative samples of subcutaneous fat provides a means of estimating overall body fatness.

slow-twitch fibers Muscle fibers that contract slowly and are highly resistant to fatigue. Red in appearance, they have the capacity to produce large quantities of ATP aerobically, making them ideally suited for low-intensity, prolonged exercise like walking or slow jogging.

specificity of training That development of muscular strength and endurance, as well as cardiorespiratory endurance, is specific to the muscle group that is exercised and the training intensity.

SPF Abbreviation for "sun protection factor." A sunscreen with an SPF of 15 provides you with 15 times more protection than unprotected skin.

spot reduction The false notion that exercise applied to a specific region of the body will result in fat loss in that region.

sprain Damage to a ligament that occurs if excessive force is applied to a joint.

starches Long chains of sugars commonly found in foods such as corn, grains, potatoes, peas, and beans. Starch is stored in the body as glycogen and is used for that sudden burst of energy often needed during physical activity.

static Stationary; in reference to muscle contractions, static is synonymous with isometric contraction.

static stretching Stretching that slowly lengthens a muscle to a point where further movement is limited.

step test A submaximal exercise test designed to evaluate cardiorespiratory fitness. The step test works on the principle that individuals with a high level of cardiorespiratory fitness will have a lower heart rate during recovery from 3 minutes of standardized exercise (bench stepping) than less-conditioned individuals.

strain Damage to a muscle that can range from a minor separation of fibers to a complete tearing of fibers.

stress A physiological and mental response to something in the environment that causes people to become uncomfortable.

stress fractures Tiny cracks or breaks in bone. Although stress fractures can occur in any leg bone, the long bones of the foot extending from the ankle to the toes are especially susceptible.

stressor A factor that produces stress.

stretch reflex Involuntary contraction of muscle that occurs due to rapid stretching of a muscle.

stroke Brain damage that occurs when the blood supply to the brain is reduced for a prolonged period of time.

stroke volume The amount of blood pumped per heart beat (generally expressed in milliliters).

sucrose; also called *table sugar* A molecule composed of glucose and fructose.

syphilis A sexually transmitted disease that can be transmitted through direct sexual contact. Syphilis is caused by a bacterial infection and can be cured by antibiotics.

systemic circuit The blood vascular system which circulates blood from the left side of the heart, throughout the body, and back to the right side of the heart.

systolic blood pressure The pressure of the blood in the arteries at the level of the heart during the contractile phase of the heart (systole).

target heart rate (THR) The range of heart rates that corresponds to an exercise intensity of approximately 50% to 85% VO_2 max. This is the range of training heart rates that results in improvements in aerobic capacity.

tendonitis Inflammation or swelling of a tendon. One of the most common exercise-related injuries.

tendons Connective tissue that connects muscles to bones.

ten percent rule A rule of training that states that the training intensity or duration of exercise should not be increased more than 10% per week.

threshold for health benefits The minimum level of physical activity required to achieve some of the health benefits of exercise.

training threshold The training intensity above which there is an improvement in cardiorespiratory fitness. This intensity is approximately 50% of VO_2 max.

triglycerides The form of fat that is broken down and used to produce energy to power muscle contractions during exercise. Triglycerides constitute approximately 95% of the fats in the diet and are the storage form of body fat.

tumor A group of cancer cells.

unsaturated A type of fatty acid that comes primarily from plant sources and is liquid at room temperature.

valsalva maneuver Breath holding during an intense muscle contraction that can reduce blood flow to the brain and cause dizziness and fainting.

veins Blood vessels that transport blood toward the heart.

venereal warts; also known as *genital warts* Warts caused by a small group of viruses called *human papilloma viruses.* Infection generally occurs through sexual contact with an infected individual; after exposure, the virus penetrates the skin or mucous membranes of the genitals or anus, and warts appear within 6 to 8 weeks.

visualization; also called *imagery* A relaxation technique that uses mental pictures to reduce stress. The idea is to create appealing mental images that promote relaxation and reduce stress.

vitamins Small molecules that play a key role in many bodily functions, including the regulation of growth and metabolism. They are classified according to whether they are soluble in water or fat.

VO$_2$ max The highest oxygen consumption achievable during exercise. Practically speaking, VO$_2$ max is a laboratory measure of the endurance capacity of both the cardiorespiratory system and exercising skeletal muscles.

waist-to-hip circumference ratio An index for determining the risk of disease associated with high body fat. The rationale for this technique is that a high percentage of fat in the abdominal region is associated with an increased risk of disease (e.g., heart disease or hypertension). Therefore, an individual with a large fat deposit in the abdominal region would have a high waist-to-hip ratio and would have a higher risk of disease than someone with a lower waist-to-hip ratio.

walk (1 mile) test A fitness test designed to evaluate cardiorespiratory fitness. The objective of the test is to complete a 1 walking mile distance (preferably on a track) in the shortest possible time.

warm-up A brief (5 to 15 minute) period of exercise that precedes the workout. The purpose of a warm-up is to elevate muscle temperature and increase blood flow to those muscles that will be engaged in the workout.

wellness A state of healthy living. This state is achieved by the practice of a healthy lifestyle, which includes regular physical activity, proper nutrition, eliminating unhealthy behaviors, and maintaining good emotional and spiritual health.

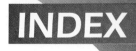

INDEX